# Endothelium, Nitric Oxide, and Atherosclerosis:
## From Basic Mechanisms to Clinical Implications

Edited by
Julio A. Panza, M.D.
Richard O. Cannon III, M.D.

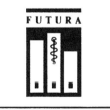

**Futura Publishing Company, Inc.**
Armonk, NY

**Library of Congress Cataloging-in-Publication Data**

Endothelium, nitric oxide, and atherosclerosis/edited by Julio A.
   Panza, Richard O. Cannon III.
        p.   cm.
     Includes bibliographical references and index.
     ISBN 0-87993-436-0
     1. Atherosclerosis—Pathophysiology.   2. Vascular endothelium.
   3. Nitric oxide—Physiological effect.   I. Panza, Julio A.
   II. Cannon, Richard O.
     [DNLM:   1. Endothelium, Vascular—physiology.   2. Cardiovascular
   Diseases—physiopathology.   3. Endothelium, Vascular—drug effects.
   4. Nitric Oxide—physiology.   WG 500 E566 1999]
   RC692.E487   1999
   616.1'3607—dc21
   DNLM/DLC
   for Library of Congress                                         99-15251
                                                                       CIP

Copyright © 1999
Futura Publishing Company, Inc.

*Published by*
Futura Publishing Company, Inc.
135 Bedford Road
Armonk, NY 10504-0418

ISBN# 0-87993-436-0

Printed in the United States of America.
This book is printed on acid-free paper.

# Contents

# PART III
## Clinical Studies of Endothelial Function and Dysfunction

# PART IV
## Therapeutic Strategies to Improve Endothelial Dysfunction

# Preface

In 1978, an experiment was performed in Robert Furchgott's laboratory in New York that would lead to his realization that the presence of the endothelium is essential for the vasodilator effect of acetylcholine (ACh). The results of the basic and clinical research conducted over the last two decades, triggered by that seemingly simple observation, constitute one of the most important recent developments in cardiovascular medicine. Twenty years after that key experiment, the Nobel prize was awarded to Dr. Furchgott (among others) for the discovery that a small molecule—nitric oxide (NO)—synthesized and released by endothelial cells plays an essential role in the regulation of vascular homeostasis. In addition, 1998 marked the 50th anniversary of the National Heart, Lung, and Blood Institute (NHLBI), the major promoter and supporter of cardiovascular research in the United States, which has funded the research endeavor of virtually every investigator who has studied the role of the endothelium in the regulation of vascular physiology. This occasion has inspired the writing of this book, which spans from Dr. Furchgott's initial observation to the most recent investigations performed in the clinical arena related to the study and treatment of endothelial dysfunction in patients.

The book is divided into four sections that include in-depth discussions of the discovery, biological roles, and regulation of endothelial NO; the basic mechanisms that lead to endothelial dysfunction in cardiovascular disease; clinical studies of impaired endothelial function in patients with different cardiovascular conditions; and the most important therapeutic strategies that have been developed to ameliorate endothelial dysfunction.

The first section of this book deals with the nature, effects, and regulation of NO. Robert F. Furchgott provides a detailed account of the sequence of experiments that led to the discovery of endothelium-derived relaxing factor (EDRF) and its subsequent identification as NO. This chapter is an invaluable historical reference for everyone interested in this field and, particularly, in the early developments that fueled the research that has contributed to our current knowledge of endothelial regulation of vascular tone. Salvador Moncada played an important part in the identification of the EDRF as NO. He and E. Anne Higgs describe the work performed in their laboratory related to the discovery of NO and its biological roles. William E. Downey and Thomas Michel review the intracellular mechanisms that regulate endothelial NO synthase (eNOS) and therefore NO activity. In particular, they explain how caveolae, small invaginations of the plasma membrane, and caveolin, a scaffolding protein, play an essential role in the initiation of intracellular mechanisms that lead to stimulation of eNOS. Paul L. Huang, Robert Gyurko, and Lin Zhang summarize experiments performed with the eNOS knockout mice that have clarified the important role of NO in the cardiovascular system, not only for the regulation of vascular tone (as demonstrated by the fact that eNOS knockout mice are hypertensive), but also for the modulation of cardiac contractility, vessel injury, and the development of atherosclerosis. Richard A. Cohen describes in detail the effect of NO on vascular smooth muscle and the molecular mediators of endothelium-dependent vascular relaxation. Timothy J. McMahon and Jonathan S. Stamler reveal another important role of NO: its participation in the respiratory cycle through its binding to hemoglobin. This is an example of how NO modulates the most important function of the vascular system (ie, the delivery of oxygen to the tissues) independently of its action on the vascular wall. Virginia M. Miller reviews the mechanisms by which sex steroid hormones modulate the production of several endothelium-derived factors, including NO. These mechanisms are both genomic and nongenomic and are dependent on the expression of cell membrane receptors. Importantly, sex steroids also may regulate the release of vasoactive factors from platelets and even the smooth muscle response to these factors.

Basic mechanisms of endothelial dysfunction are discussed in the second section of the text. Paul M. Vanhoutte reviews the evidence for reduced release of EDRF from regenerated endothelial cells following balloon injury to porcine coronary arteries. He also describes experiments showing that oxidized lipoproteins interfere with signaling mechanisms that link cell surface receptors to NOS activation. Frank T. Ruschitzka, George Noll, and Thomas F. Lüscher describe vasoconstrictor substances released from the endothelium, including free-radical molecules such as superoxide anion, prostanoids thomboxane $A_2$ and prostaglandin $H_2$, and endothelin-1 (ET-1). The potential role of ET-1 in human diseases including hypertension, atherosclerosis, coronary spasm, congestive heart failure, and pulmonary hypertension is a topic of considerable research interest, with ET receptor antagonists already in clinical trials. James K. Liao discusses the experimental evidence for the role of NO as a regulator of signaling mechanisms linking stimulation of cells with cytokines, oxidized low-density lipoproteins, and other stimuli to activation of genes that code for protein mediators of inflammation. Experimental evidence for stabilization of the proinflammatory transcription factor nuclear factor–kappa B (NF-$\kappa$B) by NO is discussed extensively. A. Maziar Zafari, David G. Harrison, and Kathy K. Griendling describe the destructive effects of superoxide anion on NO bioactivity. They found increased vascular production of superoxide anion from the endothelium of cholesterol-fed rabbits caused by xanthine oxidase activation and increased superoxide anion production in the endothelium and smooth muscle of this animal model as a consequence of activation of nicotinamide-adenine dinucleotide (NADH)- and nicotinamide-adenine-dinucleotide phosphate (NADPH)-dependent oxidases. These observations have led to experiments to reduce oxidant stress within the vessel wall with the use of direct or indirect inhibitors of these oxidase systems.

The third section is related to the study of endothelial dysfunction in patients with different cardiovascular conditions. Julio A. Panza summarizes the evidence for endothelial dysfunction in hypertension and the mechanisms that may be responsible for this abnormality. The role of diminished NO activity as part of the pathophysiology and complications of the hypertensive process is emphasized. Robert A. Vogel reviews the link between endothelial dysfunction and hypercholesterolemia. This chapter includes a detailed account of several trials that have used assessment of flow-mediated vasodilation of the brachial artery (an NO-dependent phenomenon) by means of ultrasound as a measurement of endothelial function. This technique has gained wide acceptance because of its noninvasiveness and repeatability. Arshed A. Quyyumi discusses the importance of NO activity in coronary vascular physiology. Because coronary heart disease is the most frequent cause of mortality, the processes that participate in the modulation of coronary vascular tone and in the genesis of coronary atherosclerosis assume paramount importance. Dr. Quyyumi's studies have been essential for our current understanding of how NO regulates coronary vasomotion and how abnormalities in the NO system participate in the pathophysiology of coronary artery disease. Helmut Drexler and Burkhard Hornig review the evidence for impaired endothelium-dependent vasodilation in patients with heart failure and the mechanisms that account for this defect. In particular, they discuss the role of cytokines, NO, and the renin-angiotensin system in the vascular abnormalities associated with heart failure and how these may affect the patients' exercise capacity by modulating the distribution of blood flow during exercise. Anthony M. Heagerty describes the technique of in vitro studies of human blood vessels and the insights that have been gained from these experiments in different cardiovascular conditions. This technique is particularly useful for the study of functional and morphological abnormalities of the human microvasculature.

The final section of the text describes therapeutic strategies to improve endothelial dysfunction. Scott Kinlay, Andrew P. Selwyn, and Peter Ganz review the evidence for deleterious effects of low-density lipoproteins on vascular function, especially when modified by oxidation, in patients with dyslipidemia. Endothelial dysfunction also is detected in menopause, diabetes mellitus, cigarette smoking, hypertension, and homocysteine, among other proposed risk factors for atherosclerosis. These authors discuss clinical studies in which lipid-lowering medications have improved endothelial dysfunction and relieved myocardial ischemia in patients with coronary artery disease. Other potential therapies for improving endothelial dysfunction are discussed by these authors. Mark A. Creager reports the benefit of vitamin C on endothelium-dependent vasodilator responses in patients with diabetes mellitus, cigarette smoking, hypertension, and coronary artery disease. Accordingly, antioxidant compounds may improve endothelium-dependent vasodilator responsiveness through facilitation of NOS or protection of NO from oxidative degradation. Shanthi Adimoolam and John P. Cooke present data from animal models of atherosclerosis showing improvement in endothelium-dependent dilator responsiveness and prevention of atherosclerosis with administration of the substrate for NOS, L-arginine. They provide evidence that competitive inhibitors of NOS may accumulate within the endothelium in hypercholesterolemia and that administration of L-arginine may restore appropriate substrate concentrations that increase NO synthesis. Human studies of L-arginine administration also are presented, showing favorable effects on endothelium-dependent vasodilator responsiveness in patients with hypercholesterolemia, uremia, and chronic heart failure. Richard O. Cannon III reports the effects of estrogen on NO bioactivity and endothelium-dependent dilator responsiveness in the coronary and forearm circulations of postmenopausal women. Estrogen also appears to improve other homeostatic properties of the endothelium including regulation of fibrinolysis and inflammation. G. B. John Mancini and Eric W. Hamber describe effects of angiotensin-converting enzyme inhibition on endothelium-dependent dilator responsiveness in the coronary and systemic circulations of patients with coronary artery disease. Jonathan Abrams reviews the history of nitrate use in patients with cardiovascular disease, the pharmacologic effects of nitroglycerin on smooth muscle relaxation and inhibition of platelet aggregation, and the current indications for nitrate therapy, along with the limitations of this therapy caused by nitrate tolerance.

Each chapter covers its topic in detail and usually is accompanied by an extensive list of references. We hope that this book will serve both as a comprehensive review for medical students and trainees who want to initiate themselves in the study of endothelial regulation of vascular physiology and as a stimulator of new research for established physicians and scientists who incessantly pursue the investigation of basic mechanisms and treatment of cardiovascular disease.

*Acknowledgements.* We thank Dr. Claude Lenfant, Director of NHLBI, for his interest in the production of this book and for his continued support of cardiovascular research, without which most of the work included in this volume would not have been completed. We especially acknowledge the expert editorial assistance of Judy Corbett that tremendously facilitated the preparation of this book.

Julio A. Panza, MD

Richard O. Cannon III, MD

# Contributors

**Jonathan Abrams, MD**  Department of Medicine, Cardiology Division, University of New Mexico, School of Medicine, Albuquerque, New Mexico

**Shanthi Adimoolam, PhD**  Division of Cardiovascular Medicine, Stanford University, Stanford, California

**Richard O. Cannon III, MD**  Cardiology Branch, National Heart, Lung, and Blood Institute, National Institutes of Health, Bethesda, Maryland

**Richard A. Cohen, MD**  Vascular Biology Unit, Evans Department of Medicine, Whitaker Cardiovascular Institute, Boston University School of Medicine, Boston, Massachusetts

**John P. Cooke, MD, PhD**  Division of Cardiovascular Medicine, Stanford University, Stanford, California

**Mark A. Creager, MD**  Cardiovascular Division, Brigham and Women's Hospital and Harvard Medical School, Boston, Massachusetts

**William E. Downey, MD**  Cardiovascular Divisions, Brigham and Women's Hospital and West Roxbury Veterans Affairs Medical Center, Harvard Medical School, Boston, Massachusetts

**Helmut Drexler, MD**  Cardiovascular Division, Medizinische Hochschule, Hannover, Germany

**Robert F. Furchgott, PhD, 1998 Nobel Prize Laureate for the Discovery of EDRF/Nitric Oxide**  Department of Pharmacology, State University of New York, Health Science Center at Brooklyn, Brooklyn, New York

**Peter Ganz, MD**  Cardiac Catheterization Laboratory, Brigham and Women's Hospital and Harvard Medical School, Boston, Massachusetts

**Kathy K. Griendling, PhD**  Division of Cardiology, Emory University School of Medicine, Atlanta, Georgia

**Robert Gyurko, DDS, PhD**  Cardiovascular Research Center and Cardiology Division, Massachusetts General Hospital and Harvard Medical School, Boston, Massachusettts

**Eric W. Hamber, MD**  Department of Medicine, University of British Columbia, Vancouver, British Columbia, Canada

**David G. Harrison, MD**  Emory University School of Medicine and Atlanta Veterans Administration Medical Center, Atlanta, Georgia

**Anthony M. Heagerty, MD**  Manchester Royal Infirmary, Oxford Road, Manchester, United Kingdom

**E. Annie Higgs, BSc, MSc**  The Wolfson Institute for Biomedical Research, University College London, London, United Kingdom

**Burkhard Hornig, MD**  Cardiovascular Division, Medizinische Hochschule, Hannover, Germany

**Paul L. Huang, MD, PhD**  Cardiovascular Research Center and Cardiology Division, Massachusetts General Hospital and Harvard Medical School, Boston, Massachusettts

**Scott Kinlay, MBBS, PhD**  Cardiac Catheterization Laboratory, Brigham and Women's Hospital and Harvard Medical School, Boston, Massachusetts

**James K. Liao, MD**  Department of Medicine, Atherosclerosis and Vascular Medicine Unit, Cardiovascular Division, Brigham and Women's Hospital and Harvard Medical School, Boston, Masschusetts

**Thomas F. Lüscher, MD**  Department of Cardiology, University Hospital Zürich, Cardiovascular Research and Institute of Physiology, University of Zürich-lrchel, Switzerland

**G. B. John Mancini, MD, FRCP(C), FACP**  Department of Medicine, Vancouver Hospital and Health Sciences Centre; Director, Cardiovascular Imaging Laboratory, Jack Bell Research Centre, Vancouver Hospital and Health Sciences Centre, Vancouver, British Columbia Canada

**Timothy J. McMahon, MD**  Division of Pulmonary and Critical Care, Duke University Medical Center, Durham, North Carolina

**Thomas Michel, MD, PhD**  Cardiovascular Divisions, Brigham and Women's Hospital and West Roxbury Veterans Affairs Medical Center, Harvard Medical School, Boston, Massachusetts

**Virginia M. Miller, PhD**  Department of Surgery, Mayo Clinic and Mayo Foundation, Rochester, Minnesota

**Salvador Moncada, MD**  The Wolfson Institute for Biomedical Research, University College London, London, United Kingdom

**Georg Noll, MD**  Department of Cardiology, University Hospital Zürich, Cardiovascular Research and Institute of Physiology, University of Zürich-lrchel, Switzerland

**Julio A. Panza, MD**   Cardiology Branch, National Heart, Lung, and Blood Institute, National Institutes of Health, Bethesda, Maryland

**Arshed A. Quyyumi, MD**   Cardiology Branch, National Heart, Lung, and Blood Institute, National Institutes of Health, Bethesda, Maryland

**Frank T. Ruschitzka, MD**   Department of Cardiology, University Hospital Zürich, Cardiovascular Research and Institute of Physiology, University of Zürich-lrchel, Switzerland

**Andrew P. Selwyn, MD**   Cardiac Catheterization Laboratory, Brigham and Women's Hospital and Harvard Medical School, Boston, Massachusetts

**Jonathan S. Stamler, MD**   Howard Hughes Medical Institute, Durham, North Carolina; Divisions of Pulmonary and Critical Care and Cardiovascular Medicine, Duke University Medical Center, Durham, North Carolina

**Paul M. Vanhoutte, MD**   Institut de Recherches Internationales Servier, Courbevoice Cédex, France

**Robert A. Vogel, MD**   Department of Medicine, Division of Cardiology, University of Maryland School of Medicine, Baltimore, Maryland

**A. Maziar Zafari, MD, PhD**   Emory University School of Medicine and Atlanta Veterans Administration Medical Center, Atlanta, Georgia

**Lin Zhang, MD**   Cardiovascular Research Center and Cardiology Division, Massachusetts General Hospital and Harvard Medical School, Boston, Massachusettts

# Part I

## Endothelium and the Biology of Nitric Oxide

## Chapter 1

# Discovery of Endothelium-Derived Relaxing Factor and Its Identification as Nitric Oxide

*Robert F. Furchgott, PhD*

## Some Introductory Remarks

Because this chapter is being written on the occasion of the 50th anniversary of the National Heart, Lung, and Blood Institute (NHLBI) and because research in my laboratory has been supported continuously by grants from the NHLBI (originally the NHI) for the last 40 years, I think that it is appropriate at this time to quote part of the first paragraph of the Introduction to the Research Plan in my grant application written in January, 1982:

> *It will be noted that the title of the proposal in the present Competing Continuation Application is Mechanisms of Action of Vasodilator Agents, and no longer Factors Influencing Responses to Adrenergic Drugs, as used in the previous Competing Continuation Application of five years ago. This change in title reflects changes in the project's aims that have come about during the past few years. At the beginning of the present project, in December, 1977, our experiments were largely concerned with the interactions of drugs with adrenergic receptors and with factors influencing release of catecholamines from sympathetic nerve endings and the adrenal medulla. However, toward the end of the first year we made an unexpected and exciting discovery while in the course of studying the characteristics of adrenergic beta receptors in rabbit aortic strips. This discovery was that the relaxation of isolated preparations of rabbit aorta by acetylcholine and related muscarinic agonists was eliminated if the intimal surface of the preparations was rubbed prior to testing with acetylcholine. This finding led to experiments in which we showed that the relaxation of rabbit aorta by acetylcholine was not the result of a direct action of that agent on the arterial*

The research in the author's laboratory referred to in this article was supported by grants from the National Heart, Lung, and Blood Institute of the National Institutes of Health.

From Panza JA, Cannon RO III (eds): *Endothelium, Nitric Oxide, and Atherosclerosis* ©Futura Publishing Co, Inc, Armonk, NY, 1999.

*smooth muscle, but rather the result of an indirect action in which acetyl-choline acted on muscarinic receptors of the endothelial cells, stimulating these cells to release a factor (or factors) that in turn acted on the smooth muscle cells to cause relaxation. These findings appeared to open up a very important new area in vascular physiology and pharmacology, and therefore by the end of the second year of the project [1979], our work was largely shifted from studies on adrenergic mechanisms to studies on the role of endothelial cells in the relaxation of arteries by acetylcholine and other potent relaxing agents. . . . We feel that the many novel and exciting findings that we have made in the past two or three years indicate that the shift in aims of our research was propitious. We are, naturally, very excited about continuing our new line of research in the project for which this present grant application is submitted.*

It should be noted that the NHLBI Scientific Administrator of our 1977–1982 grant, Dr. Jerry Critz, was kept aware of the shift in aims of our research and was supportive throughout.

# The Discovery of Endothelium-Derived Relaxing Factor

In 1980, our first full report was published on the obligatory role of endothelial cells in the relaxation of isolated preparations of rabbit thoracic aorta in response to acetylcholine (ACh) and other muscarinic agonists.[1] If these cells were removed either by gentle rubbing of the intimal surface or by incubation of the preparation with collagenase, relaxation in response to muscarinic agonists was lost (Figure 1). Because we have described previously in some detail how an accidental finding resulting from an error of a research assistant led to the discovery of endothelium-dependent relaxation,[2,3] it will suffice here to point out that the kind of vascular preparation developed and used for many years in the author's laboratory, namely, the helical (spiral) strip of the rabbit descending thoracic aorta,[4] had never exhibited relaxation in response to muscarinic agonists because the endothelial cells of the strip were (and unbeknown to us) rubbed off unintentionally in our standard method of preparation. Once it was recognized that ACh-induced relaxation observed in rings of aorta depended on the presence of endothelial cells, it was a simple matter of modifying the procedure for cutting strips to one in which the intimal surface was not rubbed, thus resulting in strips showing endothelium-dependent relaxation similar to that shown by rings.[1]

In our 1980 paper, we also reported that in addition to the thoracic aorta, a number of other arteries from the rabbit and various arteries from other species of laboratory animals also exhibited relaxation in response to ACh only if endothelial cells were present. Cyclooxygenase inhibitors did not interfere with the endothelium-dependent relaxation. One hypothesis to explain the obligatory role of endothelial cells was that ACh acting on a muscarinic receptor of these cells stimulates them to release a non-prostanoid substance that diffuses to and activates relaxation of the subjacent smooth muscle cells. Direct evidence for this hypothesis was obtained with the so-called "sandwich" procedure in which it was shown that a transverse strip of aorta freed of

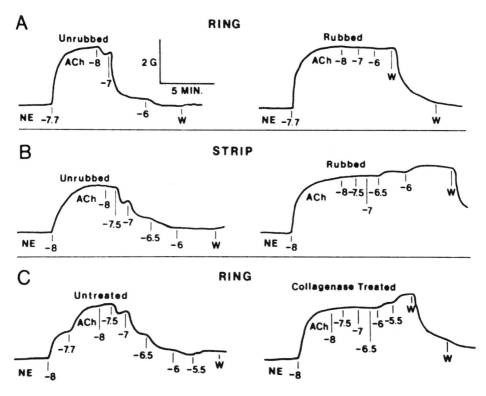

**Figure 1.** Loss of relaxing response of preparations of rabbit aorta to ACh after removal of endothelial cells by rubbing of the intimal surface or exposure to collagenase. (**A**) Recordings from the same ring before and after rubbing of the intimal surface with a small wooden stick. (**B**) Recordings from an unrubbed and rubbed transverse strip from the same aorta. (**C**) Recordings from rings of the same aorta before and after exposure of the intimal surface to 0.2% collagenase for 15 minute. Concentrations are in log molar units. Reproduced with permission from Reference 11.

endothelial cells and therefore unable to relax on exposure to ACh could be made to relax in response to ACh if it were remounted for recording with its endothelium-free intimal surface placed against the endothelium-containing intimal surface of a longitudinal strip of aorta. The ACh-induced relaxation of the sandwiched transverse strip demonstrated that ACh stimulated the release of a diffusible relaxing substance (or substances) from the endothelial cells of the longitudinal strip.[1] The relaxing substance was referred to later as endothelium-derived relaxing factor (EDRF).[5]

It is of some interest that an unintentional removal of endothelial cells in another vascular preparation used in my laboratory may have prevented the discovery of endothelium-dependent vasodilation at an earlier date. That preparation was the perfused rabbit central ear artery, which Odd Steinsland, while a graduate student in my laboratory in the early 1970s, used for investigating the inhibition by ACh and other muscarinic agonists of adrenergic neurotransmission by their action on prejunctional muscarinic inhibitory receptors. He readily demonstrated that ACh was a potent inhibitor of neurotransmission, as evidenced by its inhibition of both the release of norepineph-rine and the vasoconstriction in response to nerve stimulation.[6] To make sure that the inhibition of the vasoconstriction was caused by only inhibition of transmitter release, he tested whether infused ACh could inhibit vasoconstric-tion produced by infused norepinephrine and found that it did not.[6] About 10 years later, after endothelium-dependent relaxation by Ach had been found in a large variety of arterial preparations, we were puzzled by the earlier finding that the perfused ear artery constricted with infused norepinephrine had failed to show any vasodilation in response to ACh. Dr. Steinsland provided us with the answer. In his earlier work, he had not taken precautions to prevent gas bubbles from entering the perfusion line and passing through the ear artery. When care was now taken to avoid the occurrence of bubbles in the perfusion stream through the artery, ACh elicited good vasodilation (relax-ation) of norepinephrine-induced vasoconstriction.[7] Apparently, in the earlier work, the bubbles had removed mechanically the endothelial cells and we had been unaware of this action.

# Early Studies on
# Endothelium-Dependent Relaxation

Within a few years of the discovery that the relaxation of arteries by Ach was endothelium-dependent, a number of other agents also were found to induce relaxation of rings or strips of blood vessels from a variety of species, including man, in an endothelium-dependent manner. Among these agents were the calcium ionophore A23187, adenosine triphosphate (ATP) and aden-osine diphosphate (ADP), substance P, bradykinin, histamine, thrombin, se-rotonin, and vasopressin. (For references to first reports on endothelium-dependent relaxation by these and other agents, see reviews by Furchgott and Vanhoutte[8] and Furchgott.[9]) It should be stressed here that with many of these agents, the endothelium-dependent relaxation was found to be limited to arteries from certain species and/or to specific arteries from a given species. As an example of a difference among species, bradykinin produced endothelium-dependent relaxation of dog and human arteries but not of rabbit and cat arteries.[5] As an example of a difference among vessels in the same species, serotonin produced endothelium-dependent relaxation of canine coronary ar-teries but not of systemic arteries.[10] For other examples of differences among species and among vessels, see the review by Furchgott.[9]

Among the conditions and agents that were found to inhibit endothelium-dependent relaxation in early organ chamber experiments were anoxia and some agents that were recognized as inhibitors of the oxidation of arachidonic acid by lipoxygenase.[1] I therefore speculated that EDRF is a short-lived hy-droperoxide or free radical formed as an intermediate product in the oxidation of arachidonic acid by the lipoxygenase pathway and that this product stimu-lates guanylate cyclase (G-cyclase) of the vascular smooth muscle cells, result-ing in an increase in cyclic guanosine monophosphate (cGMP), which causes relaxation.[11] My speculation about the chemical nature of EDRF proved

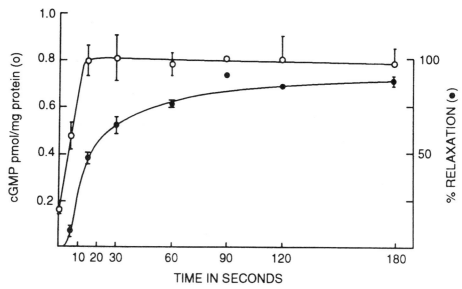

**Figure 2.** Time course of change of cGMP and of relaxation in endothelium-containing rings of rabbit aorta after addition of ACh. Norepinephrine first was added to produce a steady contraction. ACh (1 μmol/L) then was added, and the tissue was frozen after a desired period of exposure to ACh. Reproduced with permission from Reference 15.

wrong, but that about the stimulation of G-cyclase turned out to be correct. The basis for my early speculation about a key role for cGMP was that Murad et al[12] recently had shown that relaxation of tracheal smooth muscle by nitrovasodilators was accompanied by a rise in cGMP, and Ignarro and coworkers[13] had shown the same relationship in the case of relaxation of vascular smooth muscle. By 1983 Rapoport and Murad[14] clearly demonstrated that endothelium-dependent relaxation of rat thoracic aorta by ACh and other agents was correlated with an increase in cGMP, and shortly thereafter, we reported experiments on rabbit thoracic aorta in which a causal relationship was demonstrated between the increase in concentration of cGMP and endothelium-dependent relaxation in response to ACh (Figure 2).[15]

## Findings that Led to the Proposal that Endothelium-Drived Relaxing Factor Is Nitric Oxide

Between 1983 and 1985, while William Martin was working in my laboratory as a postdoctoral fellow, a number of important findings were made. Among them were that hemoglobin (Hb) (but not methemoglobin) and methylene blue (MB) were potent, very rapidly acting inhibitors of both the relaxation and the increases in cGMP produced by endothelium-dependent relaxing agents.[16] Originally, it was proposed that the inhibition by Hb was the result of its strong binding of EDRF as the latter diffused from the endothelial cells.

However, after the identification of EDRF as nitric oxide (NO), it became apparent that the scavenging of EDRF by Hb was the result of a very rapid reaction of oxygenated Hb ($HbO_2$) with NO to form metHb and $NO_3^-$. With respect to the inhibition by MB, it already was known from work of others that this agent is an inhibitor of G-cyclase. However, although agreeing that such enzyme inhibition could account for the sustained inhibition by MB developed during prolonged exposure of the aorta, we proposed that the extremely fast inhibition of endothelium-dependent relaxation immediately after addition of MB to an organ chamber resulted from some more direct inactivation of EDRF.[16] It now appears that this more direct inactivation is caused by superoxide anions generated by MB in the vascular tissue.

Through Martin, I became interested in the work that he and others had done in John Gillespie's laboratory in Glasgow in trying to identify the neurotransmitter released from so-called nonadrenergic, noncholinergic (NANC) nerves that elicits relaxation of bovine retractor penis (BRP) muscle and certain other smooth muscle preparations. I learned that both relaxation produced by NANC nerve stimulation and relaxation produced by a partly purified, acid-activated extract from the BRP muscle were both inhibited by Hb. As discussed in the paper that I presented at a symposium in Rochester, Minn, in July 1986,[17] I was struck by the similarities of the transient relaxations of the BRP muscle produced by the acid-activated extract, as found by Martin,[18] and the transient relaxations of rabbit aorta produced by acidified solutions of sodium nitrite ($NaNO_2$) (see Figure 3 and the review by Furchgott[17]). That acidified, but not neutral solutions of $NaNO_2$, produce strong transient relaxations of rabbit aorta had been found a number of years earlier in my laboratory when a new postdoctoral fellow, assigned to obtain cumulative dose-response curves for $NaNO_2$, accidentally made his standard solutions of that salt with acidified diluting fluid rather than neutral diluting fluid. At that time, I became aware that acidification of $NaNO_2$ solutions produces $HNO_2$ ($pK_a$ of 3.2), which immediately generates low concentrations of NO and $NO_2$ as a result of a reversible dismutation. However, when a solution of acidified nitrite is added to the oxygenated, well-buffered physiological salt solution used in our organ chambers, any NO present will be removed very rapidly, thus accounting for the transiency of the relaxation of the aortic rings receiving acidified nitrite.[17]

By the time we had begun to use acidified nitrite solutions as a source of NO in experiments with rabbit aorta in the spring of 1986, we also had become aware of the recent findings by Gryglewski, Palmer, and Moncada[19] and by Rubanyi and Vanhoutte[20] demonstrating that the superoxide anion ($O_2^-$) rapidly inactivates EDRF and that superoxide dismutase (SOD) protects against this inactivation. Assuming that the free radical NO might rapidly react with the free radical $O_2^-$, I began to speculate on the possibility that the acid-activatable relaxing factor in the BRP extract of Martin is inorganic nitrite and that EDRF is NO.

It should be noted here that a number of years earlier Murad et al[12] had found that NO is a very potent stimulus of G-cyclase and had proposed that a number of nitrovasodilators (eg, glyceryl trinitrate, nitroprusside, and azide) produce smooth muscle relaxation by generating NO as the proximal activator of G-cyclase; and Ignarro and coworkers[13] had found that the relaxation of a

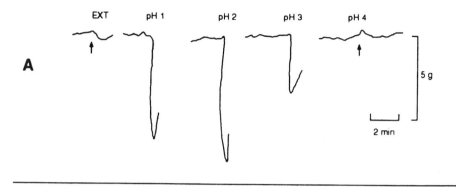

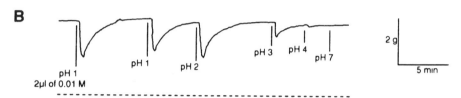

**Figure 3.** Comparison of transient relaxations of the BRP muscle produced by acidified extracts of BRP and transient relaxations of an endothelium-denuded ring of rabbit aorta produced by acidified NaNO$_2$ solutions. (**A**) BRP experiment of Martin.[18] Aliquots of BRP extract (pH 6.8) were brought to different pH levels for 10 minutes and then neutralized and quickly tested on a BRP strip. (**B**) Aorta experiment[17] Aliquots of a 10 mmol/L NaNO$_2$ solution were brought to different pH levels and then tested on an aortic ring in an organ chamber (pH 7.4 with final nitrite concentration of 1 $\mu$mol/L). Note the similarity of the pH dependence and time course of the transient relaxations with the two preparations. Reproduced with permission from Reference 17.

bovine coronary artery preparation by NO as well as nitroprusside was associated with an increase in cGMP. However, despite these early findings with NO, none of the investigators, including myself, who between 1983 and 1984 reported that endothelium-dependent relaxation was associated with an increase in cGMP (see above), hypothesized that EDRF might be the free radical NO.

My speculation in the spring of 1986 that EDRF might be NO led to a large number of experiments on rabbit aorta, carried out with the assistance of D. Jothianandan and M. T. Khan, comparing the characteristics of relaxation by EDRF (released by ACh) with the characteristics of relaxation by NO (present in acidified solutions of NaNO$_2$). The characteristics were so similar (inhibition by Hb and by MB, inhibition by superoxide generators, and protection by SOD) that I had no hesitancy proposing in the paper that I delivered at the July 1986 symposium that EDRF is NO.[17] I also proposed that the acid activatable inhibitory factor in the BRP extract of Martin and Gillespie was inorganic nitrite, and that the possibility had to be considered that the neurotransmitter of NANC nerves might also be NO.[17]

At the 1986 symposium at which I proposed that EDRF is NO, Ignarro, Byrns, and Wood,[21] on the basis of studies in their laboratory on isolated bovine pulmonary arteries, independently made the same proposal. (Unfortunately, the papers presented at that symposium were delayed in publication until 1988.) Soon after the 1986 symposium, three laboratories utilized perfusion-bioassay procedures to compare more accurately the biological and chemical characteristics of EDRF and NO. Ignarro et al,[22] using bovine pulmonary vessels, Moncada and coworkers,[23] using cultured porcine aortic endothelial cells, and Khan and myself,[24] using rabbit aorta as a source of EDRF, all found EDRF released upstream and NO infused upstream to have similar rates of decay, similar susceptibility to inhibitors like Hb and superoxide generators, similar stabilization by SOD, etc. In addition, Ignarro's laboratory obtained spectroscopic evidence that the product of the reaction of released EDRF and Hb was the same as that of NO and Hb,[22] and Moncada's laboratory showed that the amount of NO released by bradykinin (as determined by a chemiluminescence assay) could account fully for the relaxation of the bioassay strip by the EDRF released by the peptide.[23] A year later Moncada's laboratory found that the source of endothelial NO was a guanidinium nitrogen of L-arginine and that the enzyme responsible for its formation was an oxygenase [now called endothelial NO synthase (eNOS)].[25] These findings marked the beginning of a major worldwide expansion of research on the role of NO in vascular physiology and pathophysiology.

Despite the evidence for the identity of EDRF and NO, some results obtained in various laboratories in the late 1980s did not appear to be consistent completely with that conclusion. (For a review of these apparent or real inconsistencies, see the review by Furchgott, Jothianandan, and Freay[7].) Nevertheless, as of now, it generally has become accepted that EDRF is either NO or some adduct that readily releases NO or perhaps a mixture of NO and some adduct of NO. This does not preclude a contribution to endothelium-dependent relaxation in some blood vessels from the release of a non-nitric oxide endothelium-derived hyperpolarizing factor (EDHF) along with EDRF.

*Acknowledgments.* The research in the author's laboratory referred to in this article was supported by grants from the NHLBI of the National Institutes of Health.

# References

1. Furchgott RF, Zawadzki JV. The obligatory role of endothelial cells in the relaxation of arterial smooth muscle by acetylcholine. *Nature* 1980;288:373–376.
2. Furchgott RF. The discovery of endothelium-dependent relaxation. *Circulation* 1993;87(suppl V):V3–V8.4.
3. Furchgott RF. The discovery of endothelium-derived relaxing factor and its importance in the identification of nitric oxide. *J Am Med Assn* 1996;276:1186–1188.
4. Furchgott RF, Bhadrakom S. Reactions of strips of rabbit aorta to epinephrine, isopropylarterenol, sodium nitrite and other drugs. *J Pharmacol Exp Ther* 1953; 108:129–143.
5. Cherry PD, Furchgott RF, Zawadzki JV, Jothianandan D. The role of endothelial cells in the relaxation of isolated arteries by bradykinin. *Proc Natl Acad Sci U S A* 1983;79:2106–2110.
6. Steinsland OS, Furchgott RF, Kirpekar SM. Inhibition of adrenergic neurotransmission by parasympathomimetics in the rabbit ear artery. *J Pharmacol Exp Ther* 1973;184:346–356.

7. Furchgott RF, Jothianandan D, Freay AD. Endothelium-derived relaxing factor: Some old and new findings. In: Moncada S, Higgs EA, eds. *Nitric Oxide from L-Arginine: A Bioregulatory System*. Amsterdam: Elsevier; 1990:5–17.
8. Furchgott RF, Vanhoutte PM. Endothelium-derived relaxing and contracting factors. *FASEB J* 1989;3:2007–2018.
9. Furchgott RF. The Ulf von Euler Lecture. Studies on endothelium-dependent vasodilation and the endothelium-derived relaxing factor. *Acta Physiol Scand* 1990; 1989;139:257–270.
10. Cohen RA, Shepherd JT, Vanhoutte PM. 5-Hydroxytryptamine can mediate endothelium-dependent relaxation of coronary arteries. *Am J Physiol* 1983;245: H1077–1080.
11. Furchgott RF, Zawadzki JV, Cherry PD. Role of endothelium in vasodilator response to acetylcholine. In; Vanhoutte PM, Leusen I, eds. *Vasodilatation*. New York: Raven Press; 1981:49–66.
12. Murad F, Arnold WP, Mittal CK, Braughler JM. Properties and regulation of guanylate cyclase and some proposed functions of cyclc GMP. *Adv Cyclic Nucleotide Res* 1979;11:175–204.
13. Gruetter CA, Barry BK, McNamara DB, Gruetter DY, Kadowitz PJ, Ignarro LJ. Relaxation of bovine coronary artery and activation of coronary arterial guanylate cyclase by nitric oxide, nitroprusside and carcinogenic nitrosoamine. *J Cyclic Neucleotide Res* 1979;5:211–214.
14. Rapoport RM, Murad F. Agonist-induced endothelium-dependent relaxation in rat thoracic aorta may be mediated through cGMP. *Circ Res* 1983;52:352–357.
15. Furchgott RF, Cherry PD, Zawadzki JV, Jothianandan D. Endothelial cells as mediators of vasodilation of arteries. *J Cardiovasc Pharmacol* 1984;6(suppl 2): S336–334.
16. Martin W, Villani GM, Jothianandan D, Furchgott RF. Selective blockade of endothelium-dependent and glyceryl trinitrate-induced relaxation by hemoglobin and by methylene blue in the rabbit aorta. *J Pharmacol Exp Ther* 1985;232:708–716.
17. Furchgott RF. Studies on relaxation of rabbit aorta by sodium nitrite: the basis for the proposal that the acid-activatable inhibitory factor from retractor penis is inorganic nitrite and the endothelium-derived relaxing factor is nitric oxide. In: Vanhoutte PM, ed. *Vasodilatation: Vascular Smooth Muscle, Peptides, and Endothelium*. New York: Raven Press; 1988:401–418.
18. Gillespie JS, Hunter JC, Martin W. A smooth muscle inhibitory material from the bovine retractor penis and rat anococcygeus muscles. *J Physiol* 1981;309:55–64.
19. Gryglewski PJ, Palmer RMJ, Moncada SA. Superoxide anion is involved in the breakdown of endothelium-derived relaxing factor. *Nature* 1986;320:454–456.
20. Rubanyi GM, Vanhoutte PM. Superoxide anions and hyperoxia inactivate endothelium-derived relaxing factor. *Amer J Physiol* 1986;250:H822–827.
21. Ignarro LJ, Byrns RE, Wood KS. Biochemical and pharmacological properties of endothelium-derived relaxing factor and its similarity to nitric oxide radical. In: Vanhoutte PM, ed. *Vasodilatation: Vascular Smooth Muscle, Peptides and Endothelium*. New York: Raven Press; 1988:427–435.
22. Ignarro LJ, Buga GM, Wood KS, Byrns RE, Chauduri G. Endothelium-derived relaxing factor (EDRF) produced and released from artery and vein is nitric oxide. *Proc Natl Acad Sci U S A* 1987;84:9265–9269.
23. Palmer RMJ, Ferrige AG, Moncada S. Nitric oxide release accounts for the biological activity of endothelium-derived relaxing factor. *Nature* 1987;327:524–526.
24. Khan MT, Furchgott RF. Additional evidence that endothelium-derived relaxing factor is nitric oxide. In: Rand MJ, Raper C, eds. *Pharmacology*. Amsterdam: Elsevier; 1987:341–344.
25. Palmer RMJ, Ashton DS, Moncada S. Vascular endothelial cells synthesize nitric oxide from L-arginine. *Nature* 1988;333:664–666.

Chapter 2

# Discovery of Biological Roles of Nitric Oxide in the Cardiovascular System

*Salvador Moncada, MD, and E. Annie Higgs,BSc, MSc*

In 1980 Furchgott and Zawadzki demonstrated that isolated blood vessels will only relax after exposure to some vasodilators if the vascular endothelium is present.[1] Further bioassay studies showed that this phenomenon was dependent on the release of a labile substance, which was named endothelium-derived relaxing factor (EDRF). In 1985 we began to work on this substance, which was known to have a half-life of 3–5 seconds and to cause vascular relaxation via the activation of the soluble guanylate cyclase in vascular smooth muscle cells.[2]

Instead of working with freshly isolated rings or strips of vascular tissue in organ baths or cascades, as others had done, we decided to culture vascular endothelial cells on microcarrier beads, perfuse them in a modified chromatography column, and use the effluent to superfuse a series of isolated vascular strips, denuded of their endothelium, in a cascade superfusion bioassay system.[3] This allowed the simultaneous bioassay of prostacyclin and EDRF and extensive pharmacological studies as well as the characterization of the latter substance. We established that bradykinin and the $Ca^{2+}$ ionophore, A23187, release EDRF and we analyzed some of its properties, including its half-life, in our bioassay system.

These early experiments also led us to the finding that the superoxide anion ($O_2^-$) was involved in the breakdown of EDRF.[4] Later on we demonstrated that several of the disparate chemicals that had been described previously as inhibitors of EDRF, including BW755, dithiothreitol, and dihydroquinone, had a common mechanism of action because they all released $O_2^-$ in solution.[5] This differentiated them from hemoglobin, another powerful inhibitor of the actions of EDRF, which binds and, as a consequence, inactivates this molecule.[6] We further predicted and subsequently confirmed that pyrogallol, a generator of $O_2^-$ in solutions, also would be an inhibitor of EDRF.[5] All these experiments led us to suspect that EDRF might be a highly reactive radical species.

From Panza JA, Cannon RO III (eds): *Endothelium, Nitric Oxide, and Atherosclerosis* ©Futura Publishing Co, Inc, Armonk, NY, 1999.

Over the years following its discovery, several hypotheses had been put forward about the chemical structure of EDRF.[7] One of them, which suggested that this compound might be nitric oxide (NO) or a related molecule,[8,9] attracted our attention because it fitted with our hypothesis about the free-radical nature of EDRF. We decided to investigate this hypothesis critically.

In the summer of 1986 we used NO gas and a chemiluminescence technique to measure NO directly. Both the preparation of NO gas for bioassay studies as well as the adaptation of the chemiluminescence technique for the measurement of very small amounts of NO were very difficult. Nevertheless, by December 1986 we had gathered enough evidence demonstrating unequivocally that EDRF is NO.[10] Extensive pharmacological studies on vascular strips comparing EDRF released from vascular endothelial cells in culture and authentic NO demonstrated the pharmacological identity between the two compounds (Figure 1) and chemiluminescence measurements showed that NO was released from the cells in sufficient quantities to account for the actions of

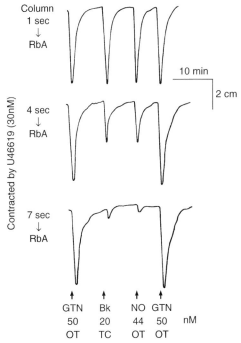

**Figure 1.**  Relaxation of rabbit aortae (RbA) by endothelium-derived relaxing factor (EDRF) and nitric oxide (NO). A column packed with porcine endothelial cells cultured on microcarriers was perfused with Krebs' buffer (5 mL min$^{-1}$). The effluent was used to superfuse three spiral strips of RbA, denuded of endothelium, in a cascade. The tissues were contracted submaximally by a continuous infusion of 9,11-dideoxy-9$\alpha$, 11$\alpha$-methano epoxy-prostaglandin F$_{2\alpha}$ (U46619; 30 nmol/L) and were separated from the cells by delays of 1, 4, and 7 seconds, respectively. The sensitivity of the bioassay tissues was standardized by administration of glyceryl trinitrate (GTN; 50 nmol/L) over the tissues (OT). The EDRF was released from the cells by a 1-minute infusion through the column (TC) of bradykinin (Bk; 20 nmol/L). The NO (0.22 nmol) was dissolved in He-deoxygenated H$_2$O and administered as a 1-minute infusion. For further details see Palmer et al.[10]

EDRF (Figure 2). Some of these experiments and those of others[11] were aided greatly by our earlier finding that superoxide dismutase enhanced the half-life of EDRF (Figure 3) and by the use of pyrogallol as an inhibitor of EDRF.

A year later, also using bioassay studies, we discovered that the amino acid L-arginine was the precursor for the biosynthesis of NO (Figure 4).[12] This was confirmed by mass spectrometry, which further identified the origin of the nitrogen of NO from the guanidino terminal(s) of the L-arginine molecule (Figure 5).[12] During these experiments we found that citrulline also could be utilized by the endothelial cells, although to a lesser extent, and that D-arginine was not a substrate. In the vascular endothelium we later demon-

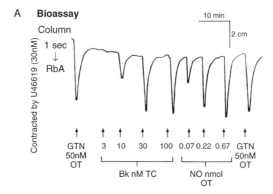

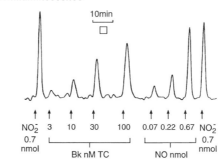

**Figure 2.** Correlation between NO measured by bioassay (**A**) and by chemiluminescence (**B**). Bioassay: relaxation of RbA by EDRF and NO. The bioassay was carried out as described in the legend to Figure 1. The bioassay tissues were relaxed in a concentration-dependent manner by EDRF released from the cells by 1-minute infusions through the column (TC) of Bk (3–100 nmol/L) and by NO (0.07–0.67 nmol, OT) dissolved in He-deoxygenated water and administered as 1-minute infusions. (**B**) Chemiluminescence: release of NO by Bk from a replicate column of the cells used in the bioassay. The amounts of NO (administered as a 1-minute infusion into the column effluent), which relaxed the bioassay tissues, also were also detectable by chemiluminescence. Effluent from the column or Krebs' buffer into which authentic NO was injected was passed continuously (5 mL/min) into a reaction vessel containing 75 mL 1.0% sodium iodide in glacial acetic acid under reflux. The NO was removed from the refluxing mixture under reduced pressure in a stream of $N_2$, mixed with ozone, and the chemiluminescent product was measured with a photomultiplier. The amounts of NO detected were quantified with reference to an $NO_2^-$ standard curve with an area equivalent to 0.22 nmol NO. For further details see Palmer et al.[10]

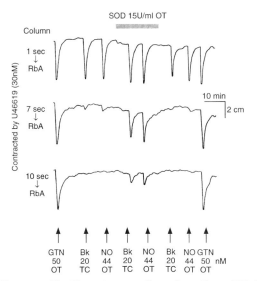

**Figure 3.** Effect of superoxide dismutase on the relaxation of RbA by EDRF and NO. The bioassay was carried out as described in the legend to Figure 1. The EDRF was released by 1-minute infusions of bradykinin (Bk, 20 nmol/L) through the column (TC). Superoxide dismutase (SOD; 15 U/mL)-infused OT caused relaxation of the tissues, the magnitude of relaxation being greater in the top tissue, and potentiated to a similar extent the relaxation induced by release of EDRF and by 1-minute infusions of NO (44 nmol/L OT).

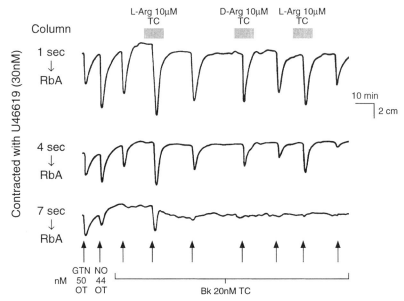

**Figure 4.** The effect of L-arginine and D-arginine on the relaxation of RbA by NO. A column, packed with porcine endothelial cells cultured on microcarriers for 24 hours in culture medium without L-arginine, was perfused with Krebs' buffer (5 mL min$^{-1}$). The effluent was used to superfuse in a cascade three spiral strips of RbA denuded of endothelium and contracted submaximally. The magnitude of the relaxations induced by NO (44 nmol/L over the tissues) declined during passage down the cascade. The NO released by a 1-minute infusion of Bk (20 nmol/L, administered through the column) caused a relaxation of the bioassay tissues, which also declined during passage down the cascade. This release was enhanced by infusion of L-arginine (10 $\mu$mol/L), but not D-arginine (10 $\mu$mol/L) through the column. For further details see Palmer et al.[17]

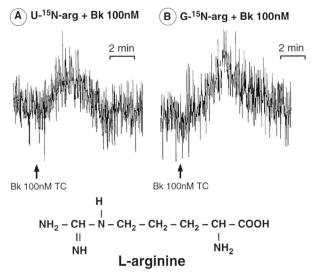

**Figure 5.** Determination of $^{15}$NO release from endothelial cells by mass spectrometry. A column of arginine-depleted cells was perfused with Krebs' buffer (5 mL min$^{-1}$) and the effluent passed continuously into a chemiluminescence reflux vessel. The $^{15}$NO was released from cells stimulated with Bk (100 nmol/L) in the presence of an infusion of universally-labeled $^{15}$N-arginine (10 $\mu$mol/L, **A**) or guanidino-labeled $^{15}$N-arginine (10 $\mu$mol/L, **B**). Comparable amounts of $^{15}$NO were released in the presence of both isotopes (2.1 $\pm$ 0.7 nmol and 2.2 $\pm$ 0.4 nmol, respectively), indicating that only the terminal guanidino nitrogen atom(s) gives rise to NO.

strated the presence of an enzyme that generated L-citrulline, which turned out to be the coproduct of the generation of NO from L-arginine.[13] This enzyme became known as NO synthase (NOS). Later, we and others showed that, in the process of generating NO, the NOS incorporates molecular oxygen at two points, first in the formation of $N$-hydroxy-arginine and second in the formation of L-citrulline.[14,15]

A significant development in our research was the finding that the L-arginine analogue $N^{G}$-monomethyl-L-arginine (L-NMMA), a compound previously shown to inhibit the generation of nitrite (NO$_2^-$) and nitrate (NO$_3^-$) in activated macrophages,[16] prevented both the endothelium-dependent relaxation and the release of NO in a competitive manner.[17] Furthermore, and more importantly, this compound induced endothelium- and dose-dependent contraction of isolated vascular rings (Figure 6), thus suggesting a continuous generation of NO, which results in a vasodilator tone.[18]

L-NMMA not only contracted vascular rings in isolated organ baths but also produced an increase in coronary perfusion pressure in isolated Langendorff-perfused hearts. This effect could be reversed by treatment with L- but not D-arginine.[19] These results led us to carry out a series of experiments in which we demonstrated that L-NMMA induces a hypertensive response in the whole animal (Figure 7).[20] This effect is accompanied by inhibition of NO synthesis in the vasculature and can be reversed by L-arginine.[20] L-NMMA and, later on, other inhibitors of the NOS, proved to constrict all vascular beds tested, including the human brachial arterial circulation (Figure 8).[21] In ad-

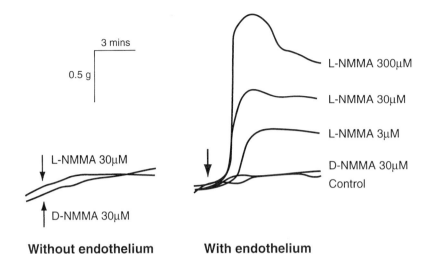

**Figure 6.** Effect of $N^G$-monomethyl-L-arginine (L-NMMA) and $N^G$-monomethyl-D-arginine (D-NMMA) on the basal tone of rabbit aortic rings precontracted with phenylephrine (750 nmol/L), with and without endothelium. For further details see Rees et al.[18]

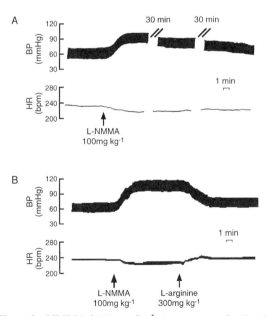

**Figure 7.** (**A**) Effect of L-NMMA [100 mg/kg[1], intravenously (i.v.)] on blood pressure (BP) and heart rate (HR) in the anesthetized rabbit. The duration of these effects of L-NMMA was between 60 and 90 minutes. (**B**) Reversal of the effect of L-NMMA (100 mg/kg[1], i.v.) on blood pressure and heart rate by L-arginine (300 mg/kg[1], i.v.). Trace is representative of three experiments. For further details see Rees et al.[20]

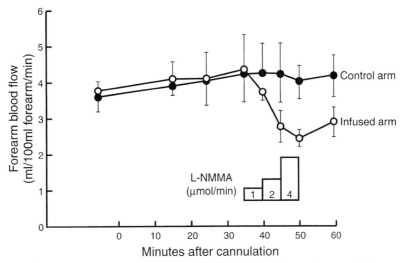

**Figure 8.** Vasoconstrictor response to L-NMMA infused into the brachial artery. The L-NMMA (1–4 µmol/min) caused a dose-dependent decrease in basal forearm blood flow. For further details see Vallance et al.[21]

dition, they induced sustained hypertension during long-term oral adminis-tration.[22] Over the next 10 years those findings were confirmed in many other laboratories around the world.

Because L-NMMA has no intrinsic constrictor activity on vascular smooth muscle and it does not affect other systems in the vascular wall, its action is entirely endothelium-dependent, and its vasoconstrictor properties result from the inhibition of an endogenous vasodilator mechanism. Therefore these ex-periments led us to suggest that an NO-dependent dilator tone is an important component of the regulatory systems of blood flow and blood pressure. Re-cently, this proposal has been strengthened by studies in mice in which the gene for endothelial NOS (eNOS) has been disrupted. Such animals lack eNOS and are of a phenotype that includes an elevated blood pressure compared with their wild-type counterparts.[23] L-NMMA, which does not affect the blood pres-sure of the eNOS mutant animals, increases the blood pressure of wild-type animals to that of the mutants (manuscript in preparation, Figure 9).

The discovery of the NO-dependent vasodilator tone indicated the exis-tence of an endogenous nitrovasodilator system, the actions of which are imitated by compounds such as glyceryl trinitrate and sodium nitroprus-side.[24,25] In addition to its vasodilator actions, NO also contributes to the control of platelet aggregation[26] and the regulation of cardiac contractility.[27] These physiological effects of NO are all mediated by activation of the soluble guanylate cyclase. Other actions of NO that relate to the cardiovascular system include inhibition of white cell activation[28] and inhibition of smooth muscle cell proliferation.[29]

NO now is known to be the mediator released in the peripheral nervous system by a widespread network of nerves, previously recognized as nonad-renergic and noncholinergic.[30–32] These nitrergic nerves, which contain neu-ronal NOS (nNOS), mediate some forms of neurogenic vasodilatation but their

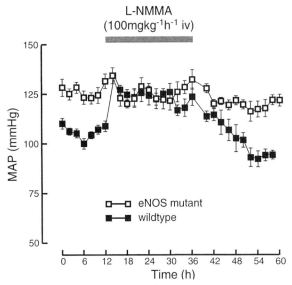

**Figure 9.** Effect of L-NMMA (100 mg/kg[1] per hour[1] i.v.) on mean arterial blood pressure in conscious wild-type and endothelia nitric oxide synthase e(NOS) mutant mice. L-NMMA increased the blood pressure of the wild-type animals to those of the eNOS mutant counterparts, without significantly affecting the blood pressure of the latter.

precise role in the regulation of blood pressure has not been established. However, recent evidence suggests that the tonic influence of vasodilator factors, in particular NO released from nitrergic nerves, is essential for the maintenance of blood supply to brain regions.[33]

Thus, NO is a physiological homeostatic regulator of the vessel wall, playing a role in the maintenance of a vasodilator tone, inhibition of platelet and white cell activation, and maintaining vascular smooth muscle in a non-proliferative state. Impaired production of NO has been implicated in several cardiovascular disorders, including hypertension, vasospasm, and atherosclerosis.[34] In humans with essential hypertension there is increasing evidence for a reduced generation of NO.[35,36] In animals, one example of experimental hypertension in which there is unequivocal evidence for an impairment in the generation of NO is the Sabra hypertension-prone (salt-sensitive) rat. We have shown that, compared with hypertension-resistant Sabra rats, vasorelaxant responses to acetylcholine are diminished in the hypertension-prone animals, the constrictor responses to L-NMMA are reduced, less eNOS is present in the vasculature, and the circulating levels of $NO_2^-$ and $NO_3^-$ (breakdown products of NO) are lower.[37] Because NO plays a role in the excretion of sodium in the kidney[38] it is likely that a reduction in production of NO leads to a dual effect, namely, an increase in vascular reactivity and reduced excretion of sodium, both of which play a role in the hypertensive state of these animals.

We have further hypothesized that in relation to NO there may be two types of hypertension. In one type, increased vasoconstrictor activity (which may be caused by different factors) leads to an increase in NO generation as a compensatory mechanism; in this situation there may be normal or increased sodium excretion. The other type may depend on a deficiency in NO generation that would be accompanied by abnormal renal sodium handling. Thus, the first type of hypertension would be associated with abnormally high vasoconstrictor levels, while in the second type, normal levels of vasoconstrictors will in effect behave as excessive because of the lack of counteracting NO-dependent vasodilator tone (Figure 10).

In rings of atherosclerotic coronary arteries, the endothelium-dependent relaxation is decreased and the responses to vasoconstrictors often are enhanced as compared with rings of normal coronary arteries.[39] Furthermore, vasodilatation induced by acetylcholine or increased blood flow is impaired in the coronary circulation of patients with atherosclerosis,[40] smokers, and children with familial hypercholesterolemia.[41] The antiatherogenic actions of NO may be attributed to many factors including inhibition of monocyte adhesion to the endothelium, inhibition of expression of vascular cell adhesion molecule 1 (VCAM-1) and monocyte chemoattractant protein 1 (MCP-1), and reduced activity of nuclear factor–kappa B (NF-κB).[42] In this context it is interesting to note that eNOS knockout mice respond to vascular damage with a greater proliferative lesion than the wild-type controls.[43]

The administration of L-arginine has been shown to exert an antiatherogenic effect because it normalizes the vascular dysfunction in patients and animals with hypercholesterolemia;[44–46] in animals the effect is accompanied by a reduction in the thickness of the intimal lesions.[45] Administration of L-arginine may be beneficial in preventing restenosis after balloon angioplasty, because it attenuates intimal hyperplasia in rabbits.[47] Whether the effects of exogenously added arginine are caused by its direct conversion into NO or the fact that the added arginine may be promoting use of the endogenous substrate is not clear. Interestingly, in a study in low-density lipoprotein (LDL) receptor knockout mice, dietary arginine supplementation markedly reduced the number of intimal lesions that these animals normally develop in response to a high-fat diet.[48] These effects were abrogated by coadministration of an inhib-

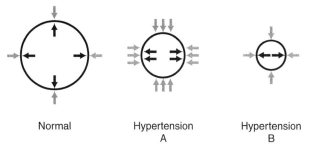

**Figure 10.** Schematic representation of two types of hypertension. In the normal situation, vasoconstrictor influences from outside the blood vessel (grey arrows) are counterbalanced by basal production of NO by eNOS (black arrows). Hypertension can occur in a situation in which vasoconstrictor activity is enhanced and more NO is produced as an attempt to compensate (type A). Alternatively, reduced synthesis of NO (type B) would lead to hypertension even in the presence of normal levels of vasoconstrictors.

itor of NOS, suggesting that they were caused by the conversion of L-arginine to NO.

The NO donors also may possess antiatherosclerotic actions, based on the down-regulation of several processes involved in the progression of this condition. Thus, for example, the NO donor SPM-5185 markedly attenuates intimal thickening in injured carotid arteries of the rat.[49]

The physiological generation of NO by eNOS is activated by a variety of chemical and physical stimuli. It may be possible to develop agonists that cause long-term activation of the L-arginine:NO pathway. Indeed, angiotensin-converting enzyme (ACE) inhibitors, besides preventing the generation of angiotensin II, act indirectly in this way by preventing the breakdown of bradykinin, which stimulates the synthesis of NO.[50] The ACE inhibitors enhance the production of NO in endothelial cells[51] and treatment of animals with inhibitors of NOS reduces the antihypertensive effect of ACE inhibitors.[50] The ability of these compounds to prevent formation of neointima after injury also is blocked by inhibitors of NOS, suggesting that these antiproliferative actions of ACE inhibitors also may be mediated, at least in part, via production of NO.[52]

In some situations the activity as well as the amount of constitutive eNOS and nNOS is increased, showing that these isoforms of the enzyme actually can be induced. We have shown that during pregnancy and treatment with estradiol mRNAs for both eNOS and nNOS are increased.[53] Since then estrogen has been shown by numerous investigators to increase NOS both in vitro and in vivo.[54] This estrogen-induced enhancement of NO synthesis could contribute to the decrease in vascular tone and contractility that occurs during pregnancy, the associated increase in gastrointestinal transit time, and the reduced incidence of heart disease in pre-menopausal women. In addition, the induction of both eNOS mRNA and protein has been demonstrated following exposure of cultured vascular endothelial cells to shear stress.[55] Shear stress-induced generation of NO accounts for the phenomenon of flow-mediated dilatation and might be a mechanism by which vessels keep shear forces constant in the face of changes in flow. Interestingly, those sites in the vasculature that are exposed to high shear stress are less prone to atherogenesis than those exposed to low shear stress. Chronic exercise also has been shown to enhance eNOS gene expression in the aortic endothelium.[55] These observations have led to the identification of consensus sites on the eNOS gene for regulation by shear stress and other stimuli.[56]

There is a different type of NOS that is inducible in many cells and tissues by immunological stimuli such as endotoxin lipopolysaccharide and cytokines and whose induction is inhibited by glucocorticoids.[57,58] This enzyme [inducible NOS (iNOS)] was identified originally in macrophages and contributes to the cytotoxic actions of these cells.[59-61] The NO produced by this enzyme in the vasculature contributes to the profound vasodilatation of septic shock and may be involved in the myocardial damage that occurs in some inflammatory conditions of the heart.[62] Endotoxin induces iNOS in the myocardium[63] and endocardium, and studies in rat myocytes in culture[64] and in isolated working hearts[65] indicate the involvement of iNOS induction in cytokine-induced myocardial contractile dysfunction. Enhanced synthesis of NO by this enzyme therefore may contribute to the cardiac dysfunction associated with endotoxemia.[66] Furthermore, the cardiac dysfunction of dilated cardiomyopathy also may be associated with induction of this enzyme. Biopsies of myocardial tissue from patients with dilated cardiomyopathy have shown that this tissue contains iNOS while tissue from nondilated ischemic hearts or from patients with dilated hearts of ischemic or valvular origin had little or no iNOS activity. Therefore the enzyme appears to be expressed only in dilated hearts of inflammatory etiology.[66] Thus, in the heart as in the vasculature, NO may have a physiological role when generated by the constitutive enzyme that is present normally in the myocardium and may become pathological, causing dilatation and tissue damage, when generated in large quantities and for long periods by the inducible enzyme. L-NMMA, when used at low doses in animals and man, reverses the hypotension and the hyporeactivity to vasoconstriction characteristic of shock.[62] Selective inhibitors of the inducible NOS may prove beneficial for the treatment of the hypotension of shock or cytokine therapy as well as provide a new approach to antiinflammatory therapy.

One potential route of NO-induced toxicity is through its interaction with other molecules, mainly superoxide anion ($O_2^-$). Originally, it was demonstrated that NO generated from vascular cells[4,67] or from leukocytes[68] interacts with $O_2^-$, leading to reduction in its vasorelaxant and platelet antiaggregatory actions. The product of the reaction between these two free radicals has been shown to be peroxynitrite anion ($ONOO^-$), which also has been shown to be formed in vitro by activated macrophages.[69,70] This powerful oxidant, when protonated, decomposes rapidly, resulting in the formation of OH· and $NO_2$, both of which are tissue-damaging agents. The formation of $ONOO^-$ has not been demonstrated directly in vivo, although 3-nitrotyrosine (which has been proposed to be a product of the interaction between tyrosine and $ONOO^-$) has been shown to be present in biological fluids[71] and in a variety of inflammatory conditions[72,73] including atherosclerosis.[74] At present it is not clear under which conditions $ONOO^-$ is formed and whether its release leads to irreversible tissue damage through nitration of proteins. Interestingly, we have shown that there are very effective detoxification mechanisms for $ONOO^-$, notably its interaction with tissue thiol, which are rapidly nitrosylated. We have postulated therefore that $ONOO^-$ may be damaging in conditions in which those mechanisms of detoxification are reduced, such as in the atherosclerotic plaque.[75]

An area of increasing interest in which NO and oxygen might be interacting is at the mitochondria where NO at physiological concentrations plays a role as a regulator of cell respiration through an action on the cytochrome c oxidase (complex IV).[76,77] Furthermore, we have demonstrated recently in vascular endothelial cells that basal production of NO maintains the cytochrome c oxidase in a down-regulated state, thus controlling oxygen consumption (Clementi et al, manuscript in preparation). It has been postulated that increasing concentrations of NO, which may inhibit cytochrome c oxidase for long periods, may lead to the generation of $O_2^-$ in the redox chain and thus to the formation of $ONOO^-$.[78] Peroxynitrite may inhibit other complexes in the mitochondria in an irreversible manner.[79,78] Interestingly, some recent results suggest that while NO-induced inhibition of mitochondrial complex IV is always reversible even after long-term exposure, NO induces persistent inhibition of mitochondrial complex I. This only occurs following a decrease in intracellular glutathione.[80] Whether decreases in glutathione favor the formation of $O_2^-$ in the redox chain, leading to localized generation of $ONOO^-$ in complex I, remains to be established.

Thus, the discovery of the L-arginine:NO pathway has had a great impact in our understanding of the physiology and pathophysiology of the cardiovascular system. It is likely that this knowledge will lead to novel therapies for the treatment and prevention of cardiovascular disease.

# References

1. Furchgott RF, Zawadzki JV. The obligatory role of endothelial cells in the relaxation of arterial smooth muscle by acetylcholine. *Nature* 1980;288:373–376.
2. Furchgott RF. The 1989 Ulf von Euler lecture; studies on endothelium-dependent vasodilation and the endothelium-derived relaxing factor. *Acta Physiol Scand* 1990; 139:257–270.
3. Gryglewski RJ, Moncada S, Palmer RM. Bioassay of prostacyclin and endothelium-derived relaxing factor (EDRF) from porcine aortic endothelial cells. *Br J Pharmacol* 1986;87:685–694.
4. Gryglewski RJ, Palmer RM, Moncada S. Superoxide anion is involved in the breakdown of endothelium-derived vascular relaxing factor. *Nature* 1986;320:454–456.
5. Moncada S, Palmer RM, Gryglewski RJ. Mechanism of action of some inhibitors of endothelium-derived relaxing factor. *Proc Natl Acad Sci U S A* 1986;83:9164–9168.
6. Martin W, Smith JA, White DG. The mechanisms by which haemoglobin inhibits the relaxation of rabbit aorta induced by nitrovasodilators, nitric oxide, or bovine retractor penis inhibitory factor. *Br J Pharmacol* 1986;89:563–571.
7. Furchgott RF. The role of endothelium in the responses of vascular smooth muscle to drugs. *Annu Rev Pharmacol Toxicol* 1984;24:175–197.
8. Furchgott RF. Studies on relaxation of rabbit aorta by sodium nitrite: The basis for the proposal that the acid-activatable inhibitory factor from retractor penis is inorganic nitrite and the endothelium-derived relaxing factor is nitric oxide. In: Vanhoutte PM, ed. *Vasodilatation: Vascular Smooth Muscle, Peptides, Autonomic Nerves, and Endothelium.* New York: Raven Press, 1988:401–414.
9. Ignarro LJ, Byrns RE, Wood KS. Biochemical and pharmacological properties of endothelium-derived relaxing factor and its similarity to nitric oxide radical. In: Vanhoutte PM, ed. *Vasodilatation: Vascular Smooth Muscle. Peptides. Autonomic Nerves and Endothelium.* New York: Raven Press, 1988:427–436.
10. Palmer RM, Ferrige AG, Moncada S. Nitric oxide release accounts for the biological activity of endothelium-derived relaxing factor. *Nature* 1987;327:524–526.
11. Furchgott RF, Jothianandan D, Freay AD. Endothelium-derived relaxing factor: some old and new findings. In: Moncada S, Higgs EA, eds. *Nitric Oxide from L-Arginine: A Bioregulatory System.* New York: Elsevier Science Publishers (Biomedical Division), 1990:5–17.
12. Palmer RM, Ashton DS, Moncada S. Vascular endothelial cells synthesize nitric oxide from L-arginine. *Nature* 1988;333:664–666.
13. Palmer RM, Moncada S. A novel citrulline-forming enzyme implicated in the formation of nitric oxide by vascular endothelial cells. *Biochem Biophys Res Commun* 1989;158:348–352.
14. Kwon NS, Nathan CF, Gilker C, et al. L-citrulline production from L-arginine by macrophage nitric oxide synthase. The ureido oxygen derives from dioxygen. *J Biol Chem* 1990;265:13442–13445.

15. Leone AM, Palmer RM, Knowles RG, et al. Constitutive and inducible nitric oxide synthases incorporate molecular oxygen into both nitric oxide and citrulline. *J Biol Chem* 1991;266:23790–23795.

16. Hibbs JB, Jr, Taintor RR, Vavrin Z. Macrophage cytotoxicity: Role for L-arginine deiminase and imino nitrogen oxidation to nitrite. *Science* 1987;235:473–476.

17. Palmer RM, Rees DD, Ashton DS, et al. L-arginine is the physiological precursor for the formation of nitric oxide in endothelium-dependent relaxation. *Biochem Biophys Res Commun* 1988;153:1251–1256.

18. Rees DD, Palmer RM, Hodson HF, et al. A specific inhibitor of nitric oxide formation from L-arginine attenuates endothelium-dependent relaxation. *Br J Pharmacol* 1989;96:418–424.

19. Amezcua JL, Palmer RM, de Souza BM, et al. Nitric oxide synthesized from L-arginine regulates vascular tone in the coronary circulation of the rabbit. *Br J Pharmacol* 1989;97:1119–1124.

20. Rees DD, Palmer RM, Moncada S. Role of endothelium-derived nitric oxide in the regulation of blood pressure. *Proc Natl Acad Sci U S A* 1989;86:3375–3378.

21. Vallance P, Collier J, Moncada S. Effects of endothelium-derived nitric oxide on peripheral arteriolar tone in man. *Lancet* 1989;2:997–1000.

22. Gardiner SM, Compton AM, Bennett T, et al. Regional haemodynamic changes during oral ingestion of NG-monomethyl-L-arginine or NG-nitro-L-arginine methyl ester in conscious Brattleboro rats. *Br J Pharmacol* 1990;101:10–12.

23. Huang PL, Huang Z, Mashimo H, et al. Hypertension in mice lacking the gene for endothelial nitric oxide synthase. *Nature* 1995;377:239–242.

24. Moncada S, Palmer RM, Higgs EA. The discovery of nitric oxide as the endogenous nitrovasodilator. *Hypertension* 1988;12:365–372.

25. Feelisch M, Stamler J. Donors of nitrogen oxides. In: Feelisch M, Stamler JS, eds. *Methods in Nitric Oxide Research*. New York: John Wiley & Sons, 1996:71–115.

26. Radomski MW, Moncada S. Biological role of nitric oxide in platelet function. In: Moncada S, Higgs EA, et al, *Clinical Relevance of Nitric Oxide in the Cardiovascular System*. Madrid: EDICOMPLET. 1991:45–56.

27. Kelly RA, Balligand JL, Smith TW. Nitric oxide and cardiac function. *Circ Res* 1996;79:363–380.

28. Kubes P, Suzuki M, Granger DN. Nitric oxide: An endogenous modulator of leukocyte adhesion. *Proc Natl Acad Sci U S A* 1991;88:4651–4655.

29. Garg UC, Hassid A. Nitric oxide-generating vasodilators and 8-bromo-cyclic guanosine monophosphate inhibit mitogenesis and proliferation of cultured rat vascular smooth muscle cells. *J Clin Invest* 1989;83:1774–1777.

30. Gillespie JS, Liu X, Martin W. The neurotransmitter of the non-adrenergic non-cholinergic inhibitory nerves to smooth muscle of the genital system. In: Moncada S, Higgs EA, eds. *Nitric Oxide from L-Arginine: A Bioregulatory System*. Amsterdam: Elsevier Science Publishers BV, 1990:147–164.

31. Rand MJ. Nitrergic transmission: Nitric oxide as a mediator of non-adrenergic, non-cholinergic neuro-effector transmission. *Clin Exp Pharmacol Physiol* 1992;19: 147–169.

32. Toda N. Nitric oxide and the regulation of cerebral arterial tone. In: Vincent S, ed. *Nitric Oxide in the Nervous System*. Orlando: Academic Press Ltd, 1995:207–225.

33. Toda N, Okamura T. Cerebral vasodilators. *Jpn J Pharmacol* 1998;76:349–367.

34. Moncada S, Higgs A. The L-arginine-nitric oxide pathway. *N Engl J Med* 1993;329: 2002–2012.

35. Calver A, Collier J, Moncada S, et al. Effect of local intra-arterial NG-monomethyl-L-arginine in patients with hypertension: The nitric oxide dilator mechanism appears abnormal. *J Hypertens* 1992;10:1025–1031.

36. Panza JA, Garcia CE, Kilcoyne CM, et al. Impaired endothelium-dependent vasodilation in patients with essential hypertension. Evidence that nitric oxide abnormality is not localized to a single signal transduction pathway. *Circulation* 1995; 91:1732–1738.

37. Rees D, Ben Ishay D, Moncada S. Nitric oxide and the regulation of blood pressure in the hypertension-prone and hypertension-resistant Sabra rat. *Hypertension* 1996;28:367–371.
38. Lahera V, Salom MG, Miranda Guardiola F, et al. Effects of NG-nitro-L-arginine methyl ester on renal function and blood pressure. *Am J Physiol* 1991;261:F1033–F1037.
39. Forstermann U. Properties and mechanisms of production and action of endothelium-derived relaxing factor. *J Cardiovasc Pharmacol* 1986;8(suppl 10):S45–S51.
40. Cox DA, Vita JA, Treasure CB, et al. Atherosclerosis impairs flow-mediated dilation of coronary arteries in humans. *Circulation* 1989;80:458–465.
41. Celermajer DS, Sorensen KE, Gooch VM, et al. Non-invasive detection of endothelial dysfunction in children and adults at risk of atherosclerosis. *Lancet* 1992;340:1111–1115.
42. Cooke JP, Tsao PS. Arginine: A new therapy for atherosclerosis? *Circulation* 1997;95:311–312.
43. Moroi M, Zhang L, Yasuda T, et al. Interaction of genetic deficiency of endothelial nitric oxide, gender, and pregnancy in vascular response to injury in mice. *J Clin Invest* 1998;101:1225–1232.
44. Drexler H, Zeiher AM, Meinzer K, et al. Correction of endothelial dysfunction in coronary microcirculation of hypercholesterolaemic patients by L-arginine. *Lancet* 1991;338:1546–1550.
45. Cooke JP, Tsao P. Cellular mechanisms of atherogenesis and the effects of nitric oxide. *Curr Opin Cardiol* 1992;7:799–804.
46. Creager MA, Gallagher SJ, Girerd XJ, et al. L-Arginine improves endothelium-dependent vasodilation in hypercholesterolemic humans. *J Clin Invest* 1992;90:1248–1253.
47. McNamara DB, Bedi B, Aurora H, et al. L-Arginine inhibits balloon catheter-induced intimal hyperplasia. *Biochem Biophys Res Commun* 1993;193:291–296.
48. Aji W, Ravalli S, Szabolcs M, et al. L-Arginine prevents xanthoma development and inhibits atherosclerosis in LDL receptor knockout mice. *Circulation* 1997;95:430–437.
49. Lefer AM, Lefer DJ. Therapeutic role of nitric oxide donors in the treatment of cardiovascular disease. *Drugs Future* 1994;19:665–672.
50. Cachofeiro V, Sakakibara T, Nasjletti A. Kinins, nitric oxide, and the hypotensive effect of captopril and ramiprilat in hypertension. *Hypertension* 1992;19:138–145.
51. Grafe M, Bossaller C, Graf K, et al. Effect of angiotensin-converting-enzyme inhibition on bradykinin metabolism by vascular endothelial cells. *Am J Physiol* 1993;264:H1493–H1497.
52. Farhy RD, Carretero OA, Ho KL, et al. Role of kinins and nitric oxide in the effects of angiotensin converting enzyme inhibitors on neointima formation. *Circ Res* 1993;72:1202–1210.
53. Weiner CP, Lizasoain I, Baylis SA, et al. Induction of calcium-dependent nitric oxide synthases by sex hormones. *Proc Natl Acad Sci U S A.* 1994;91:5212–5216.
54. Nathan L, Chaudhuri G. Estrogens and atherosclerosis. *Annu Rev Pharmacol Toxicol.* 1997;37:477–515.
55. Sessa WC. The nitric oxide synthase family of proteins. *J Vasc Res* 1994;31:131–143.
56. Nathan C, Xie QW. Regulation of biosynthesis of nitric oxide. *J Biol Chem* 1994;269:13725–13728.
57. Nathan CF, Hibbs JB, Jr. Role of nitric oxide synthesis in macrophage antimicrobial activity. *Curr Opin Immunol* 1991;3:65–70.
58. Nussler AK, Billiar TR. Inflammation, immunoregulation, and inducible nitric oxide synthase. *J Leukocyte Biol* 1993;54:171–178.
59. Hibbs JB, Jr, Taintor RR, Vavrin Z, et al. Nitric oxide: A cytotoxic activated macrophage effector molecule [published erratum appears *in Biochem Biophys Res Commun* 1989 Jan 31;158:624]. *Biochem Biophys Res Commun* 1988;157:87–94.

60. Marletta MA, Yoon PS, Iyengar R, et al. Macrophage oxidation of L-arginine to nitrite and nitrate: Nitric oxide is an intermediate. *Biochemistry* 1988;27:8706–8711.
61. Stuehr DJ, Gross SS, Sakuma I, et al. Activated murine macrophages secrete a metabolite of arginine with the bioactivity of endothelium-derived relaxing factor and the chemical reactivity of nitric oxide. *J Exp Med* 1989;169:1011–1020.
62. Vallance P, Moncada S. Role of endogenous nitric oxide in septic shock. *New Horiz* 1993;1:77–86.
63. Schulz R, Nava E, Moncada S. Induction and potential biological relevance of a Ca(2+)-independent nitric oxide synthase in the myocardium. *Br J Pharmacol* 1992;105:575–580.
64. Ungureanu Longrois D, Balligand JL, Kelly RA, et al. Myocardial contractile dysfunction in the systemic inflammatory response syndrome: Role of a cytokine-inducible nitric oxide synthase in cardiac myocytes. *J Mol Cell Cardiol* 1995;27:155–167.
65. Schulz R, Panas DL, Catena R, et al. The role of nitric oxide in cardiac depression induced by interleukin-1 beta and tumour necrosis factor-alpha. *Br J Pharmacol* 1995;114:27–34.
66. de Belder A, Moncada S. Cardiomyopathy: A role for nitric oxide? *Int J Cardiol* 1995;50:263–268.
67. Rubanyi GM, Vanhoutte PM. Superoxide anions and hyperoxia inactivate endothelium-derived relaxing factor. *Am J Physiol* 1986;250:H822–H827.
68. McCall TB, Boughton Smith NK, Palmer RM, et al. Synthesis of nitric oxide from L-arginine by neutrophils. Release and interaction with superoxide anion. *Biochem J* 1989;261:293–296.
69. Blough NV, Zafirious OC. Reaction of superoxide with nitric oxide to form peroxonitrite in alkaline aqueous solution. *Inorg Chem* 1985;24:3504–3505.
70. Beckman JS, Beckman TW, Chen J, et al. Apparent hydroxyl radical production by peroxynitrite: Implications for endothelial injury from nitric oxide and superoxide. *Proc Natl Acad Sci U S A* 1990;87:1620–1624.
71. Ischiropoulos H, Zhu L, Beckman JS. Peroxynitrite formation from macrophage-derived nitric oxide. *Arch Biochem Biophys* 1992;298:446–451.
72. Miller MJ, Thompson JH, Zhang XJ, et al. Role of inducible nitric oxide synthase expression and peroxynitrite formation in guinea pig ileitis. *Gastroenterology* 1995;109:1475–1483.
73. Kooy NW, Royall JA, Ye YZ, et al. Evidence for in vivo peroxynitrite production in human acute lung injury. *Am J Respir Crit Care Med* 1995;151:1250–1254.
74. Beckmann JS, Ye YZ, Anderson PG, et al. Extensive nitration of protein tyrosines in human atherosclerosis detected by immunohistochemistry. *Biol Chem Hoppe-Seyler* 1994;375:81–88.
75. Moro MA, Darley Usmar VM, Goodwin DA, et al. Paradoxical fate and biological action of peroxynitrite on human platelets. *Proc Natl Acad Sci U S A* 1994;91:6702–6706.
76. Brown GC, Cooper CE. Nanomolar concentrations of nitric oxide reversibly inhibit synaptosomal respiration by competing with oxygen at cytochrome oxidase. *FEBS Lett* 1994;356:295–298.
77. Cleeter MW, Cooper JM, Darley Usmar VM, et al. Reversible inhibition of cytochrome c oxidase, the terminal enzyme of the mitochondrial respiratory chain, by nitric oxide. Implications for neurodegenerative diseases. *FEBS Lett* 1994;345:50–54.
78. Lizasoain I, Moro MA, Knowles RG, et al. Nitric oxide and peroxynitrite exert distinct effects on mitochondrial respiration which are differentially blocked by glutathione or glucose. *Biochem J* 1996;314:877–880.
79. Radi R, Rodriguez M, Castro L, et al. Inhibition of mitochondrial electron transport by peroxynitrite. *Arch Biochem Biophys* 1994;308:89–95.
80. Clementi E, Brown GC, Feelisch M, et al. Persistent inhibition of cell respiration by nitric oxide: Crucial role of *S*-nitrosylation of mitochondrial complex I and protective action of glutathione. *Proc Natl Acad Sci U S A* 1998;95:7631–7636.

## Chapter 3

# Molecular Mechanisms of Intracellular Endothelial Nitric Oxide Synthase Regulation

*William E. Downey, MD, and Thomas Michel MD, PhD*

## Introduction

The endothelial isoform of nitric oxide synthase (eNOS) modulates diverse biological responses in different tissues. Originally characterized in aortic endothelium, eNOS now is known to be expressed in cardiac myocytes,[1] blood platelets,[2] hippocampal neurons,[3] pulmonary epithelium,[4] renal epithelium,[5] and other tissues. In the vascular wall, eNOS plays a key role in vasodilation, and also may regulate vascular smooth muscle cell proliferation, platelet adherence and activation, leukocyte adherence, and chemokine production. In cardiac myocytes, eNOS plays a key role in the modulation of autonomic control of contractility and heart rate. A principal point for the control of NO synthesis in these tissues involves the regulation of eNOS by posttranslational modifications and by cell-specific protein-protein interactions. This chapter will review some of the principal molecular mechanisms for the cellular regulation of eNOS in the cardiovascular system.

## Regulation of Endothelial Nitric Oxide Synthase Production

The eNOS gene is located on human chromosome 7 and contains 26 exons spanning 22 kilobases. Although eNOS originally was characterized as a "constitutive" enzyme, being stably expressed in its characteristic tissues, numerous subsequent reports have documented that transcription of the eNOS gene is regulated in a variety of physiological and pathophysiological conditions. Indeed, the putative promoter region of the eNOS gene contains

From Panza JA, Cannon RO III (eds): *Endothelium, Nitric Oxide, and Atherosclerosis* ©Futura Publishing Co, Inc, Armonk, NY, 1999.

consensus sequences for a wide variety of transacting factors, including nuclear factor–kappa B (NF-$\kappa$B), interleukin 6 (IL-6), AP-1, AP-2, phenethyl alcohol 3 (PEA-3), and NF-1, among others (see review by Förstermann et al[6]). In most cases, the relevance of these regulatory sequences to the in vivo regulation of the eNOS gene remains less well understood. However, transcriptional regulation of the eNOS gene has been documented in response to changes in a number of stimuli, including hemodynamic shear stress and hypoxia. Harrison and colleagues[7] demonstrated a dose-dependent increase in eNOS gene transcription in response to shear stress in cultured bovine aortic endothelial cells. In cultured endothelial cells, hypoxia is associated with a decrease in mRNA stability and decreased eNOS transcript levels.[8] By contrast, in animal models, chronic hypoxia appears to be associated with an increase in eNOS mRNA transcript levels[9]; such differences between cultured cells and animal models point to the challenges in extrapolating from in vitro systems to pathophysiological processes in intact animals. Other perturbations shown to affect the quantity of the eNOS transcript are chronic exercise, cell proliferation, sex steroids, lipoproteins, angiotensin II, and inflammatory mediators such as tumor necrosis factor $\alpha$ (TNF-$\alpha$) and transforming growth factor $\beta$ (TGF-$\beta$).[6] The mechanisms whereby these factors modulate eNOS production in cells, as well as their relationships to pathophysiological states, are under active investigation.

# Regulation of Endothelial Nitric Oxide Synthase Activity

## Protein–Protein Interactions: Calmodulin

All three NOS isoforms depend on binding of $Ca^{2+}$-calmodulin for enzyme activation. Although calmodulin is an essential allosteric activator for all NOS isoforms, the inflammatory cell-related inducible NOS (iNOS) isoform is fully active at the intracellular calcium levels ($[Ca^{2+}]_i$) characteristic of unstimulated cells. In contrast, eNOS and neuronal NOS (nNOS) are inactive at basal $[Ca^{2+}]_i$, likely reflecting the higher $K_A$ for calmodulin binding by these isoforms at ambient intracellular calcium levels. Increase in $[Ca^{2+}]_i$, stimulated by hemodynamic shear stress or by the activation of G-protein–coupled cell surface receptors, represents the key mechanism whereby intracellular regulation of eNOS is achieved. However, another key inhibitory protein-protein interaction, that between eNOS and caveolin, directly affects the allosteric activation of eNOS by calmodulin.

## Reversible Targeting: Interactions with Caveolin and Caveolae

Caveolae are small invaginations of the plasma membrane characterized by a distinctive lipid composition, being highly enriched in glycosphingolipids and cholesterol, and are distinguished by the presence of the transmembrane protein caveolin, which appears to serve as the scaffold for assembly of this organelle. Caveolae are abundant in endothelial cell membranes, and also are an essential component of the cardiac myocyte T-tubular system. Originally, they were characterized as sites for transcytosis and endocytosis, but studies over the past several years have identified a key role for caveolae in signal transduction. In addition to eNOS, caveolae may contain G-protein–coupled receptors, growth factor receptors, G-proteins, protein kinases, as well as diverse membrane-targeted proteins involved in calcium homeostasis and signaling.[9] Some of these signaling proteins are targeted dynamically to caveolae, with different receptor stimuli or alterations in cellular lipids leading to their disappearance or reappearance in this organelle. Two distinct G-protein–coupled receptors known to stimulate NO production, B2 bradykinin and M2 muscarinic cholinergic receptors, are targeted to caveolae on agonist stimulation.[10,11] The eNOS targeting to caveolae also is regulated dynamically by agonists: treatment of endothelial cells with bradykinin promotes the reversible translocation of eNOS from caveolae to an intracellular compartment,[12] a process dependent on the agonist-induced increase in intracellular calcium. This reversible association of eNOS with caveolae (the organelle) appears to be enhanced by the dynamic association of eNOS with caveolin (the protein).

Caveolin, the characteristic structural protein of plasmalemmal caveolae, plays a central role in the regulation of eNOS. Endothelial cells contain the caveolin isoform caveolin-1, while cardiac myocytes express the muscle-specific isoform caveolin-3; in both cell types, eNOS directly interacts with caveolin,[13–15] with profound effects on the enzyme's targeting and activity. Other signaling proteins, including G-protein $\alpha$-subunits, Ha-Ras, Src family kinases, and eNOS all directly interact with caveolin-1.[16] A specific sequence within caveolin, termed the caveolin scaffolding domain, appears to modulate the interactions between caveolin and its associated proteins. The diverse proteins that interact with caveolin share no obvious similarities in overall structure, but a putative consensus caveolin-binding motif has been proposed.[16] This putative caveolin-binding motif is found within eNOS, and also is present in G-protein $\alpha$-subunits and in many protein kinases thought to interact with caveolin. The most direct experimental validation of this caveolin-binding consensus sequence is based on mutagenesis studies within this region in eNOS.[15] However, it has been shown that the regulation of eNOS reductase activity by caveolin occurs independently of this putative caveolin-binding site.[17] Clearly, much remains to be understood in identifying the domains of eNOS involved in its interactions with caveolin.

The binding of eNOS to caveolin-1 both facilitates targeting of the enzyme to caveolae and dynamically regulates eNOS activity. The direct association of caveolin-1 with eNOS markedly attenuates enzyme activity.[13,14] This inhibitory interaction is reversed by $Ca^{2+}$-calmodulin: calmodulin has the dual roles of reversing eNOS inhibition by caveolin and directly activating the enzyme. In resting cells, eNOS is complexed to caveolin; increases in intracellular calcium promote binding of calmodulin to eNOS concomitant with caveolin dissociation.[13] Following prolonged agonist stimulation, concomitant with return of $[Ca^{2+}]_i$ to basal levels, eNOS reassociates with caveolin, once again inhibiting the enzyme.[18]

In cardiac myocytes, which contain caveolin-3 rather than caveolin-1, eNOS is associated quantitatively with caveolin-3 via a scaffolding domain similar to that found in caveolin-1. As does the binding to caveolin-1 in endothelial cells, this association of eNOS with caveolin-3 in cardiac myocytes markedly inhibits eNOS activity.[19,20] This inhibitory action of the caveolins on signaling is not limited to the eNOS system: caveolin appears to inhibit the tyrosine kinase activity of c-Src and may also suppress guanosine diphosphate (GDP)-guanosine triphosphate (GTP) exchange for some heterotrimeric G-proteins.[16] Taken together, these findings suggest that caveolin may function both to bind and to inhibit the tonic activity of diverse signaling protein. This inhibition, at least in the case of eNOS and caveolin-1, is readily reversible, allowing activation of the enzyme when appropriate stimuli are present.

## Other Protein Partners of Endothelial Nitric Oxide Synthase

Stimulation of endothelial cells by bradykinin has been shown to promote the association of eNOS with a 90-kd protein, originally termed ENAP-1,[21] and subsequently shown to be the molecular chaperone protein Hsp90.[22] Hsp90 is a molecular chaperone that can interact with a variety of signaling proteins including methylethyl ketone (MEK), Src family members, Raf, and G-protein $\beta\gamma$-subunits. A fraction of the eNOS in resting endothelial cells appears to coimmunoprecipitate with Hsp90, and stimuli known to activate eNOS promote the formation of an eNOS–Hsp90 heterocomplex.[17] Other recent studies have shown that eNOS and the bradykinin B2 receptor are associated physically.[23] The interaction of the B2 receptor with eNOS is reversed by agonist occupation of the receptor as well as by treatment of cells with $Ca^{2+}$ ionophore.[23] Studies using purified proteins and peptides suggest that the B2 receptor and eNOS may interact in vitro to attenuate directly eNOS enzyme activity. Although these eNOS–B2 receptor interactions have not been shown yet to regulate dynamically eNOS in cells, this discovery may represent a novel mechanism for eNOS regulation and may suggest the existence of still other protein partners for eNOS.

## Covalent Modifications: Acylation and Phosphorylation

The eNOS is unique among the NOS isoforms in being dually acylated by myristate and palmitate (see review by Sase and Michel.[24]). During translation, the 14-carbon saturated fatty acid myristate is linked covalently via an amide bond to an N-terminal glycine within the consensus sequence MGxxxS.[25] Like myristoylation of other proteins, this modification of eNOS essentially is irreversible. After translation, the 16-carbon fatty acid palmitate is added to two cysteine residues near the protein's N-terminus (Cys-15 and Cys-26). These palmitoylated cysteines flank a (Gly-Leu)$_5$ repeat not previously described in the protein sequence database. As has been described for a number of other dually acylated proteins, including the Src family of kinases and several G-protein α-subunits, a myristoylation-deficient eNOS mutant also fails to be palmitoylated. The palmitoylation-deficient mutant eNOS still undergoes myristoylation, but its targeting to plasmalemmal caveolae is attenuated.[26]

In contrast with the myristoylation of eNOS, the enzyme's palmitoylation is readily reversible. For a number of other signaling proteins, palmitoylation is regulated dynamically and can modulate subcellular localization and function. For example, activation of G-protein $\alpha_s$ appears to promote its depalmitoylation and subsequent redistribution from the membrane to cytosolic subcellular fractions. This translocation away from the membrane may be associated with a decreased ability to interact with downstream effectors.[25] In similar fashion, agonist activation of endothelial cells by bradykinin promotes the depalmitoylation of eNOS,[27] associated with enzyme translocation[12] and phosphorylation.[28] Thus, the same enzyme activating stimuli that promote eNOS dissociation from caveolin and association with $Ca^{2+}$-calmodulin seem to trigger the removal of its palmitate. Exactly how agonist-induced depalmitoylation and the subsequent repalmitoylation of eNOS are regulated at the molecular level remains poorly understood; identifying the molecular pathways coordinating the reversible palmitoylation of signaling proteins represents an important area of investigation in signal transduction.

Like the other NOS isoforms, eNOS can be phosphorylated in vitro by purified serine/threonine and tyrosine kinases and can be isolated as a phosphoprotein from cultured cell systems. In intact endothelial cells, eNOS is reversibly phosphorylated on serine residues in response to diverse agonists and hemodynamic shear stress.[28,29] Tyrosine phosphorylation of eNOS was detected in intact endothelial cells treated with the phosphatase inhibitor sodium orthovanadate.[30] However, no physiological agonists for the tyrosine phosphorylation of eNOS have been identified, and other reports have failed to document any tyrosine phosphorylation of eNOS.[29] Treatment of cultured endothelial cells with phorbol esters has been shown to diminish NO production, suggesting that serine/threonine phosphorylation may be associated with inhibition of eNOS activity. Thus, there are a variety of intriguing but inconclusive data suggesting that eNOS is regulated via phosphorylation by both serine/threonine and tyrosine kinases.

## Putting It All Together— Receptor Activation, Reversible Acylation, and Caveolin and Endothelial Nitric Oxide Synthase Signaling

The best-characterized mechanisms for the molecular regulation of eNOS are derived from studies carried out in cellular reconstitution systems in which individual components of this signaling pathway can be recombined functionally and manipulated. The relative roles of eNOS phosphorylation and of other eNOS protein-protein interactions remain less well understood in this biological context. Cellular reconstitution studies have identified a central role for reversible eNOS–caveolin interactions and for eNOS acylation in modulating the physiological response to receptor activation.

One such cellular reconstitution studied the role of wild-type and mutant eNOS cDNA constructs transfected back into cardiac myocytes isolated from mice with targeted disruption of the eNOS gene (*eNOS*[null] mice). This gene "knock-in" approach permitted the study of components of the eNOS signaling system to be characterized in their physiological milieu. Myocytes isolated from *eNOS*[null] mice had been used to show that eNOS has a key role coupling muscarinic receptor activation to the control of myocyte beating rate.[31] The phenotype of *eNOS*[null] myocytes could be rescued by transfecting these cells with cDNA constructs encoding wild-type but not acylation-deficient eNOS.[20] Thus, in *eNOS*[null] myocytes expressing recombinant wild-type eNOS, the muscarinic cholinergic agonist carbachol elicited a strong negative chronotropic response and markedly activated cyclic guanosine monophosphate (cGMP) production, while in eNOS[null] myocytes transfected with the acylation-deficient eNOS mutant transfected myocytes, there was no response whatsoever to carbachol stimulation. Acylation-deficient eNOS is uncoupled from the muscarinic receptor because of the mutant's aberrant subcellular localization and its failure to target to caveolae. Furthermore, the expression of exogenous caveolin in this system completely abrogated the cGMP-dependent negative chronotropic effect of carbachol observed in myocytes transfected with wild-type eNOS.[20] Acylation of eNOS thus is required for coupling the enzyme's physiological stimulus (muscarinic cholinergic activation) to its physiological response (eg, negative chronotropic effect), but acylation also leads to the attenuation of eNOS by caveolin in resting cells. Thus, the caveolar compartmentalization of eNOS plays an apparently paradoxical role, both tonically repressing basal eNOS activity by the enzyme's interactions with caveolin, but also ensuring the efficient activation of the enzyme on agonist stimulation. It is plausible that pathological conditions might lead to a modulation of caveolin expression or function and thereby modulate NO-dependent physiological processes both in cardiac myocytes and in vascular endothelium.

# Conclusions

Work over the past several years has revealed eNOS at the center of a complex web of regulatory interactions within and beyond plasmalemmal caveolae. Through a variety of experimental approaches, we are beginning to understand the outlines of an eNOS regulatory cycle wherein the dually acylated eNOS is targeted to caveolae where it is inhibited tonically by its association with caveolin in resting cells. Activation of upstream signals that result in an increase in $[Ca^{2+}]_i$, which promotes the binding of $Ca^{2+}$-calmodulin to eNOS, thereby displacing caveolin, and the enzyme begins to produce NO. After prolonged agonist stimulation, but probably before $[Ca^{2+}]_i$ falls back to basal levels, eNOS translocates to an intracellular compartment coincident with its depalmitoylation. Finally, the enzyme becomes repalmitoylated and associates once again with caveolin, returning to plasmalemmal caveolae to await another round of agonist activation. The diverse points of regulation of this complex signaling pathway provide for complex effects of pathophysiological states on NO-dependent signaling in the vascular wall and in the heart.

# References

1. Balligand JL, Kobzik L, Han X, et al. Nitric oxide-dependent parasympathetic signaling is due to activation of constitutive endothelial (type III) nitric oxide synthase in cardiac myocytes. *J Biol Chem* 1995;270:14582–14586.
2. Sase K, Michel T. Expression of constitutive nitric oxide synthase in human blood platelets. *Life Sci* 1995;57:2049–2055.
3. Dinerman JL, Dawson TM, Schell MJ, et al. Endothelial nitric oxide synthase localized to hippocampal pyramidal cells: Implications for synaptic plasticity. *Proc Natl Acad Sci U S A* 1994;91:4214–4218.
4. Shaul PW, North AJ, Wu LC, et al. Endothelial nitric oxide synthase is expressed in cultured human bronchiolar epithelium. *J Clin Inv* 1994;94:2231–2236.
5. Tracey WR, Pollock JS, Murad F, et al. Identification of a type III (endothelial-type) particulate nitric oxide synthase in LLC-PK1 kidney tubular cells. *Am J Physiol* 1994;266(pt 1):C22—C28.
6. Förstermann U, Boissel JP, Kleinert H. Expressional control of the "constitutive" isoforms of nitric oxide synthase (NOS I and NOS III). *FASEB J* 1998;12:773–790.
7. Harrison DG, Sayegh H, Ohara Y, et al. Regulation and expression of the endothelial cell nitric oxide synthase. *Clin Exp Pharmacol Physiol* 1996;23:251–255. Review.
8. McQuillan LP, Leung GK, Marsden PA, et al. Hypoxia inhibits expression of endothelial nitric oxide synthase via transcriptional and post-transcriptional mechanisms. *Am J Physiol* 1994;267:H1921–H1927.
9. Shaul PW, North AJ, Brannon TS, et al. Prolonged in vivo hypoxia enhances nitric oxide synthase type I and type III gene expression in adult rat lung. *Am J Respir Cell Biol* 1995;13:167–174.
10. de Weerd WFC, Leeb-Lundberg LMF. Bradykinin sequesters B2 bradykinin receptors and the receptor-coupled $G\alpha$ subunits $G\alpha q$ and $G\alpha i$ in caveolae in $DDT_1$ MF-2 smooth muscle cells. *J Biol Chem* 1997;272:17858–17866.
11. Feron O, Smith TW, Michel T, et al. Dynamic targeting of the agonist-stimulated M2 muscarinic acetylcholine receptor to caveolae in cardiac myocytes. *J Biol Chem* 1997;272:17744–17748.
12. Prabhakar P, Thatte HS, Goetz RM, et al. Receptor-regulated translocation of endothelial nitric oxide synthase. *J Biol Chem* 1998;273:27383–27388.
13. Michel JB, Feron O, Sacks D, et al. Reciprocal regulation of endothelial nitric oxide synthase by $Ca^{2+}$-calmodulin and caveolin. *J Biol Chem* 1997;272:15583–15586.
14. Ju H, Zou R, Venema VJ, et al. Direct interaction of endothelial nitric oxide synthase and caveolin-1 inhibits synthase activity. *J Biol Chem* 1997;272:18522–18525.
15. García-Cardeña G, Martasek P, Masters NS, et al. Dissecting the interaction between nitric oxide synthase and caveolin. Functional significance of the NOS caveolin binding domain in vivo. *J Biol Chem* 1997;272:25437–25440.
16. Okamoto T, Schlegel A, Scherer PE, et al. Caveolins, a family of scaffolding proteins for organizing "preasssembled signaling complexes" at the plasma membrane. *J Biol Chem* 1998;273:5419–5422. Review.
17. Ghosh S, Gachui R, Crooks C, et al. Interaction between caveolin-1 and the reductase domain of endothelial nitric oxide synthase. *J Biol Chem* 1998;273:22267–22271.
18. Feron O, Saldana F, Michel JB, et al. The endothelial nitric oxide synthase-caveolin regulatory cycle. *J Biol Chem* 1998;273:3125–3128.

19. Feron O, Behassen L, Kobzik L, et al. Endothelial nitric oxide synthase targeting to caveolae. *J Biol Chem* 1996;271:22810–22810.
20. Feron O, Dessy C, Opel DJ, et al. Modulation of the endothelial nitric oxide synthase-caveolin interaction in cardiac myocytes:Implications for the autonomic regulation of heart rate. *J Biol Chem* 1998;273:30249–30254.
21. Venema VJ, Marrero MB, Venema RC. Bradykinin-stimulated protein tyrosine phosphorylation promotes endothelial nitric oxide synthase translocation to the cytoskeleton. *Biochem Biophy Res Commun* 1996;226:703–710.
22. García-Cardeña G, Fan R, Shah V, et al. Dynamic activation of endothelial nitric oxide synthase by Hsp90. *Nature* 1998;392:821–824.
23. Ju H, Venema VJ, Marrero MB, et al. Inhibitory interactions of the bradykinin B2 receptor with endothelial nitric oxide synthase. *J Biol Chem* 1998;273:24025–24029.
24. Sase K, Michel T. Expression and regulation of endothelial nitric oxide synthase. *Trends Cardiovasc Med* 1997;7:28.
25. Wedegaertner PB, Wilson PT, Bourne HR. Lipid modification of trimeric G proteins. *J Biol Chem* 1995;270:503–506. Review.
26. Shaul PW, Smart EJ, Robinson LJ, et al. Acylation targets endothelial nitric oxide synthase to plamalemmal caveolae. *J Biol Chem* 1996;271:6518–6522.
27. Robinson LJ, Busconi L, Michel T. Agonist-modulated palmitoylation of endothelial nitric oxide synthase. *J Biol Chem* 1995;270:995–998.
28. Michel T, Li GK, Buskoni L. Phosphorylation and subcellular translocation of nitric oxide synthase. *Proc Natl Acad Sci U S A* 1993;90:6252–6256.
29. Corson MA, James NC, Latta SE, et al. Phosphorylation of endothelial nitric oxide synthase in response to fluid shear stress. *Circ Res* 1996;79:984–991.
30. García-Cardeña G, Fan R, Stern D, et al. Endothelial nitric oxide synthase is regulated by tyrosine phosphorylation and interacts with caveolin-1. *J Biol Chem* 1996;271:27237–27240.
31. Han X, Kubota I, Feron O, et al. Muscarinic cholinergic regulation of cardiac myocyte ICa-L is absent in mice with targeted disruption of endothelial nitric oxide synthase. *Proc Natl Acad Sci U S A* 1998;95:6510–6515.

## Chapter 4

# Cardiovascular Effects of Nitric Oxide:

## Lessons Learned from Endothelial Nitric Oxide Synthase Knockout Mice

*Paul L. Huang, MD, PhD, Robert Gyurko, DDS, PhD, and Lin Zhang, MD*

## Introduction

Targeted disruption of genes to create gene knockout mice has helped elucidate the function of many genes. In studying the nitric oxide synthases (NOS), a genetic approach has been particularly useful to complement pharmacological studies.[1] The three known NOS isoforms share L-arginine as substrate and have similar enzymatic mechanisms, so their sensitivities to pharmacological inhibitors overlap.[2] This makes it difficult to distinguish the roles of the individual NOS isoforms. Moreover, most tissues contain more than one NOS isoform. In addition to NOS that may be present in the parenchymal cells of the tissue itself, the blood vessels, nerves, and circulating cells may contain various NOS isoforms.

The genes for each of the three major isoforms of NOS have been disrupted in mice. Neuronal NOS (nNOS) knockout mice lack nNOS in the brain as well as in nonadrenergic, noncholinergic autonomic nerves of the peripheral nervous system.[3] They have enlarged stomachs and serve as an animal model for the human disorder infantile hypertrophic pyloric stenosis. This phenotype is caused by a defect in the inhibitory junction potential of stomach smooth muscle that requires nNOS.[4] Surprisingly, the neuroanatomy of the brain in nNOS knockout mice appears preserved. Several inducible NOS (iNOS) knockout mice have been reported.[5-7] These animals do not become hypotensive in response to lipopolysaccharide, an effect normally mediated by NO made by iNOS. Endothelial NOS (eNOS) knockout mice are hypertensive and lack endothelium-derived relaxing factor (EDRF) activity.[8,9]

There are several important concerns for any studies that involve gene knockouts. First, because knockout mice develop without the disrupted gene,

From Panza JA, Cannon RO III (eds): *Endothelium, Nitric Oxide, and Atherosclerosis* ©Futura Publishing Co, Inc, Armonk, NY, 1999.

any developmental roles normally served by the gene may be absent, or they may be served by other genes. Second, other genes that function in parallel with the deleted gene may compensate for its absence. The nNOS knockout mice show several examples of physiological compensation. The cerebral blood flow increase that occurs in response to hypercapnia is blunted by NOS inhibitors in wild-type mice, consistent with a role for NO in its mediation. In the nNOS knockout mice, the response is quantitatively normal, but it is no longer blocked by NOS inhibitors.[10] Thus, other parallel pathways for cerebral vasodilation compensate for the absence of nNOS to maintain a normal response. Other examples of physiological compensation in the nNOS knockout mice include the cerebral blood flow response to whisker stimulation,[11] the nociceptive response to pain,[12] and the dose response to volatile anesthetics.[13] Another concern for knockout studies relates to genetic background effects.[14] Embryonic stem cells used to generate the knockout mice often are derived from a genetic background particularly suited to maintain pluripotency. The chimeric mice that result then are mated with mice of a second genetic background, so that resulting knockout mice have contributions from more than one genetic background. Therefore it is important to ensure that any differences between knockout mice and control mice are caused by the disrupted gene and not the genetic background differences. Repeated backcrossing of the knockout mice to a standard mouse strain such as C57BL/6 will lead to mice that are congenic with C57BL/6 except for the gene disruption. Knockouts of each of the NOS isoforms have been or are being backcrossed to the C57BL/6 strain.

# Nitric Oxide Synthase Isoforms and Cerebral Ischemia

Levels of NO in the brain rise several orders of magnitude following cerebral ischemia.[15] Potential sources of NO in the brain include neurons, vascular endothelium, glial cells, astrocytes, vascular smooth muscle, and perivascular nerves. Autoradiography studies with [³H] labeled nitro L-arginine (L-NA) show that the bulk of NOS in the brain is nNOS, although eNOS clearly is detectable as well.[16] Some eNOS is in cerebral blood vessels and some is expressed by neurons.[17,18] The nNOS knockout mice have lower basal levels of cyclic guanosine monophophosphate (cGMP) and NOS activity than do wild-type mice. They also fail to show a marked increase in cGMP and NO production by electron spin trapping methods in response to cerebral ischemia that are observed in wild-type mice.[19] Thus, nNOS is responsible not only for most of the NOS in the brain, but also for the marked increase in NO generated following ischemia.

The effect of NOS inhibitors on the outcome of cerebral ischemia has been controversial.[20] Some of the variation in results may be caused by differential effects of NOS inhibitors on nNOS and eNOS isoforms, which may have opposing roles following cerebral ischemia. On the one hand, excess neuronal production of NO may be toxic and may contribute to tissue damage by virtue of peroxynitrite formation, activation of polyadenosine diphosphate (polyADP) ribose polimerase, and generation of free radicals. On the other hand, vascular NO production may be protective by vasodilation (with consequent improved blood flow), inhibition of thrombosis, and inhibition of leukocyte adhesion. The nNOS and eNOS knockout mice were ideal genetic tools to test the hypothesis that nNOS and eNOS isoforms mediate toxic and protective effects, respectively.

Neuronal NOS knockout mice are resistant to cerebral ischemia. They develop smaller infarcts and have better neurologic function than wild-type mice following middle cerebral artery occlusion (MCAO), a model of focal ischemia.[19] The nNOS knockouts showed resistance to both transient[21] and permanent focal ischemia. These effects are not mediated by differences in the hemodynamic effect of MCAO, because laser Doppler flowmetry shows equivalent reductions in relative cerebral blood flow (rCBF) from MCAO in both the core infarct zone and the ischemic penumbra. The nNOS knockout mice also are resistant to global ischemia induced by bilateral carotid artery and basilar artery occlusion, with preservation of cytoarchitecture and reduced neuronal dropout in the hippocampus.[22] These results confirm that nNOS contributes to the damage seen following stroke.

In contrast, eNOS knockout mice develop larger strokes following MCAO than wild-type mice.[23] By laser Doppler flowmetry, these effects in fact are caused by differences in blood flow. Recordings over the penumbra show more marked reduction in rCBF from MCAO in eNOS knockout mice than in wild-type mice. This vascular effect has been confirmed independently by functional computed tomography (CT) imaging.[24] After intravenous injection of the contrast agent iodohexol, the kinetics of its appearance and disappearance were determined in individual pixels. Each pixel in a coronal slice can be mapped by kinetics of blood flow, from one extreme of no blood flow (no contrast agent), to the other extreme of normal blood flow (contrast agent appears and disappears with normal kinetics), with gradations of abnormal blood flow (contrast agent appears and disappears with slower than normal kinetics). In Figure 1 (see page 56A), normal blood flow is mapped as green, absent blood flow is mapped as black, and abnormal blood flow is mapped as shades of red. The area of normal blood flow (green) is the same in the eNOS knockout mice as in wild-type mice. However, the core ischemic territory (no blood flow, black) is larger in the eNOS knockout mice than wild-type mice, and the ischemic penumbra (abnormal but present blood flow, red) is correspondingly smaller. These results show that eNOS normally serves a protective role following ischemia by vasodilation as the brain attempts to maintain normal perfusion in the ischemic penumbra.

## Endothelial Nitric Oxide Synthase and Blood Pressure Regulation

To test whether disruption of the eNOS gene abolishes EDRF activity, rings of aorta from eNOS knockout mice were studied in an organ bath. As shown in Figure 2, the vessel rings of wild-type mice, but not eNOS knockout

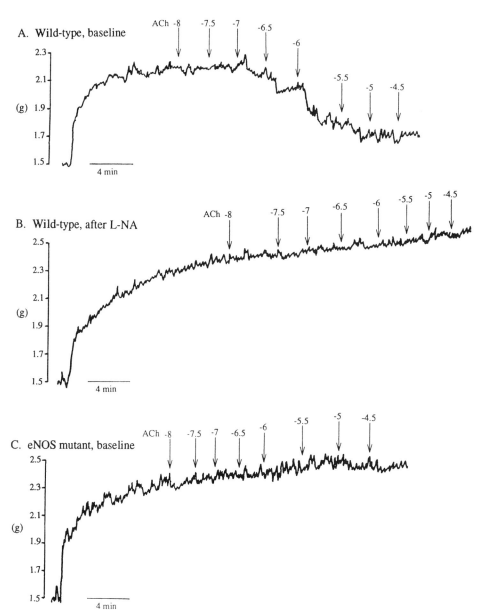

**Figure 2.** Dose-dependent effect of acetylcholine (ACh) on aortic rings in vitro. Wild-type aorta at baseline (**A**) relaxes in response to increasing doses of ACh, shown as log *M* concentration. Wild-type aorta treated with nitro L-arginine (L-NA) (**B**) no longer relaxes in response to ACh. The eNOS knockout aorta (**C**) even at baseline fails to relax in response to ACh. These results show that disruption of the eNOS gene results in absence of endothelium-derived relaxing factor (EDRF) activity. Reproduced with permission from Reference 8.

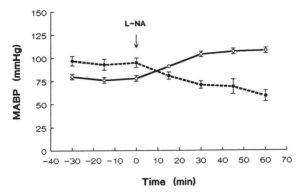

**Figure 3.** Paradoxic response of eNOS knockout mice to L-NA treatment. Mean arterial blood pressure (MABP) of wild-type (solid lines) and eNOS knockout (dotted lines) mice are shown. L-NA infusion at time 0 results in a rise in blood pressure of wild-type mice, consistent with basal production of NO in setting vascular tone. The L-NA infusion results in a drop in the blood pressure of eNOS knockout mice, implicating nonendothelial isoforms of NOS in maintaining or raising blood pressure. Reproduced with permission from Reference 8.

mice, relax in response to acetylcholine in an endothelium-dependent manner.[8] This provides genetic evidence that expression of the eNOS gene is required for EDRF activity.

The eNOS knockout mice are hypertensive with mean arterial blood pressures that are 20–30 mmHg over values seen in wild-type littermate animals.[8] This difference originally was observed in anesthetized animals using invasive measurements, but persisted with different types of anesthesia. It was later confirmed using noninvasive measurements in an independently generated line of eNOS knockout mice.[9] The NOS inhibitors normally raise the blood pressure by blocking basal endothelial production of NO in many species, including mice. Because they lack eNO production, eNOS knockout mice might be expected to have no response to NOS inhibitors. However, as seen in Figure 3, they have a paradoxic response; the blood pressure of eNOS knockout mice drops in response to L-NA.[8] This suggests that other remaining isoforms of NOS (most likely nNOS) may serve important roles in maintaining blood pressure. These effects likely are small in magnitude and in wild-type animals may be outweighed by the effect of eNOS in maintaining basal levels of vasodilation.

# Nitric Oxide Synthase Isoforms in Cardiac Function

Pharmacological blockade of NOS activity suggests that NO plays a significant role in regulating cardiac contractility.[25–28] Among the three NOS enzymes, the eNOS isoform is the most abundant in the heart. The eNOS knockout mice offer an opportunity to study the contribution of the eNOS-derived NO in modulating cardiac physiology and potential compensatory mechanisms. Anesthetized mice were instrumented with Millar catheters introduced retrogradely into the left ventricle and femoral arterial and venous catheters. Left ventricular pressure measurements were recorded and analyzed for indices of systolic contractility ($dP/dt_{max}$) and diastolic relaxation (time constant of relaxation $\tau$).

Although the eNOS mutant mice are hypertensive, other cardiovascular parameters such as heart rate and baseline cardiac contractility are similar to those of wild-type mice. As seen in Figure 4A, intravenous isoproterenol increases cardiac contractility in wild-type mice in a dose-dependent manner. The response of the eNOS knockout mice is increased significantly compared with wild-type mice, consistent with a role for eNOS-derived NO in attenuating the increased contractility to $\beta$-adrenergic stimulation. Wild-type mice

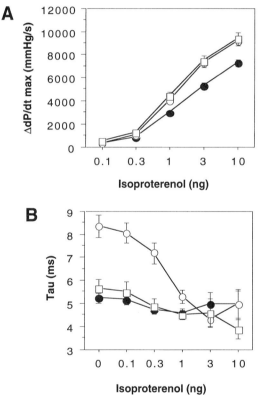

**Figure 4.** Systolic and diastolic responses of wild-type and eNOS knockout mice to isoproterenol. (**A**) Dose-dependent increase in $dP/dt_{max}$ caused by isoproterenol in wild-type (solid circles), wild-type treated with L-NA (open circles), and eNOS knockout mice (open squares). Increases in contractility are more marked in eNOS knockout mice and wild-type mice treated with L-NA than in wild-type mice. (**B**) Dose-dependent change in the ventricular time constant of relaxation $\tau$ in wild-type (solid circles), wild-type treated with L-NA (open circles), and eNOS knockout mice (open squares). Both eNOS knockout and wild-type mice have values of $\tau$ between 5 and 6 milliseconds. The L-NA treatment of wild-type mice raises wild-type (solid circles), wild-type treated with L-NA (open circles), and eNOS knockout mice (open squares) to over 8 milliseconds. Isoproterenol lowers $\tau$ in a dose-dependent manner.

pretreated with the NOS inhibitor L-NA similarly have an augmented response to isoproterenol. Thus, the effect of pharmacologic blockade with L-NA is the same as that of eNOS gene deletion.

In these studies, heart rate and preload do not influence the contractility measurements. The heart rate and end-diastolic left ventricular pressure of eNOS knockout mice and wild-type mice were similar, both at baseline and following isoproterenol infusion. To address potential effects of afterload, the experiment was repeated in wild-type mice whose blood pressure was raised to levels seen in eNOS knockout mice using the α-adrenergic agonist phenylephrine. Despite the acute increase in afterload, no increase in contractility is observed. Thus, the afterload itself cannot account for the increased contractile response in the eNOS knockout mice. Indeed, animal models of increased afterload such as aortic banding generally diminish, not augment, contractility.[29]

Left ventricular relaxation was assessed by calculating the time constant of relaxation τ from the left ventricular pressure tracing. As seen in Figure 4B, the value of τ is similar in wild-type and eNOS mutant mice, and it declines moderately with increasing doses of isoproterenol. However, L-NA treatment of wild-type mice prolongs ventricular relaxation and increases τ by 60%. The impaired relaxation of the ventricle is corrected by β-adrenergic stimulation, as indicated by the merger of the two dose-response curves at higher isoproterenol doses. In terms of diastolic relaxation response, the L-NA–treated wild-type mice do not behave like eNOS knockout mice, even though the systolic response of L-NA–treated wild-type mice were similar to those of the eNOS knockouts. These results suggest that parallel mechanisms present in the eNOS knockout mice compensate for absence of eNOS to mediate ventricular relaxation. These mechanisms do not involve other NOS enzymes, because L-NA does not affect ventricular relaxation in the eNOS knockout mice.

Results from hemodynamic measurements in eNOS knockout mice establish that the eNOS isoform modulates cardiac contractility under physiological conditions. Furthermore, NO has distinct and separable effects on systolic function and diastolic relaxation. Both systolic and diastolic function may be perturbed in heart failure but to differing degrees in different patients and with markedly different symptomatology. The results in wild-type and eNOS knockout mice suggest that there are important differences in the response of systolic and diastolic function to chronic absence of eNOS.

# Endothelial Nitric Oxide Synthase and Vessel Injury

The endothelium serves important functions, including modulating the vascular response to mechanical stress, hormonal and chemical mediators, and vessel injury. The eNO regulates vascular tone, inhibits platelet aggregation,[30] inhibits leukocyte adhesion to vessel walls,[31–34] and suppresses vascular smooth muscle proliferation.[35,36] Some of these effects are mediated by stabilization of inhibitory nuclear factor–kappa B (IκB), effectively suppressing the expression of nuclear factor–kappa B (NF-$\kappa$B)–dependent genes like vascular cell adhesion molecule-1 (VCAM-1), intercellular adhesion molecule-1 (ICAM-1).[37] Atherosclerosis, hypertension, diabetes mellitus, hypercholesterolemia, and normal aging are associated with endothelial dysfunction and reduced eNO levels. Under these conditions, the physiological protective roles of NO may be diminished with resulting vasoconstriction, increased propensity to thrombosis, increased leukocyte activation and adhesion, and increased vascular smooth muscle proliferation.

Reductions in endothelial NO may be caused by down-regulation of eNOS expression,[38,39] decreased substrate availability, or increased destruction of endothelial NO.[40] Under conditions where the substrate L-arginine is limiting, eNOS may not be able to form NO, but forms superoxide instead. Superoxide reacts with NO in a nearly diffusion-limited reaction to form peroxynitrite.[41] This reaction is extremely rapid and functionally may dispose of NO so it is not available to mediate its physiological vascular functions. It also may lead to additional consequences because peroxynitrite anion is reactive and can nitrosylate tyrosine residues in proteins.

Intimal proliferation plays a critical role in the development of atherosclerotic lesions.[42] It occurs as a common response to arterial injury of many types. Animal models of intimal proliferation include adventitial cuff injury models, and intraluminal filament or balloon injury models.[43] Cuff models may be especially useful to study the role of individual endothelial products like NO because they do not involve direct damage to or removal of the endothelium.[44,45] The endpoint of the cuff model is development of neointima, which can be quantitated by morphometry. The ratio of the intimal volume to the medial volume reflects the degree of neointimal cellular proliferation.

To test the role of eNOS in suppression of vascular smooth muscle cell proliferation, the eNOS knockout mice were subjected to a cuff model of vessel injury.[46] At baseline, mice do not have intima and no intima developed in any sham-operated animals. Following cuff injury, the eNOS knockout mice develop significantly more intima than do wild-type mice (Figure 5 see page 56A). Male eNOS knockout mice have an intima/muscle (I/M) ratio of 0.70, as compared with male wild-type mice with an I/M ratio of 0.31. Female eNOS knockout mice have an I/M ratio of 0.42, as compared with female wild-type mice with an I/M ratio of 0.17. These results indicate that eNOS deficiency is associated with a more pronounced neointimal proliferative response and are consistent with a physiological role for eNOS in suppressing these responses. Neointimal proliferation was associated with increased 5-bromodeoxyuridine (BrdU) uptake in the media, indicating that medial cells may proliferate and migrate through the internal elastic lamina to form the intima. Immunohistochemical studies show that the cells in the neointima, like cells in the media, stain for smooth muscle $\alpha$-actin. Cells in the neointima do not stain for the endothelial markers CD31 and von-Willebrand factor.

The reduced intimal proliferation in female animals as compared with male animals is a general feature of vessel injury models.[47–49] These gender differences are thought to reflect the protective effects of estrogens. Estrogen may suppress atherosclerosis by increasing eNOS expression, by direct effects on vascular smooth muscle and by altering the lipid profile.[50] In acute injury models like the cuff model described, lipid levels are not likely to play a major role and short-term cholesterol measurements are unaltered by ovarectomy, gender, or hormone replacement. As indicated by BrdU labeling, indices of cellular proliferation correlate with the degree of neointimal formation, so effects of estrogen on vascular smooth muscle growth are likely to be important. Although some effects of estrogen may be mediated by increased eNOS expression, the results in the eNOS knockout mice indicate that eNOS cannot mediate all of the effects of estrogens. If it did, then there would be no difference between the responses of male and female eNOS knockout mice.

An unexpected finding was that pregnant mice developed almost no intima at all after cuff placement. This effect overrode the effect of even eNOS gene deletion, in that pregnant eNOS knockout mice had extremely low I/M ratios and essentially no intima. To study the basis for gender and pregnancy effects, we ovarectomized female mice and implanted subcutaneous pumps for hormone administration. As observed in other models of vessels injury, ovarectomy obliterates the protective effect of female gender but estrogen replacement restores it. We have found that chorionic gonadotropin (CG), an important hormone produced during pregnancy, reduces the neointimal response of intact (nonovarectomized) female mice, but not of ovarectomized mice (L. Zhang, M. C. Fishman, and P. L. Huang, preliminary results). Thus, CG does not act directly on vascular smooth muscle to suppress proliferation. Estrogen levels suggest that ovarian estrogen production mediates the protective effect of CG and pregnancy.

# Endothelial Nitric Oxide Synthase Expression and 3-Hydroxy-3-methylglutaryl Coenzyme A Reductase Inhibitors

Several large clinical studies have shown an association between the use of 3-hydroxy-3-methylglutaryl coenzyme A (HMG-CoA) reductase inhibitors— the statins—and reduction in incidence of stroke.[51,52] These effects were independent of cholesterol lowering, suggesting that these drugs may act by more than one mechanism. The statins up-regulate eNOS expression by prolonging eNOS mRNA.[53] They also increase aortic NO production and endothelium-dependent relaxation. To test whether these effects may underlie the reduction in incidence of stroke, statins were administered to animals subjected to MCAO model of focal ischemia. Statins reduced the cerebral infarct size in a dose-dependent manner. However, when they were administered to eNOS knockout mice, there was no effect. These results indicate that the majority, if not all, of the protective effect of statins is mediated by eNOS.[54]

# References

1. Huang PL, Fishman MC. Genetic analysis of NOS isoforms: Targeted mutation in mice. *J Mol Med* 1996;74:415–421.

2. Nathan C, Xie QW. Nitric oxide synthases: Roles, tolls, and controls. *Cell* 1994;78: 915–918.

3. Huang PL, Dawson TM, Bredt DS, et al. Targeted disruption of the neuronal nitric oxide synthase gene. *Cell* 1993;75:1273–1286.

4. Mashimo H, He XD, Huang PL, et al. Neuronal constitutive nitric oxide synthase is involved in murine enteric inhibitory neurotransmission. *J Clin Invest* 1996;98:8–13.

5. MacMicking, JD, Nathan,C, Hom G, et al. Altered responses to bacterial infection and endotoxic shock in mice lacking inducible nitric oxide synthase. *Cell* 1995;81: 641–650.

6. Laubach VE, Shesely EG, Smithies O, et al. Mice lacking inducible nitric oxide synthase are not resistant to lipopolysaccaride-induced death. *Proc Natl Acad Sci U S A* 1995;92:10688–10692.

7. Wei, XQ, Charles, IG, Smith, A, et al. Altered immune responses in mice lacking inducible nitric oxide synthase. *Nature.* 1995;375:408–411.

8. Huang PL, Huang Z, Mashimo H, et al. Hypertension in mice lacking the gene for endothelial nitric oxide synthase. *Nature* 1995;377:239–242.

9. Shesely EG, Maeda N, Kim HS, et al. Elevated blood pressures in mice lacking endothelial nitric oxide synthase. *Proc Natl Acad Sci U S A* 1996;93:13176–13181.

10. Irikura K, Huang PL, Ma J, et al. Cerebrovascular alterations in mice lacking neuronal nitric oxide synthase gene expression. *Proc Natl Acad Sci U S A* 1995; 92:6823–6827.

11. Ma J, Ayata C, Huang PL, et al. Regional cerebral blood flow response to vibrissal stimulation in mice lacking type I NOS gene expression. *Am J Physiol* 1996;270: H1085–H1090.

12. Crosby G, Marota JJA, Huang PL. Intact nociception-induced neuroplasticity in transgenic mice deficient in neuronal nitric oxide synthase. *Neuroscience* 1995;69: 1013–1017.

13. Ichinose F, Huang PL, Zapol WM. Effects of targeted neuronal nitric oxide synthase gene disruption and nitroG-L-arginine methylester on the threshold for isoflurane anesthesia. *Anesthesiology* 1995;83:101–108.

14. Gerlai R. Gene targeting studies of mammalian behavior: Is it the mutation or the background genotype? *Trends Neurosci* 1996;19:177–181.

15. Malinski T, Bailey F, Zhang ZG, et al. Nitric oxide measured by a porphyrinic microsensor in rat brain after transient middle cerebral artery occlusion. *J Cereb Blood Flow Metab* 1993;13:355–358.

16. Hara H, Waeber C, Huang PL, et al. Brain distribution of nitric oxide synthase in neuronal or endothelial nitric oxide synthase mutant mice using [3H]L-NG-nitro-arginine autoradiography. *Neuroscience.* 1996;75:881–890.

17. Dinerman JL, Dawson,TM, Schell MJ, et al. Endothelial nitric oxide synthase localized to hippocampal pyramidal cells: Implications for synaptic plasticity. *Proc Natl Acad Sci U S A* 1994;91:4214–4218.

18. O'Dell TJ, Huang PL, Dawson TM, et al. Endothelial NOS and the blockade of LTP by NOS inhibitors in mice lacking neuronal NOS. *Science* 1994;265:542–546.

19. Huang Z, Huang PL, Panahian N, et al. Effects of cerebral ischemia in mice deficient in neuronal nitric oxide synthase. *Science* 1994;265:1883–1885.

20. Iadecola C, Pelligrino DA, Moskowitz MA, et al. Nitric oxide synthase inhibition and cerebrovascular regulation. *J Cereb Blood Flow Metab* 1994;14:175–192.

21. Hara H, Huang PL, Panahian N, et al. Reduced brain edema and infarction volume in mice lacking the neuronal isoform of nitric oxide synthase after transient MCA occlusion. *J Cereb Blood Flow Metab* 1996;16:605–611.

22. Panahian N, Yoshida T, Huang PL, et al. Attenuated hippocampal damage after global cerebral ischemia in knock-out mice deficient in neuronal nitric oxide synthase. *Neuroscience* 1996;72:343–354.

23. Huang Z, Huang PL, Ma J, et al. Enlarged infarcts in endothelial nitric oxide synthase knockout mice are attenuated by nitro-L-arginine. *J Cereb Blood Flow Metab* 1996;16:981–987.

24. Lo E, Hara H, Rogowska J, et al. Temporal correlation mapping analysis of the hemodynamic penumbra in mutant mice deficient in endothelial nitric oxide synthase gene expression. *Stroke* 1996;27:1381–1385.

25. Balligand JL, Kelly RA, Marsden PA, et al. Control of cardiac muscle function by an endogenous nitric oxide signaling system. *Proc Natl Acad Sci U S A* 1993;90:347–351.

26. Balligand JL, Kobzik L, Han X, et al. Nitric oxide-dependent parasympathetic signaling is due to activation of constitutive endothelial (type III) nitric oxide synthase in cardiac myocytes. *J Biol Chem* 1995;270:14582–14586.

27. Hare JM, Loh E, Creager MA, et al. Nitric oxide inhibits the positive inotropic response to β-adrenergic stimulation in humans with left ventricular dysfunction. *Circulation* 1995;92:2198–2203.

28. Kelly RA, Balligand JL, Smith TW. Nitric oxide and cardiac function. *Circ Res* 1996;79:363–380.

29. Dorn GW, Robbins J, Ball N, et al. Myosin heavy chain regulation and myocyte contractile depression after LV hypertrophy in aortic-banded mice. *Am J Physiol* 1994;267:H400–H405.

30. Radomski MW, Palmer RM, Moncada S. Modulation of platelet aggregation by an L-arginine-nitric oxide pathway. *Trends Pharmacol Sci.* 1991;12:87–88.

31. Davenpeck KL, Gauthier TW, Lefer AM. Inhibition of endothelial-derived nitric oxide promotes P-selectin expression and actions in the rat microcirculation. *Gastroenterology* 1994;107:1050–1058.

32. De Caterina R, Libby P, Peng HB, et al. Nitric oxide decreases cytokine-induced endothelial activation. Nitric oxide selectively reduces endothelial expression of adhesion molecules and proinflammatory cytokines. *J Clin Invest* 1995;96:60–68.

33. Gauthier TW, Davenpeck KL, Lefer AM. Nitric oxide attenuates leukocyte-endothelial interaction via P-selectin in splanchnic ischemia-reperfusion. *Am J Physiol* 1994;267:G562–G568.

34. Gauthier TW, Scalia R, Murohara T, et al. Nitric oxide protects against leukocyte-endothelium interactions in the early stages of hypercholesterolemia. *Arterioscler Thromb Vasc Biol* 1995;15:1652–1659.

35. Mooradian DL, Hutsell TC, Keefer LK. Nitric oxide (NO) donor molecules: Effect of NO release rate on vascular smooth muscle cell proliferation in vitro. *J Cardiovasc Pharmacol* 1995;25:674–678.

36. Hansson GK, Geng YJ, Holm J, et al. Arterial smooth muscle cells express nitric oxide synthase in response to endothelial injury. *J Exp Med* 1994;180:733–738.

37. Peng HB, Libby P, Liao JK. Induction and stabilization of I-kappa B alpha by nitric oxide mediates inhibition of NF-kappa B. *J Biol Chem* 1995;270:14214–14219.

38. Liao JK, Shin WS, Lee WY, et al. Oxidized low density lipoprotein decreases the expression of endothelial nitric oxide synthase. *J Biol Chem* 1995;270:319–324.

39. Yoshizumi M, Perrella MA, Burnett JC, et al. Tumor necrosis factor downregulates an endothelial nitric oxide synthase mRNA by shortening its half-life. *Circ Res* 1993;73:205–209.

40. Mugge A, Elwell JH, Peterson TE, et al. Release of intact endothelium-derived relaxing factor depends on endothelial superoxide dismutase activity. *Am J Physiol* 1991;260:219–225.

41. Beckman JS, Ye YZ, Anderson, PG, et al. Extensive nitration of protein tyrosines in human atherosclerosis detected by immunohistochemistry. *Biol Chem Hoppe-Seyler* 1994;375:81–88.

42. Benditt EP, Benditt JM. Evidence for a monoclonal origin of human atherosclerotic plaques. *Proc Natl Acad Sci U S A* 1973;70:1753–1756.

43. Schwartz SM, DeBlois B, O'Brien ERM. The intima: Soil for atherosclerosis and restenosis. *Circ Res* 1995;77:445–465.

44. Booth RFG, Martin JF, Honey AC, et al. Rapid development of atherosclerotic lesions in the rabbit carotid artery induced by perivascular manipulation. *Atherosclerosis* 1989;76:257–268.

45. Kockx MM, De Meyer GRY, Andires LJ, et al. The endothelium during cuff-induced neointima formation in the rabbit carotid artery. *Arterioscler Thromb Vasc Biol* 1993;13:1874–1884.
46. Moroi, M, Zhang, L, Yasuda, T, et al. Interaction of genetic deficiency of endothelial nitric oxide, gender, and pregnancy in vascular response to injury in mice. *J Clin Invest* 1998;101:1225–1232.
47. Akishita M, Ouchi Y, Miyoshi H, et al. Estrogen inhibits cuff-induced intimal thickening of rat femoral artery: Effects on migration and proliferation of vascular smooth muscle cells. *Atherosclerosis* 1997;130:1–10.
48. Chen SJ, Li H, Durand J, et al. Estrogen reduces myointimal proliferation after balloon injury of rat carotid artery. *Circulation* 1996;93:577–584.
49. Sullivan TR, Karas RH, Aronovitz M, et al. Estrogen inhibits the response to injury in a mouse carotid artery model. *J Clin Invest* 1995;96:2482–2488.
50. White CR, Darley-Usmar V, Oparil S. Gender and cardiovascular disease; recent insights. *Trends Cardiovasc Med* 1997;7:94–100.
51. Sacks FM, Pfeffer MA, Moye LA, et al. The effect of pravastatin on coronary events after myocardial infarction in patients with average cholesterol levels. Cholesterol and recurrent events trial investigators. *N Engl J Med* 1996;335:1001–1009.
52. Blauw GJ, Lagaay AM, Smelt AH, et al. Stroke, statins, and cholesterol. A meta-analysis of randomized, placebo-controlled double-blind trials with HMG-CoA reductase inhibitors. *Stroke* 1997;28:946–950.
53. Laufs U, Fata VL, Liao JK. Inhibition of 3-hydroxy-3-methylglutaryl (HMG)-CoA reductase blocks hypoxia-mediated down-regulation of endothelial nitric oxide synthase. *J Biol Chem* 1997;272:31725–31729.
54. Endres M, Laufs U, Huang Z, et al. Stroke protection by 3-hydroxy-3-methylglutaryl (HMG)-CoA reductase inhibitors mediated by endothelial nitric oxide synthase. *Proc Natl Acad Sci U S A* 1998;95:8880–8885.

## Chapter 5

# Nitric Oxide Signaling Mediating Relaxation of Vascular Smooth Muscle

*Richard A. Cohen, MD*

## Introduction

Decreased bioactivity of nitric oxide (NO) is a feature of vascular diseases of diverse etiologies including those associated with hypercholesterolemia, diabetes, and hypertension.[1] Both clinical studies and animal models demonstrate impaired relaxant or vasodilator responses to endothelium-dependent vasodilators such as acetylcholine (ACh). Except in advanced disease, it commonly has been noted that vasodilation to nitrovasodilators, including sodium nitroprusside and nitroglycerin, are normal. This has been interpreted to mean that abnormal endothelium-dependent vasodilation is caused by abnormal release of NO from the endothelium. However, recent studies indicate that this interpretation may be invalid. For instance, in hypercholesterolemic rabbit aorta in which vasodilation caused by sodium nitroprusside is normal, the vasodilation to exogenous authentic NO is impaired nearly to the same extent as that to ACh (Figure 1).[2] Furthermore, the abnormality of smooth muscle responsiveness to NO is maintained in culture.[2] This suggests that a principal cause of impaired endothelium-dependent vasodilation is impaired responsiveness of smooth muscle to NO. The difference between endothelium-dependent vasodilation mediated by NO and the response to nitrovasodilators is interesting and certainly therapeutically important with respect to the use of nitrovasodilators. The contrast in function may depend on the fact that nitrovasodilators release NO intracellularly and act on smooth muscle differently than the vasodilator released endogenously from the endothelium, which diffuses to the smooth muscle. In any case, these observations indicate that in order to understand abnormal endothelium-dependent vasodilation, one should attempt to understand the abnormal responsiveness of diseased vascular smooth muscle to NO. This chapter briefly summarizes recent studies

The author gratefully acknowledges support by the National Institutes of Health, National Lung and Blood Institute through Grants HL-31607, HL-55620, HL-55993, and HL-55854.

From Panza JA, Cannon RO III (eds): *Endothelium, Nitric Oxide, and Atherosclerosis* ©Futura Publishing Co, Inc, Armonk, NY, 1999.

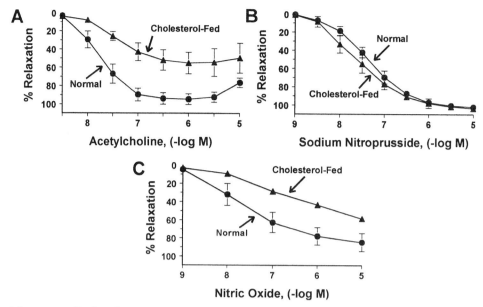

**Figure 1.** Reduced responsiveness to nitric oxide (NO) in hypercholesterolemic rabbit thoracic aorta. Relaxation to acetylcholine (ACh), sodium nitroprusside, and authentic NO was determined in phenylephrine contracted rings of thoracic aorta from rabbits fed a 0.5% cholesterol diet for 10–12 weeks. Relaxation to ACh and NO was impaired indicating impaired responsiveness of the smooth muscle to the endogenous vasodilator. Responses to sodium nitroprusside were normal, indicating that the smooth muscle had the capability to respond normally to a nitrovasodilator. Reproduced with permission from Reference 2.

directed toward a more complete understanding of the mechanisms underlying endothelium-dependent vasodilation.

## Nitric Oxide Is the Principal Mediator of Endothelium-Dependent Hyperpolarization and Relaxation

Although the point has been debated and alternative forms of NO proposed, the physical and chemical properties of the principal vasodilator released from endothelium most closely resemble those of authentic NO.[3] In addition to causing relaxation, endothelium-dependent vasodilators also cause hyperpolarization of the underlying vascular smooth muscle. For several reasons, a mediator other than NO has been sought as the mediator of this response. Among the candidates have been prostacyclin and other prostanoids, hydroxyeicosatetraenoic acids, epoxyeicosatrienoic acids, and adenosine triphosphate (ATP).[4] The following are the arguments that a mediator other than NO plays a role. (1) Nitric oxide synthase (NOS) inhibitors incompletely inhibit endothelium-dependent vasodilation and hyperpolarization. (2) Endothelium-dependent vasodilators apparently do not depend on cyclic guanosine monophosphate (cGMP), which is thought to be the essential signaling mechanism by which NO exerts its actions. (3) Exogenous nitrovasodilators poorly mimic the hyperpolarization caused by endothelium-dependent vasodilators.[4] However, the following discussion indicates that these points may be explained by the poorly understood properties of NO released from the endothelium and that the primary mediator of endothelium-dependent vasodilation and hyperpolarization is NO.

Collaborative studies of the isolated rabbit carotid artery were conducted to better understand these issues.[5] When the changes in smooth muscle cell membrane potential were measured in contracted arteries, hyperpolarization was correlated highly with the relaxation to acetylcholine (ACh). The amount of NO released from the endothelium, measured by two independent techniques, also correlated with both responses. High concentrations of L-arginine

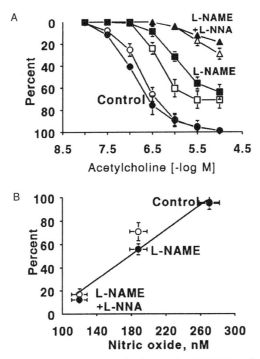

**Figure 2.** Effect of nitro-L-arginine methylester (L-NAME) and $N^G$-nitro-L-arginine (L-NNA on ACh-induced hyperpolarization, relaxation, and NO release rings of rabbit carotid artery were mounted for isometric tension measurement and membrane potential was recorded with a microelectrode inserted from the adventitial aspect. Rings were untreated or pretreated with L-NAME or L-NNA, prior to contracting and depolarizing with phenylephrine and administering ACh. (**A**) ACh-evoked relaxations (open symbols) and repolarizations (closed symbols) under control conditions (circles), after treatment with L-NAME ($3 \times 10^{-5}$ mol/L squares), or after treatment with L-NAME ($3 \times 10^{-5}$ mol/L) together with L-NNA ($3 \times 10^{-4}$ mol/L, triangles). (**B**) Close correlation between the maximal relaxation (filled circles) or repolarization (open circles) and the release of NO from rabbit carotid arteries caused by ACh ($3 \times 10^{-6}$ mol/L) measured with a porphyrinic microsensor under control conditions or after treatment with the same concentrations of L-NAME, or L-NAME combined with L-NNA. Reproduced with permission from Reference 5.

derivative NOS inhibitors decreased but did not eliminate the responses to ACh, but the correlation between the quantity of NO released and the response remained (Figure 2). Even with the highest concentrations of the inhibitors used, up to 40% of a controlled amount of NO was released. An exogenous NO donor that released NO in the same concentration range as that from the endothelium also caused coordinated relaxation and hyperpolarization. Thus, the persistent release of NO, rather than another endothelial cell–derived substance, accounted for the vasoactive response. The inability of NOS inhibitors to block NO release demonstrated in this study likely accounts for the vasodilation demonstrated to occur in a number of vascular beds after treatment with NOS inhibitors.[4]

# Cyclic Guanosine Monophosphate-Dependent and -Independent Actions of Nitric Oxide

Another striking finding was made in the course of these studies of the rabbit carotid artery. In contrast to the ACh-stimulated release of NO, which persists in the presence of NOS inhibitors, the elevation of cGMP was blocked effectively by the inhibitors.[6] Further studies[7] have confirmed that both ACh-induced relaxation and hyperpolarization persist when cGMP production is blocked with H-(1,2,4) oxadiazolo(4,3-$a$) quinoxallin-1-one (ODQ), a guanylyl cyclase inhibitor (Figure 3). Indeed, exogenous NO also persists in mediating a similar degree of relaxation and hyperpolarization in the presence of ODQ, despite having prevented increases in cGMP[7] or activation of protein kinase G (personal communication from P. Komalavilas and T. Lincoln, 1998). Thus, the actions of NO, released from the endothelium, or administered exogenously do not depend strictly on cGMP.[8] Obviously, cGMP participates in the actions of endothelium-derived NO: cGMP levels are increased by NO, the cyclic nucleotide activates protein kinase G, and most of the actions of NO can be mimicked by exogenous membrane permeable analogues of cGMP. Indeed, in contrast to authentic NO, the actions of some donors of NO, such as molsidomine,[7] sodium nitroprusside, and nitroglycerin, are blocked completely by ODQ. (R. Cohen, unpublished observations, 1998) are blocked completely by ODQ. In the case of molsidomine, which also causes coordinated relaxation and hyperpolarization, these actions apparently are dependent entirely on cGMP.[7] This also suggests that authentic NO is a better mimic of the endogenous nitrovasodilator released from the endothelium than are other NO donors. One possibility to explain cGMP-independent actions of NO are the interactions it is known to have with redox-sensitive thiol groups demonstrated to modulate the activity of several ion channels including the calcium-dependent potassium channel[9] and the ryanodine receptor channel.[10]

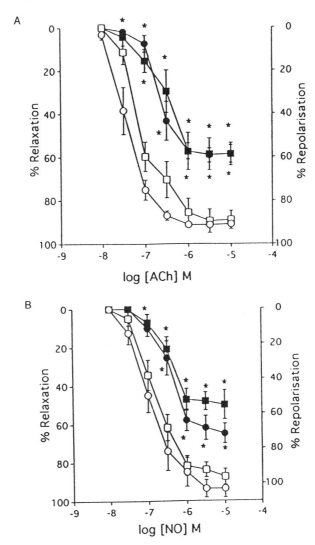

**Figure 3.** Effect of H-(1,2,4) oxadiazolo(4,3-$a$) quinoxallin-1-one (ODQ) on the response of rabbit carotid artery to ACh and NO. Artery rings were pretreated for 10 minutes with ODQ ($10^{-5}$ mol/L) and contracted and depolarized with phenylephrine. ACh (**A**) or NO (**B**) were administered in increasing concentrations (indicated as the logarithm). Both NO-dependent agonists caused complete relaxation (circles) and repolarization (squares). Although ODQ (solid symbols) significantly reduced relaxation and repolarization to ACh and NO relative to vehicle (open symbols), significant responses persisted. Under these conditions, ODQ completely prevented the increase in cGMP and protein kinase G activation stimulated by ACh or NO[7] (R. Cohen, unpublished observations, 1998). Reproduced with permission from Reference 7.

# Regulation of Intracellular Calcium and Membrane Potential by Nitric Oxide

Many molecular targets of NO have been proposed to mediate its effects in vascular smooth muscle. The best substantiated of these are guanylyl cyclase, potassium and calcium channels, and ion transporters including the plasma membrane calcium ATPase and sodium-calcium exchanger, the sarcoplasmic reticulum calcium ATPase, the sodium-potassium ATPase, and myosin light chain kinase and phosphatase (see review by Lincoln and Cornwell[11]). Aside from the above discussion of cGMP, the relative importance of these targets to endothelium-dependent vasodilation is not known. Figure 4 diagrams the regulation of vascular smooth muscle calcium by NO. Of importance in understanding the response to NO is that NO does not affect smooth muscle contractility unless it is first increased. Agonists or membrane depolarization activate the two major mechanisms that increase intracellular calcium in vascular smooth muscle and cause contraction. First, membrane depolarization activates L-type calcium channels admitting calcium to the cell. Second, receptor-dependent agonists such as catecholamines, 5-hydroxytryptamine, or angiotensin II increase intracellular calcium by store-operated or capacitative calcium entry mechanisms in addition to membrane depolarization. Store-

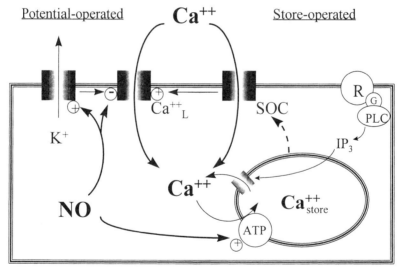

**Figure 4.** NO regulates two types of calcium entry pathways in vascular smooth muscle. Shown are potential operated, depolarization-dependent L-type ($Ca_L^{2+}$) channels and store-operated cation (SOC) channels, which mediate calcium influx in smooth muscle. NO inhibits (−) $Ca^{2+}$ entry through $Ca_L^{2+}$ by cGMP-dependent effects on the channel itself as well as by cGMP-dependent and -independent hyperpolarization mediated by its stimulation (+) of $K^+$ channels. Store-operated calcium entry through SOC is initiated by inositol trisphosphate ($IP_3$)–mediated release of $Ca^{2+}$ from the stores. NO increases (+) uptake into stores via the sarcoplasmic reticulum $Ca^{2+}$ ATPase pump (ATP). By refilling $Ca^{2+}$ stores, NO indirectly inhibits store-operated calcium entry.

operated calcium entry, described in a variety of cell types, depends on the inositol trisphosphate–induced emptying of intracellular calcium stores, which induces the entry of calcium through membrane ion channels that as yet are defined poorly.[12] The contribution to the contraction mediated by different agonists is heterogeneous among different blood vessels. This implies that the inhibition of contraction caused by NO also occurs by heterogeneous mechanisms.

Recent studies indicate that NO regulates both calcium entry mechanisms to reduce calcium entry and intracellular calcium levels. The depolarization-induced activation of L-type calcium channels is inhibited by NO through a cGMP-dependent inhibition of the channels themselves.[13] In addition, NO activates potassium channels both directly[9] and via cGMP[14] and by the hyperpolarization induced, prevents the activation of L-type calcium channels. The regulation by NO of agonist-induced calcium entry is understood poorly, but our recent studies indicate that NO regulates store-operated calcium entry. These studies suggest that NO accelerates the reuptake of calcium into intracellular stores via the sarcoplasmic reticulum calcium ATPase. By increasing the quantity of calcium in the stores, NO inhibits the store-operated influx of extracellular calcium.[15] Additional studies would indicate that the regulation of calcium stores by NO is via both cGMP-dependent and cGMP-independent mechanisms.[8] Thus, NO inhibits the two major mechanisms of calcium entry into cells by different mechanisms.

## Conclusions

NO is, by far, the major mediator of endothelium-dependent vasodilation. In experimental studies designed to determine its role, it is important to realize that agonist-induced stimulation of NO release is inhibited poorly by L-arginine analog inhibitors of NOS. In addition, nitrovasodilator drugs may demonstrate substantially different properties from endogenous NO, both with regard to the role of the intracellular mechanism of action as well as with the influence of vascular diseases on their efficacy. Perhaps through evolutionary pressures diverse mechanisms have evolved to mediate the response of vascular smooth muscle to NO. In terms of its effects on contraction mediated via changes in intracellular calcium, NO regulates both membrane depolarization-induced activation of L-type calcium channels and store-operated calcium entry in vascular smooth muscle. These diverse mechanisms may be affected by vascular diseases differently.

## References

1. Cohen RA. The role of nitric oxide and other endothelium-derived vasoactive substances in vascular disease. *Prog Cardiovasc Dis* 1995;38:105–128.
2. Weisbrod RM, Griswold MC, Du Y, et al. Reduced responsiveness of hypercholesterolemic rabbit aortic smooth muscle cells to nitric oxide. *Arterioscler Thromb Vasc Biol* 1997;17:394–402.

3. Feelisch M, te Poel M, Zamora R, et al. Understanding the controversy over the identity of EDRF. *Nature* 1994;368:62–65.
4. Cohen RA, Vanhoutte PM. Endothelium-dependent hyperpolarization: Beyond nitric oxide and cyclic GMP. *Circulation* 1995;92:3337–3349.
5. Cohen RA, Plane F, Najibi S, et al. Nitric oxide is the mediator of both endothelium-dependent relaxation and hyperpolarization of the rabbit carotid artery. *Proc Natl Acad Sci U S A* 1997;94:4193–4198.
6. Cowan CL, Palacino JJ, Najibi S, et al. Potassium channel mediated relaxation to acetylcholine in rabbit arteries. *J Pharmacol Exp Ther* 1993;266:1482–1489.
7. Plane F, Wiley KE, Jeremy JY, et al. Evidence that different mechanisms underlie smooth muscle relaxation to nitric oxide and nitric oxide donors in the rabbit isolated carotid artery. *Br J Pharmacol* 1998;123:1351–1358.
8. Weisbrod RM, Griswold MC, Yaghoubi M, et al. Evidence that additional mechanisms to cyclic GMP mediate the decrease in intracellular calcium and relaxation of rabbit aortic smooth muscle to nitric oxide. *Br J Pharmacol* 1998;125:1695–1707.
9. Bolotina VM, Najibi S, Palacino JJ, et al. Nitric oxide directly activates calcium-dependent potassium channels in vascular smooth muscle cells. *Nature* 1994;368:850–853.
10. Xu L, Eu JP, Meissner G, et al. Activation of the cardiac calcium release channel (ryanodine receptor) by poly-S-nitrosylation. *Science* 1998;279:234–237.
11. Lincoln TM, Cornwell TL. Intracellular cyclic GMP receptor proteins. *FASEB J* 1993;7:328–338.
12. Thomas AP, Bird GSJ, Hajnoczky G, et al. Spatial and temporal aspects of cellular calcium signalling. *FASEB J* 1996;10:1505–1517.
13. Campbell DL, Stamler JS, Strauss HD. Redox modulation of L-type calcium channels in ferret ventricular myocytes. *J Gen Physiol* 1996;108:277–293.
14. Taniguchi J, Furukawa KI, Shigekawa M. Maxi $K^+$ channels are stimulated by cyclic guanosine monophosphate-dependent protein kinase in canine coronary artery smooth muscle cells. *Pflugers Arch Eur J Physiol* 1993;423:167–172.
15. Bolotina VM, Weisbrod RM, Gericke M, et al. Novel mechanism of nitric oxide-induced relaxation: Accelerated refilling of intracellular calcium stores and inhibition of store-operated calcium influx. *Circulation* 1997;96:I448. Abstract.

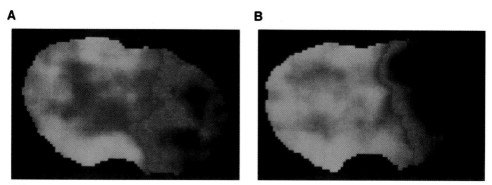

**A**        **B**

**Figure 1.** Temporal correlation mapping images of hemodynamic deficits in wild-type (**A**) and endothelial nitric oxide synthase (eNOS) knockout (**B**) micefollowing middle cerebral artery occlusion (MCAO). Normal hemodynamic status is indicated as shades of green. Abnormal hemodynamic status is indicated as shades of red to black, with black indicating absence of blood flow. The hemodynamic penumbra is red, and the core infarct zone is black. Thirty minutes following ischemia, there is a substantial penumbra in wild-type mice, while the core infarct zone is larger in the eNOS knockout mice and the penumbra is correspondingly smaller. Reproduced with permission from Reference 24.

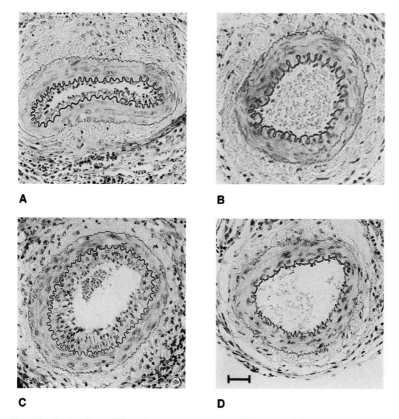

**A**        **B**

**C**        **D**

**Figure 5.** Neointimal proliferation response to cuff injury of femoral artery. Wild-type mice develop reproducible amounts of intima on the cuffed artery (**A**) but not sham-operated artery (**B**). The eNOS knockout mice develop increased amount of intima on the cuffed artery (**C**), while the sham-operated side shows no intima. Both wild-type and eNOS knockout mice were male in this case. Reproduced with permission from Reference 46.

56A

## Chapter 6

# Hemoglobin-Bound Nitric Oxide Participates in the Mammalian Respiratory Cycle

*Timothy J. McMahon, MD, and Jonathan S. Stamler, MD*

## Introduction

Human hemoglobin (Hb) is the most extensively studied protein in biology. Yet despite all that is known about this essential $O_2$-transport molecule, fundamental questions have persisted regarding its structure and function. For example, chemical modification of the evolutionarily conserved Cys$\beta$93 residues in human Hb increases $O_2$ affinity. However, the physiological counterpart of such modification and its role have remained elusive.

On another front, the emergence of nitric oxide (NO) as a critical signaling molecule in vascular biology has raised difficult questions about the role of Hb. Iron-containing heme groups in proteins represent an important point in signal transduction for the numerous biological activities of NO. The enzyme soluble guanylate cyclase (SGC) in the vasular smooth muscle cell is prototypical of such NO-responsive hemoproteins. The binding of NO by the heme moiety in SGC induces a conformational change that up-regulates enzyme activity. Increased production of cyclic guanosine monophosphate (cGMP) (among other pathways) then leads to vasodilation; in the platelet, the same pathway leads to the inhibition of platelet aggregation. By contrast, the tight binding of NO by the heme centers of hemoglobin classically has been considered irreversible. The functional correlate of this binding is to block the activation of SGC. Therefore, it is not obvious how endothelium-derived NO dilates blood vessels in vivo because the addition of Hb to blood vessels in vitro constricts them.

Kinetic models have been constructed in attempts to explain NO behavior in vivo. Assuming a steady-state NO concentration of $10^{-8}$ mol/L (a conservative estimate), blood Hb concentration of $3 \times 10^{-3}$ mol/L, circulating blood

From Panza JA, Cannon RO III (eds): *Endothelium, Nitric Oxide, and Atherosclerosis* ©Futura Publishing Co, Inc, Armonk, NY, 1999.

volume of 5 L (for a 70-kg human), and an Hb–NO binding reaction constant of $10^7$ mol/L$^{-1}$ per second (the dissociation constant is negligible), one would predict approximately 100 mol of NO to be consumed by Hb over a 24-hour period.[1] However, estimates of the rates of total body synthesis of NO for a 70-kg individual are on the order of 1.68 mmol per 24-hour period.[2] This disparity (by a factor of $10^5$!) between the rates of total NO production and the rates of predicted NO consumption by Hb strongly suggests that rather than acting simply as a passive sink for NO (in accordance with the classic view), Hb actively participates in the delivery of NO to target sites in the circulation.

Here we explain how Hb cycles NO, which thereby participates in the respiratory cycle. Specifically, we review recent studies showing that (1) NO may bind to both the hemes and the reactive thiols of Hb, (2) NO binding to hemes or thiols depends on the protein's conformation, (3) binding to thiols is favored in the high-affinity oxy (R; relaxed)-structure, and (4) the peripheral release of vasodilator $S$-nitrosothiol (SNO) from Hb takes place in such a way as to optimize $O_2$ delivery.

## Hemoglobin Conformation and Function

Human Hb, a tetramer consisting of $2\alpha$- and $2\beta$-subunits, assumes one of two quaternary structures: the R-structure, which has high affinity for ligand, or the deoxy (T; tense)-conformation, which has low affinity.[3,4] The Hb exhibits cooperativity in both loading and delivering $O_2$.

## Oxygen and Hemoglobin in the Respiratory Cycle: The Paradox

DeoxyHb moves from the venous circulation into the lung in the low-affinity T-structure, carrying $CO_2$ molecules on its $\alpha$-amino termini. The binding of $O_2$ elicits a conformational change to the R-structure, liberating $CO_2$. OxyHb in R-structure then enters the microcirculation where it encounters an $O_2$ gradient and high concentrations of allosteric effectors ($H^+/CO_2$), which together promote the allosteric transition and consequent release of $O_2$.[4] However, this model does not integrate NO and is not compatible with NO binding/dissociation kinetics; specifically, as pointed out above, Hb would constrict blood vessels by scavenging NO and thus oppose $O_2$ delivery.

## Interactions of Nitric Oxide with Hemoglobin

NO and related molecules such as SNO bind to Hb in a conformation-dependent manner. Specifically, NO binding to Hb's reactive thiols is favored in the R-structure (Figure 1) and binding to its heme groups is favored in the

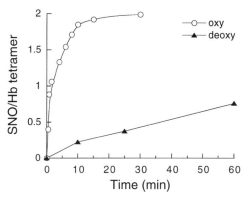

**Figure 1.** Allosteric regulation of hemoglobin (Hb) S-nitrosylation (SNO). Rates of Hb SNO (SNO/Hb tetramer) by *S*-nitrosocysteine are faster in the oxy (R) $Hb[FeII]O_2)$-structure than in the deoxy (T) Hb[FeII]) conformation. Incubations of Hb [aerated 2% borate, 0.5 mmol/L ethylenediaminetetraacetic acid (EDTA)] with 10-fold molar excess CysNO were performed either in air or in a tonometer rigorously evacuated of $O_2$ (deoxy). Samples were analyzed for SNO content at the times indicated.[6] ($n = 5$).

T-structure.[5,6] Conversely, under anaerobic conditions, the rate of denitrosylation of Hb is accelerated relative to the rate in air (data not shown). The SNOs, in contrast with NO, react only with Hb's reactive thiols and do not bind to its heme centers.[6]

## Hemoglobin-Bound Nitric Oxide and Oxygen Affinity

The $O_2$ binding curve for deoxygenated blood incubated with supraphysiological concentrations of NO is shifted to the right (ie, blood $O_2$ affinity is lowered).[7] Electron spin resonance spectroscopy measurements demonstrate that this fall in $O_2$ affinity is accompanied by formation of T-structure–reinforcing, 5-coordinate a-heme-NO adducts.[7] Whether similar NO-heme dynamics play any role in shaping the $O_2$-binding characteristics of human blood exposed to physiological concentrations of (endothelium-derived) NO is entirely uncertain. However, these observations at least raise the possibility that under conditions characterized by the overproduction of NO (eg, in septic shock), or with the therapeutic use of NO donors such as systemic nitroglycerin or inhaled NO, blood $O_2$ affinity may be diminished in the peripheral circulation.

Still, less is known of how the binding of NO to Hb's reactive thiol groups may affect $O_2$ affinity. Although heme nitrosylation reinforces the T-structure of Hb, S-nitrosylation is expected to promote the R-structure and thus augment $O_2$ affinity. Our preliminary data demonstrate that, indeed, the $O_2$-binding curve for SNO–Hb is shifted to the left in a parallel manner relative to unmodified Hb, consistent with a greater $O_2$ affinity and no significant change in cooperativity (T. J. M. McMahon and J. S. Stamler, unpublished observations, 1998). Further studies will be needed to confirm these findings and to explore their mechanism and significance.

# Measurements In Vivo: Endogenous Mammalian S-Nitrosothiols–Hemoglobin and Nitrosylhemoglobin

Arterial and central venous blood was drawn from anesthetized Sprague–Dawley rats, first while the animals were exposed to room air and then during exposure to 100% $O_2$ and 3 atmospheres of absolute (ATA) pressure in a hyperbaric chamber.[8] In these experiments, the mean $O_2$ saturation of venous room air blood was 69% and arterial room air blood was 93% saturated. Venous and arterial blood drawn from animals breathing 100% $O_2$ in 3 ATA was 93% and 100% saturated, respectively. Nitrosylhemoglobin (Hb[FeII]NO) was found to predominate in venous blood from rats breathing 21% $O_2$ (Hb $O_2$ saturation 69%), while in room air arterial blood (93% saturation), SNO–Hb was present in significant amounts (Figure 2).[6,8] By contrast, in both venous and arterial blood from animals breathing 100% $O_2$ in 3 ATA (ie, where the microvascular $O_2$ gradient was eliminated effectively; 93% and 100% saturations, respectively), SNO–Hb predominated (Figure 2). The presence of SNO–Hb has been demonstrated in human fetal blood, where the placenta subserves the role of the adult lung in synthesizing SNO (Table 1).[9] Levels of SNO–Hb were greater in oxygenated (umbilical venous) than deoxygenated (umbilical arterial) blood (Table 1).[9] However, extending these observations will require meticulous efforts to control the oxygen environment of the samples.

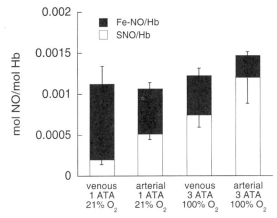

**Figure 2.**   Levels of endogenous SNO—Hb and Hb[FeII]NO in mammalian blood: influence of the $O_2$ tension. Blood was drawn via indwelling arterial and venous catheters from rats exposed first to room air (21% $O_2$) and then to 100% $O_2$ + 3 atmospheres of absolute (ATA) in a hyperbaric chamber. See review by Stamler et al[8] for methods and resulting $O_2$ saturations.

Table 1

**Measurements of S-Nitrosylation of Hemoglobin
(SNO–Hb) in Human Fetal (Umbilical Cord)
Arterial and Venous Blood**

| Sample | $n$ | [SNO]/[Hb] |
|---|---|---|
| Arterial (deoxy) | 19 | 0.00145 ± 0.00066 |
| Venous (oxy) | 19 | 0.00219 ± 0.00022 |

SNO content was determined by the modified Saville method and corrected for the Hb concentration. Levels of SNO-Hb were significantly higher in umbilical venous than in umbilical arterial blood ($P < 0.001$ for the paired $t$ test), while total plasma $NO_x$ levels did not differ significantly between artery and vein.[3] $n = 19$. Values are means ± SD.

# Dynamic Equilibrium Between *S*-Nitric Oxide–Hemoglobin and Nitrosylhemoglobin

Measurements of Hb-bound NO in mammalian (rat) blood suggest that SNO–Hb is in an $O_2$-dependent equilibrium with Hb[FeII]NO.Indeed, exposure of partially nitrosylated Hb[FeII]NO to $O_2$—mimicking the experience of erythrocytes entering the lung—results in NO migrating from the heme to the thiol. In this respect, Hb is exemplary of a novel class of protein capable of supporting S-nitrosylation and containing a consensus sequence centered around a reactive cysteine residue.[10] Conversely, deoxygenation of SNO–Hb results in formation of Hb[FeII]NO. Allosteric transitions in Hb thus are coupled with NO exchange between heme and thiol.

# Role of Oxygen Tension in Nitric Oxide Cycling by Hemoglobin

The preferred site of NO's binding to Hb in vivo reflects the $O_2$ tension in the two limbs of the circulation. Changes in $O_2$ concentration thus translate directly into circulatory alterations in the level of NO binding. For example, when animals breathing 100% $O_2$ were studied in a hyperbaric chamber set to 3 ATA pressure (conditions under which the longitudinal $O_2$ gradient in arterioles is eliminated), the arterial–venous differences in the concentrations of SNO–Hb and Hb[FeII]NO were no longer seen (Figure 2).[8] In addition, when venous human blood samples are processed in room air for the simultaneous measurement of SNO–Hb and Hb[FeII]NO, conditions that artifactually elevate the $PO_2$ of the samples, the levels of SNO–Hb are greater than those measured from simultaneous processing of paired samples in an oxygen-controlled ("glove box") environment (T. J. McMahon and J. S. Stamler, unpublished observations, 1998).

# Hemoglobin and Oxygen Delivery

Oxygen delivery ($VO_2$) is the product of tissue blood flow ($Q$) and the oxygen content ($CaO_2$) of circulating blood (see Equation 1).

$$VO_2 = (Q)(CaO_2) \tag{1}$$

$$CaO_2 \sim [Hb](SO_2) \tag{2}$$

Blood oxygen content is, in turn, primarily a product of the Hb concentration and the fractional oxygen saturation of Hb (Equation 2); under normal circumstances, dissolved oxygen contributes a negligible amount. The NO–Hb interactions are poised to influence oxygen delivery mainly through regulation of resistance vessel tone.

# Hemoglobin-Bound Nitric Oxide Participates in the Respiratory Cycle

We propose the following revised model of the respiratory cycle. Venous blood entering the lung contains partially heme-nitrosylated deoxyHb (Hb[FeII]NO) in T-structure. Exposure there to high $PO_2$ elicits an allosteric transition in Hb (from T- to R-structure) that is coupled to S-nitrosylation: SNO–$HbO_2$ thus is formed during venous–arterial transit. When SNO–$HbO_2$ encounters the longitudinal $O_2$ gradient in systemic arterioles that control resistance, SNO is released allosterically from T-structured molecules, increasing blood flow.

# S-Nitrosothiols–Hemoglobin and Hypoxic Vasodilation

In the respiratory cycle, Hb delivers to the peripheral tissues only one of the four $O_2$ molecules it carries; that is, Hb leaves the lung 100% saturated, while venous Hb typically is ~65%–75% saturated. This cycle might appear poorly suited to the efficient off-loading of $O_2$, because Hb does not assume the low-affinity T-structure at such high levels of $O_2$ saturation. In point of fact, $O_2$ saturation at the level of the capillaries is 40%–50%, as a result of a functional shunt between arterial and venous vessels. Thus, an allosteric transition in Hb from the R- to the T-conformation occurs in microvessels serving the peripheral tissues.[11] As Hb/SNO–Hb undergoes the allosteric transition in precapillary resistance vessels, SNO is released and elicits vasodilation. Regional blood flow thereby is increased in those regions that are most hypoxic. Conversely, increases in blood flow by SNO–Hb are abolished when the longitudinal oxygen gradient is eliminated by the concomitant adminstration of hyperbaric oxygen[8]; that is, hemoglobin is designed to bring blood flow back in line with the demand for oxygen.

# References

1. Kharitonov VG, Bonaventura J, Sharma VS. Interactions of nitric oxide with heme proteins using UV-vis spectroscopy. In: Feelisch M, Stamler JS, eds. *Methods in Nitric Oxide Research.* Chichester, England: John Wiley & Sons; 1996.
2. Castillo L, Beaumier L, Ajami AM, et al. Whole body nitric oxide synthesis in healthy men determined from [$^{15}$N]-arginine-to-[$^{15}$N-]citrulline labelling. *Proc Natl Acad Sci U S A* 93;1996:11460–11465.
3. Antonini E, Brunori M. *Hemoglobin and Myoglobin in Their Reactions with Ligands.* New York: Elsevier; 1971.
4. Perutz M. Molecular anatomy, physiology, and pathology of hemoglobin. In: Stammatayanopoulos G, ed. *Molecular Basis of Blood Diseases.* Philadelphia, PA: WB Saunders; 1987.
5. Gow AG, Stamler JS. Nitric oxide/hemoglobin reactions reexamined under physiological conditions. *Nature* 1998:391:169–173.
6. Jia L, Bonaventura C, Bonaventura J, et al. *S*-Nitrosohaemoglobin: A dynamic activity of blood involved in vascular control. *Nature* 1996;380:221–226.
7. Kosaka H, Seiyama A. Physiological role of nitric oxide as an enhancer of oxygen transfer from erythrocytes to tissues. *Biochem Biophys Res Commun* ;1996;218: 749–752.
8. Stamler JS, Jia L, Eu JP, et al. Blood flow regulation by *S*-nitrosohemoglobin in the physiological oxygen gradient. *Science* 1997;276:2034–2037.
9. Funai EF, A Davidson, SP Seligman, et al. *S*-Nitrosohemoglobin in the fetal circulation may represent a cycle for blood pressure regulation. *Biochem Biophys Res Commun* 1997;239:875–877.
10. Stamler JS, Toone EJ, Lipton SA, et al. S-Nitrosylation: Translocation, consensus motif, and functional consequences. *Neuron* 1997;18;691–696.
11. McMahon TJ, Stamler JS. Concerted nitric oxide/oxygen delivery from hemoglobin. *Methods Enzymol* 1999;301:99–114.-

## Chapter 7

# Hormonal Regulation of Endothelium-Derived Factors

*Virginia M. Miller, PhD*

## Introduction

Epidemiological studies indicate that the incidence of coronary artery disease is less in premenopausal women compared with age-matched men but increases in women at menopause to levels comparable with age-matched men.[1] Estrogen replacement reduces the incidence of coronary artery disease in postmenopausal women,[2–5] suggesting that this female sex steroid is important in maintaining physiological functions of the cardiovascular system, which reduce and/or limit the onset of disease. Mechanisms by which hormones in general and estrogens in particular alter vascular function are multifactorial affecting all components of the blood vessel wall including the endothelium,[6–9] smooth muscle,[10,11] and peripheral adrenergic nerve endings.[12]

Endothelial cells produce diffusible factors that limit processes implicated in development of coronary arterial disease including platelet aggregation,[13,14] leukocyte adhesion,[8,15,16] and proliferation of vascular smooth muscle.[17] Therefore, understanding how sex steroids affect endothelial functions may lead to new therapeutic strategies to reduce vascular disease in both men and women. This chapter will review experimental data that estrogens modulate production and release of endothelium-derived factors and response of vascular smooth muscle to those factors.

## Hormones and Endothelium-Derived Nitric Oxide

Augmentation of endothelium-dependent relaxations to acetylcholine in femoral arteries isolated from estrogen-treated ovariectomized rabbits (Figure

This work was supported in part by Grants HL-51736 and HL-07111 from the National Heart, Lung and Blood Institute and grants from the Mayo Clinic and Mayo Foundation.
From Panza JA, Cannon RO III (eds): *Endothelium, Nitric Oxide, and Atherosclerosis* ©Futura Publishing Co, Inc, Armonk, NY, 1999.

1) was the first observation that estrogen replacement could modulate production and/or release of endothelium-derived relaxing factors (EDRFs).[6] At that time, the exact nature of EDRF was not known. Metabolites of arachidonic acid by cyclooxygenase could be excluded as contributing to the response as experiments were conducted in the presence of indomethacin.[6] The augmentation of relaxations to acetylcholine in femoral arteries from those estrogen-treated rabbits was modest. However, subsequently, others verified estrogenic modulation of endothelium-dependent responses in vitro by incubation of isolated aortic rings from experimental animals with estrogen.[18] Also, in vivo experiments with acute infusion of estrogen into coronary arteries of nonhuman primates[19,20] and humans[21–24] and brachial arteries of postmenopausal women identified increases in vasodilatation following estrogen treatment.[25,26] With the identification of nitric oxide (NO) as a major component of EDRF(s),[27,28] direct measures of total oxidized products of NO (NO$_x$) began to identify changes in production/release of NO with hormonal status. For example, basal release of NO is greater from aorta of female compared with male rabbits.[29] Observations from humans and experimental animals indicate that plasma NO$_x$ increases with endogenous increases in estrogen associated with the normal menstrual/reproductive cycle.[7,30,31] In addition, increasing circulating estrogen either by administration of exogenous estrogen (transdermal or

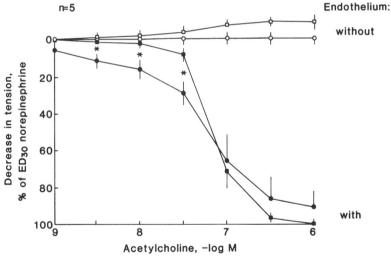

**Figure 1.**   Effect of estradiol-17$\beta$ (100 $\mu$g intramuscularly for 4 days) on relaxations evoked by acetylcholine in rings of femoral arteries of ovariectomized rabbits, contracted with norepinephrine (ED$_{30}$), in the presence of indomethacin ($10^{-5}$ mol/L). Rings with endothelium are shown as closed symbols and those without endothelium as open symbols. The estrogen-treated group is designated by circles and the untreated group by squares. Data are expressed as percent of the response to norepinephrine and are shown as means $\pm$ SEM; $n = 5$ in each group. The asterisk denotes that the relaxations of the estrogen-treated group with endothelium are significantly different from those of the untreated group and rings without endothelium by Scheffe's test ($P < 0.05$). At concentrations greater than $3 \times 10^{-8}$ mol/L, relaxations of rings with endothelium in both treatment groups are different from the relaxations of rings without endothelium. Reproduced with permission from Reference 6.

oral administration) or decreasing endogenous prolactin (by bromocryptine) consistently increased plasma $NO_x$ in postmenopausal or premenopausal, amenorrheic women (Table 1).

The mechanisms by which estrogens modulate production/release of NO are controversial. One mechanism may be through the antioxidant properties of estrogen increasing the bioavailability of a fixed quantity of NO.[32] Alternatively, estrogens may act genomically to increase production of NO synthase (NOS). The gene for endothelial (type III) NOS contains 15-half palindrome regions for the estrogen receptor.[33,34] Estrogen-treatment increased mRNA for type III NOS in tissue homogenates of brain and skeletal muscle of guinea pigs.[35] Because type III NOS may occur in cells other than endothelial, it is difficult to account for the increases in NOS as occurring only in endothelium. In cultured endothelial cells from humans (sex not specified) 48 hours of estrogen treatment increased mRNA for type III NOS, which is coincident with increases in $NO_x$ in the culture media.[36] These observations suggest that estrogen can modulate type III NOS genomically involving transcription. However, increases in media $NO_x$ occur rapidly in the presence of transcription inhibition, suggesting nongenomic regulation of NOS.[9] With endogenous fluctuations of estrogen, mRNA for type III NOS was not greater in aortic endothelial cells from gonadally intact female pigs with high-circulating estrogen compared with those with low-circulating estrogen or ovariectomized animals even though plasma $NO_x$ was elevated in the high-estrogen females.[7] Neither total quantity of enzyme (by Western blot) nor activity of isolated enzyme (by arginine to citrulline assay) was elevated in assays of aortic endothelial cells from the high-estrogen pigs.[7] Collectively, these observations suggest that estrogen may modulate production of NO by mechanisms not requiring transcription or translation of the NOS gene. Whether or not estrogens modulate

Table 1

**Plasma $NO_X$ and Estrogen in Postmenopausal and Premenopausal, Amenorrheic Women**

| Replacement | Duration | Number of Subjects | $NO_X$ ($\mu$m/L) | | Reference |
|---|---|---|---|---|---|
| | | | Before | After | |
| Transdermal estradiol 100 $\mu$g/d (Estraderm 0.1) | 24 h | 10 | 21.0 ± 5.7 | 37.3 ± 7.6 | Cicinelli et al[58] |
| Oral Bromocriptin 2.5 mg b.i.d. | 6 wk | 25 | 18.4 ± 2.5 | 36.5 ± 5.2 | Shaarawy et al[59] |
| Oral estradiol-17$\beta$ 2 mg/d (Estrace) | 6 mo | 15 | 27.5 ± 13.1 | 34.7 ± 18.3 | Best et al[44] |
| Oral estradiol valerate 2 mg/d (Progynova) | 6 mo 12 mo | 26 26 | 20.1 ± 1.6 20.1 ± 1.6 | 23.2 ± 2.3 30.0 ± 3.7 | Imthurn et al[43] |

NOS activity by affecting cellular localization of the enzyme, substrate, or cofactor availability remains to be determined.

The conclusion that estrogens modulate production of NO by nongenomic mechanisms is consistent with the rapidity by which acute administration of estrogen modulates vasodilatation in vivo[19,20,26] and release of $NO_x$ from human female endothelial cells in vitro.[9] Modulation of NO may require estrogen receptors. For example, estrogen-stimulated release of NO from cultured human female umbilical arterial cells could be blocked by the estrogen receptor antagonist ICI 164,384.[36] In addition, in male mice lacking estrogen receptors [estrogen receptor knockout (ERKO) mice], basal release of NO from aortas as measured by contraction to an arginine analog was less than in aortas from wild-type mice.[37] However, agonist-stimulated release of endothelium-derived factors (presumably NO) by acetylcholine was the same in aortas from wild-type and ERKO male mice. Therefore, association of estrogen receptors with production of NO may not be the same for agonist-stimulated versus basal or flow-mediated release. For example, flow-mediated release of NO as measured by hyperemic response in the brachial artery was absent in a man lacking functional estrogen receptors. However, vasodilation to sublingual estradiol was still observed. These observations validate in part association of expression of estrogen receptors and endothelial function.[38] The importance of estrogen receptors in affecting endothelial function and subsequent development of atherosclerotic disease is emphasized by the observation that few estrogen receptors are observed in atherosclerotic human arteries compared with nondiseased human arteries.[39] Other associations between estrogen receptors and endothelial function need to be clarified.

It is unlikely that estrogens modulate responsiveness of arterial smooth muscle to NO. Both the sensitivity [effective dose $(ED_{50})$] to exogenously administered NO and the magnitude of relaxations were similar between rings of coronary arteries from estrogen-replete or -deplete experimental animals.[11,40,41] Also, estrogen replacement did not modify vasodilator responses to sodium nitroprusside, a measure of smooth muscle sensitivity to NO-induced vasodilation in perimenopausal women.[25,42]

Hormones other than estrogen may modulate production/release of NO. In experimental animals, pharmacologic concentrations of progesterone given in conjunction with estrogen negate the stimulatory effects of estrogen on expression of endothelium-dependent relaxations to an $\alpha_2$-adrenergic agonist, a response mediated by NO.[41] However, in humans, intermittent treatment with progestins in conjunction with estrogens does not seem to reverse increases in plasma $NO_x$ or vasodilator functions observed in subjects treated with estrogens alone.[4,43,44] Effects of testosterone alone or estrogen-testosterone interactions are less well described. Gender differences in expression of endothelium-dependent relaxations are documented. In gonadally intact male pigs, circulating concentrations of estrogen are greater than in gonadally intact female pigs probably because of testosterone being converted to estrogens by aromatase in the adipose tissue.[7] However, even with high-circulating estrogen, plasma $NO_x$ tends to be less in males compared with females and differences in endothelium-dependent relaxations mediated by agents other than NO are observed.[7,11,40] Therefore, future studies examining relationships among hormones may be important in identifying gender-specific approaches to management of cardiovascular disease.

# Hormones and Other Endothelium-Derived Factors

NO is only one of several vasoactive/antimitogenic factors produced by endothelial cells, which may be regulated by sex steroid hormones. Another general class of endothelium-derived factors is the eicosanoids, a term applied to any of the metabolites of arachidonic acid. Arachidonic acid is produced by both vascular endothelium and smooth muscle usually in response to ligand stimulation of a receptor or ion channel. Arachidonic acid can be metabolized by one of three distinct enzymatic pathways all resulting in vasoactive end products: cyclooxygenase, lipoxygenases, or cytochrome P450. Some products, particularly those of the cyclooxygenase pathway (thromboxane $A_2$, and prostacyclin), in addition to being vasoactive also may affect smooth muscle mitogenesis and platelet aggregation, processes contributing to progression of vascular occlusive disease, and atherosclerosis.[45]

How hormonal status affects basal-stimulated production of eicosanoids compared with agonist-stimulated production of eicosanoids is not understood completely. Whether estrogen increases or decreases production of a particular end product will be determined by sex of the tissue (male or female); type of preparation (in vitro or in vivo); and type, dose, and duration of hormone treatment.[45] For example, endothelium-dependent relaxations to an $\alpha_2$-adrenergic agonist are greater in coronary arteries from sexually mature female pigs compared with male pigs. Incubation of rings with an inhibitor of cyclooxygenase increased relaxations only in rings from male pigs, suggesting that contractile prostanoids may be produced preferentially by endothelium of male pigs (Figure 2).40 Estrogen may alter production or sensitivity of the smooth muscle to prostanoids in smooth muscle.[46]

Gender and/or hormonal status may affect eicosanoid production in extravascular tissue like platelets. Release of thromboxane $A_2$ is greater from aggregating platelets of sexually mature male pigs compared with female pigs.[47] Becuse thromboxane $A_2$ is mitogenic to smooth muscle as well as causing vasoconstriction, conditions that cause platelet aggregation would be more likely to produce local ischemia and proliferation in coronary arteries of males compared with females. If similar conditions apply in human arteries, these results could explain in part the effectiveness of aspirin treatment to reduce incidence of coronary artery disease in humans.[48]

Another endothelium-derived factor that may be regulated by hormonal status and that both relaxes arterial smooth muscle and inhibits formation of vascular lesions is C-type natriuretic peptide (CNP).[49–51] The CNP is the most highly conserved member of the family of natriuretic peptides.[52] It is not known whether or not production of CNP by endothelial cells is modulated by gender and/or estrogen. However, coronary arterial smooth muscle from female pigs is more sensitive to inhibition by CNP than that from male pigs.[11]

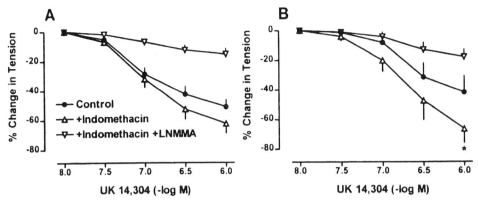

**Figure 2.** Concentration-response curves to the $\alpha_2$-adrenergic agonist UK-14304 in rings or right coronary arteries with endothelium from female (**A**) and male (**B**) sexually mature pigs in the absence (control) or presence of indomethacin ($10^{-5}$ mol/L) or of indomethacin ($10^{-5}$ mol/L) plus the arginine analog $N^{G}$-monomethyl-L-arginine (L-NMMA, $10^{-4}$ mol/L). Data are expressed as percent change in tension from a contraction to prostaglandin $F_{2\alpha}$ ($2 \times 10^{-6}$ mol/L). All data represent means $\pm$ SEM. The asterisks represents significant difference in maximal relaxation between control and indomethacin-treated arteries from male pigs (analysis of variance, $P < 0.05$). Reproduced with permission from Reference 40.

This gender difference in sensitivity to CNP reflects differences in activity of the natriuretic clearance receptors, activity of low conductance $Ca^{2+}$-activated $K^{+}$ channels, and activity of phosphodiesterases.[11]

Endothelin-1 (ET-1) is an endothelium-derived vasoconstrictor and smooth muscle mitogen whose production and receptor may be affected by gender and/or hormonal status. Circulating concentrations of ET-1 decreased in the same group of postmenopausal women who showed increases in plasma $NO_x$ with estrogen replacement.[44] It is unclear whether or not this represents a direct effect of estrogen on transcriptional or posttranscriptional regulation of production of ET-1 or an indirect effect related to increases in production of NO. The NO regulates production/release of ET-1 independent of hormonal status.[53,54] Decreases in plasma concentrations of ET-1 with estrogen treatment of male-female transsexuals and increases with testosterone-treatment of female–male transsexuals further supports that production of this endothelium-derived peptide may be regulated by sex steroid hormones.[55] Regulation of this peptide by estrogen may be important in limiting progress of atherosclerotic disease, because ET-1 is prominent in atherosclerotic plaques in humans.[56]

Affinity of high-affinity ET receptors was enhanced with increasing concentrations of endogenous estrogen in coronary arteries of sexually mature pigs.[10] How changes in affinity of ET receptors relate to responses of the smooth muscle to the peptide remains to be clarified. Although contractions to ET-1 applied exogenously are greater in arteries without endothelium from female pigs compared with male pigs, the magnitude of the increase was not related to estrogen status.[10] Affinity of the receptors may represent modulation of calcium mobilization necessary for functions other than contraction,

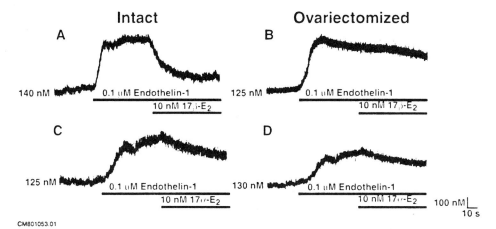

**Figure 3.**   Changes in intracellular calcium in fluo-3-loaded, freshly dispersed coronary arterial smooth muscle cells from sexually mature (**Intact, left panels**) and ovariectomized (**right panels**) female pigs. Cells were exposed to endothelin-1 (ET-1; 0.1 $\mu$mol/L) and the response allowed to stabilize. The estradiol-17$\beta$ (10 $\mu$mol/L; 17$\beta$-E$_2$) was added acutely to the preparation. A rapid decrease in intracellular calcium was observed only in cells from sexually mature animals with intact ovaries. This decrease was not observed with $\alpha$-isomers of the steroid (lower panels) and was blocked by the estrogen receptor antagonist ICI 182,780 (1 $\mu$mol/L, not shown).

such as mitogenesis.[57] In freshly dissociated smooth muscle cells from coronary arteries of sexually mature female pigs, estradiol-17$\beta$ promotes calcium extrusion from cells stimulated with ET-1 (Figure 3). This effect of estradiol-17$\beta$ requires estrogen receptors, as decreases in calcium signal caused by the steroid were blocked by the estrogen receptor antagonist ICI 182,780 and were not observed in cells of arteries from ovariectomized animals, which have decreased numbers of estrogen receptors. The association between expression of estrogen receptors and production and response to other endothelium-derived factors will be important to define in future experiments.

# Summary

Sex steroid hormones modulate production of several endothelium-derived factors including NO, metabolites of arachidonic acid, and ET-1. Mechanisms by which hormones modulate endothelium-derived factors are beginning to be defined. Both genomic and nongenomic actions of the steroids requiring binding to receptors may be required. In addition, sex steroids affect release of vasoactive factors from platelets and responses of the smooth muscle to endothelium-derived factors (Figure 4). Gender and hormone-associated differences in smooth muscle also may be associated with expression of estrogen receptors and involve regulation of ET and natriuretic clearance receptors, phosphodiesterases, and K$^+$- and Ca$^{2+}$-activated ion channels. The integrated actions of sex steroids on all components of the blood vessel will affect development of arterial disease. Future experiments that account carefully for

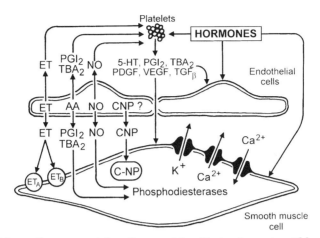

**Figure 4.**   Schematic summarizing the possible effects of sex steroid hormones on the vascular wall. Hormones affect production of and release of NO, metabolites of arachidonic acid, and ET-1 from endothelial cells. They also may modulate production and release of vasoactive and growth factors from extravascular cells like platelets. Changes in production of factors from the endothelium may contribute to vasospasm and proliferative disease indirectly by regulating platelet aggregation or directly by affecting vasomotion and proliferation of the underlying smooth muscle. Sex steroids also affect functions in the smooth muscle, which are required for responsiveness to endothelium- and platelet-derived factors. Abbreviations: AA, arachidonic acid; C-NP; natriuretic peptide clearance receptor; CNP, C-type natriuretic factor; ET, endothelin-1; $ET_{A,B}$, endothelin-A and-B, receptors; 5-HT, 5-hydroxytryptamine; NO, nitric oxide; PDGF, platelet-derived growth factor; $PGI_2$, prostacyclin; $TBA_2$, thromboxane $A_2$; $TGF_\beta$, transforming growth factor $\beta$; VEGF, vascular endothelial growth factor.

differences in gender, expression of steroids receptors, dose response, and type of steroid replacement are necessary for development of novel therapies to reduce the incidence of coronary artery diseases in men and women.

# References

1. Barrett-Connor E, Bush TL. Estrogen and coronary heart disease in women. *JAMA* 1991;265:1861–1867.
2. Eaker ED, Chesebro JH, Sacks FM, et al. AHA medical/scientific statement: Cardiovascular disease in women. *Spec Rep Circ* 1993;88:1999–2009.
3. Stampfer MJ, Colditz GA. Estrogen replacement therapy and coronary heart disease: A quantitative assessment of the epidemiologic evidence. *Prev Med* 1991;20:47–63.
4. Grodstein F, Stampfer MJ, Manson JE, et al. Postmenopausal estrogen and progestin use and the risk of cardiovascular disease. *N Engl J Med* 1996;335:453–461.
5. Chow MS. Benefit/risk of estrogen therapy in cardiovascular disease: Current knowledge and future challenges. *J Clin Pharmacol* 1995;35(suppl):11S–17S.
6. Gisclard V, Miller VM, Vanhoutte PM. Effect of 17B-estradiol on endothelium-dependent responses in the rabbit. *J Pharmacol Exp Ther* 1988;244:19–22.
7. Wang X, Barber DA, Lewis DA, et al. Gender and transcriptional regulation of NO synthase and ET-1 in porcine aortic endothelial cells. *Am J Physiol* 1997;273(pt 2):H1962–H1967.

8. Caulin-Glaser T, Watson CA, Pardi R, et al. Effects of 17β-estradiol on cytokine-induced endothelial cell adhesion molecule expression. *J Clin Invest* 1996;98:36–42.

9. Caulin-Glaser T, Garcia-Cardena G, Sarrel P, et al. 17 beta-estradiol regulation of human endothelial cell basal nitric oxide release, independent of cytosolic $Ca^{2+}$ mobilization. *Circ Res* 1997;81:885–892.

10. Barber DA, Sieck GC, Fitzpatrick LA, et al. Endothelin receptors are modulated in association with endogenous fluctuations in estrogen. *Am J Physiol* 1996;271(pt 2):H1999–H2006.

11. Barber DA, Burnett JC Jr, Fitzpatrick LA, et al. Gender and relaxation to C-type natriuretic peptide in porcine coronary arteries. *J Cardiovasc Pharmacol* 1998;32:5–11.

12. Hamlet MA, Rorie DK, Tyce GM. Effects of estradiol on release and disposition of norepinephrine from nerve endings. *Am J Physiol* 1980;239:H450–H456.

13. Cohen RA, Shepherd JT, Vanhoutte PM. Inhibitory role of the endothelium in the response of isolated coronary arteries to platelets. *Science* 1983;221:273–274.

14. Alheid U, Frolich JC, Forstermann U. Endothelium-derived relaxing factor from cultured human endothelial cells inhibits aggregation of human platelets. *Thromb Res* 1987;47:561–571.

15. Gaboury JP, Woodman RC, Granger DN, et al. Nitric oxide prevents leukocyte adherence: Role of superoxide. *Am J Physiol* 1993;265(pt 2):H862–H867.

16. Butcher EC. Leukocyte-endothelial cell adhesion as an active, multi-step process: A combinatorial mechanism for specificity and diversity in leukocyte targeting. In: Gupta S, Waldmann TA, eds. *Mechanisms of Lymphocyte Activation and Immune Regulation IV. Cellular Communications.* New York: Plenum Press; 1992:181–194.

17. Scott-Burden T, Vanhoutte PM. The endothelium as a regulator of vascular smooth muscle proliferation. *Circulation* 1993;87:V51–V55.

18. Bell DR, Rensberger HJ, Koritnik DR, et al. Estrogen pretreatment directly potentiates endothelium-dependent vasorelaxation of porcine coronary arteries. *Am J Physiol* 1995;268:H377–H383.

19. Williams JK, Adams MR, Klopfenstein HS. Estrogen modulates responses of atherosclerotic coronary arteries. *Circulation* 1990;81:1680–1687.

20. Williams JK, Adams MR, Herrington DM, et al. Short-term administration of estrogen and vascular responses of atherosclerotic coronary arteries. *J Am Coll Cardiol* 1992;20:452–457.

21. Collins P, Rosano GMC, Sarrel PM, et al. 17β-Estradiol attenuates acetylcholine-induced coronary arterial constriction in women but not men with coronary heart disease. *Circulation* 1995;92:24–30.

22. Blumenthal RS, Heldman AW, Brinker JA, et al. Acute effects of conjugated estrogens on coronary blood flow response to acetylcholine in men. *Am J Cardiol* 1997;80:1021–1024.

23. Reis SE, Gloth ST, Blumenthal RS, et al. Ethinyl estradiol acutely attenuates abnormal coronary vasomotor responses to acetylcholine in postmenopausal women. *Circulation* 1994;89:52–60.

24. Guetta V, Quyyumi AA, Prasad A, et al. The role of nitric oxide in coronary vascular effects of estrogen in postmenopausal women. *Circulation* 1997;96:2795–2801.

25. Tagawa H, Shimokawa H, Tagawa T, et al. Short-term estrogen augments both nitric oxide-mediated and non-nitric oxide-mediated endothelium-dependent forearm vasodilation in postmenopausal women. *J Cardiovasc Pharmacol* 1997;30:481–488.

26. Gilligan DM, Badar DM, Panza JA, et al. Acute vascular effects of estrogen in postmenopausal women. *Circulation* 1994;90:786–791.

27. Furchgott RF. Studies on relaxation of rabbit aorta by sodium nitrite: The basis for the proposal that the acid-activatable inhibitory factor from bovine retractor penis is inorganic nitrite and the endothelium-derived relaxing factor is nitric oxide. In: Vanhoutte PM, ed. *Vasodilatation.* New York: Raven Press; 1998:401–414.

28. Ignarro LJ. Biosynthesis and metabolism of endothelium-derived nitric oxide. *Annu Rev Pharmacol Toxicol* 1990;30:535–560.
29. Hayashi T, Fukuto JM, Ignarro LJ, et al. Basal release of nitric oxide from aortic rings is greater in female rabbits than in male rabbits: Implications for atherosclerosis. *Proc Natl Acad Sci U S A* 1992;89:11259–11263.
30. Cicinelli E, Ignarro LJ, Lograno M, et al. Circulating levels of nitric oxide in fertile women in relation to the menstrual cycle. *Fertil Steril* 1996;66:1036–1038.
31. Rosselli M, Imthurm E, Macas E, et al. Circulating nitrite/nitrate levels increase with follicular development: Indirect evidence for estrogen mediated NO release. *Biochem Biophys Res Commun* 1994;202:1543–1552.
32. Niki E, Nakano M. Estrogens as antioxidants. *Methods Enzymol* 1990;186:330–333.
33. Venema RC, Nishida K, Alexander RW, et al. Organization of the bovine gene encoding the endothelial nitric oxide synthase. *Biochim Biophys Acta* 1994;1218:413–420.
34. Marsden PA, Heng HHQ, Scherer SW, et al. Structure and chromosomal localization of the human constitutive endothelial nitric oxide synthase gene. *J Biol Chem* 1993;268:17478–17488.
35. Weiner CP, Lizasoain I, Baylis SA, et al. Induction of calcium-dependent nitric oxide synthases by sex hormones. *Proc Natl Acad Sci U S A* 1994;91:5212–5216.
36. Hayashi T, Yamada K, Esaki T, et al. Estrogen increases endothelial nitric oxide by a receptor-mediated system. *Biochem Biophys Res Commun* 1995;214:847–855.
37. Rubanyi GM, Freay AD, Kauser K, et al. Vascular estrogen receptors and endothelium-derived nitric oxide production in the mouse aorta. Gender difference and the effect of estrogen receptor gene distruption. *J Clin Invest* 1997;99:2429–2437.
38. Sudhir K, Chou TM, Messina LM, et al. Endothelial dysfunction in a man with disruptive mutation in oestrogen-receptor gene. *Lancet* 1997;349:1146–1147.
39. Losordo DW, Kearney M, Kim EA, et al. Variable expression of the estrogen receptor in normal and atherosclerotic coronary arteries of premenopausal women. *Circulation* 1994;89:1501–1510.
40. Barber DA, Miller VM. Gender differences in endothelium-dependent relaxations do not involve NO in porcine coronary arteries. *Am J Physiol* 1997;273(pt 2):H2325–H2332.
41. Miller VM, Vanhoutte PM. Progesterone and modulation of endothelium-dependent responses in canine coronary arteries. *Am J Physiol* 1991;261(pt 2):R1022–R1027.
42. Sudhir K, Jennings GL, Funder JW, et al. Estrogen enhances basal nitric oxide release in the forearm vasculature in perimenopausal women. *Hypertension* 1996;28:330–334.
43. Imthurn B, Rosselli M, Jaeger AW, et al. Differential effects of hormone-replacement therapy on endogenous nitric oxide (nitrite/nitrate) levels in postmenopausal women substituted with 17β-estradiol valerate and cyproterone acetate or medroxyprogesterone acetate. *J Clin Endocrinol Metab* 1997;82:388–394.
44. Best PJM, Berger PB, Miller VM, et al. The effect of estrogen replacement therapy on plasma nitric oxide and endothelin-1 levels in postmenopausal women. *Ann Intern Med* 1998;128:285–288.
45. Barber DA, Miller VM. Endothelium-dependent vasoconstrictors. In: Rubanyi G, ed. *Endothelial Cell Research.* Berkshire, U.K.: Harwood Academic Publishers; 1998:167–185.
46. Miller VM, Vanhoutte PM. 17B-Estradiol augments endothelium-dependent contractions to arachidonic acid in rabbit aorta. *Am J Physiol* 1990;258(pt 2):R1502–R1507.
47. Miller VM, Lewis DA, Barber DA. Gender differences and endothelium- and platelet-derived factors in the coronary circulation. *Clin Exp Pharmacol Physiol* 1999;26:132–136.

48. Hennekens CH, Dyken ML, Fuster V. Aspirin as a therapeutic agent in cardiovascular disease: A statement for healthcare professionals from the American Heart Association. *Circulation* 1997;96:2751–2753.
49. Stingo AJ, Clavell AL, Heublein DM, et al. Presence of C-type natriuretic peptide in cultured human endothelial cells and plasma. *Am J Physiol* 1992;263(pt 2): H1318–H1321.
50. Suga S-I, Itoh H, Komatsu Y, et al. Cytokine-induced C-type natriuretic peptide (CNP) secretrion from vascular endothelial cells: Evidence for CNP as a novel autocrine/paracrine regulator from endothelial cells. *Endocrinology* 1993;133: 3038–3041.
51. Shinomiya M, Tashiro J, Saito Y, et al. C-type natriuretic peptide inhibits intimal thickening of rabbit carotid artery after balloon catheter injury. *Biochem Biophys Res Commun* 1994;205:1051–1056.
52. Tawaragi Y, Fuchimura K, Tanaka S, et al. Gene and precursor structures of human C-type natriuretic peptide. *Biochem Biophys Res Commun* 1991;175:645–651.
53. Boulanger CM, Luscher TF. Release of endothelin from the porcine aorta. *J Clin Invest* 1990;85:587–590.
54. Flowers MA, Wang Y, Stewart RJ, et al. Reciprocal regulation of endothelin-1 and endothelial constitutive NOS in proliferating endothelial cells. *Am J Physiol* 1995; 269(pt 2):H1988–H1997.
55. Polderman KH, Stehouwer CDA, van Kamp GJ, et al. Influence of sex hormones on plasma endothelin levels. *Ann Intern Med* 1993;118:429–432.
56. Lerman A, Edwards BS, Hallett JW Jr, et al. Circulating and tissue endothelin immunoreactivity in advanced atherosclerosis. *N Engl J Med* 1991;325:997–1001.
57. Moraghan T, Antoniucci DM, Grenert JP, et al. Differential response in cell proliferation to β-estradiol in coronary artery vascular smooth muscle cells obtained from mature female versus male animals. *Endocrinology* 1996;137:5174–5177.
58. Cicinelli E, Ignarro LJ, Lograno M, et al. Acute effects of transdermal estradiol administration on plasma levels of nitric oxide in postmenopausal women. *Fertil Steril* 1997;67:63–66.
59. Shaarawy M, Nafei S, Abul-Nasr A, et al. Circulating nitric oxide levels in galactorrheic, hyperprolactinemic, amenorrheic women. *Fertil Steril* 1997;68:454–459.

# Part II

## Basic Mechanisms
## of Endothelial Dysfunction

## Chapter 8

# Endothelial Dysfunction and Vascular Disease

*Paul M. Vanhoutte, MD*

## Introduction

The discovery by Furchgott and Zawadzki[1] of the obligatory role played by the endothelial cells in relaxations of isolated arteries in response to acetylcholine (Ach),[1] has initiated a major exploration of the pivotal role of the endothelium in contributing to the normal physiological function of the vascular wall. Endothelium-dependent responses are mediated by the release of several diffusible substances [endothelium-derived relaxing factors (EDRFs) and -derived constricting factors (EDCFs)] from the endothelial cells. This brief review focuses on experiments performed in the author's laboratory that have examined how the secretion by endothelial cells of vasodilator substances brings about moment-to-moment changes in the tone of the underlying vascular smooth muscle cells and how dysfunction of the endothelial cells may underly or accompany several major vascular diseases. For more exhaustive references, the reader is referred to several similar overviews.[2–12]

## Endothelium-Derived Relaxing Factors

### Endothelium-Derived Nitric-Oxide

The labile diffusible, nonprostanoid substance that mediates the endothelium-dependent relaxation to ACh described by Furchgott and Zawadzki[1] has been identified as nitric oxide (NO) or a closely related compound (see Chapters 1 and 2). The NO is formed from the guanidine-nitrogen terminal of L-arginine, by an enzyme called NO synthase (NOS), which is constitutive (NO synthase III) in endothelial cells. The activation of this NOS depends on the intracellular concentration of calcium ions in the endothelial cells, is calmodulin dependent, and requires reduced

From Panza JA, Cannon RO III (eds): *Endothelium, Nitric Oxide, and Atherosclerosis* ©Futura Publishing Co, Inc, Armonk, NY, 1999.

nicotinamide-adenine-dinucleotide phosphate (NADPH) and 5,6,7,8-tetra-hydrobiopterin (BH4) for optimal activity. The enzyme can be inhibited competitively by L-arginine analogs such as $N^G$-monomethyl-L-arginine (L-NMMA) or $N^G$-nitro-L-arginine methylester (L-NAME). The NO diffuses to the vascular smooth muscle cells and relaxes them by stimulating a cytosolic enzyme, soluble guanylate cyclase, that leads to an increase in cyclic $3'5'$-guanosine monophosphate (cGMP; see Figure 1). The latter increase is

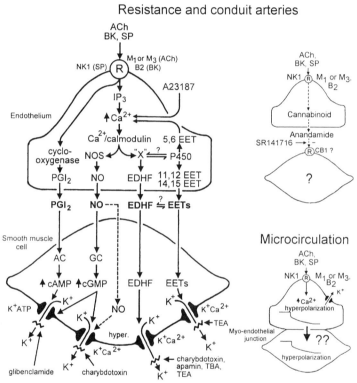

**Figure 1.**   Activation of endothelial receptors (R) induces an increase in intracellular calcium in the cytoplasm of the endothelial cell. This activates nitric oxide synthase (NOS) and cyclooxygenase and leads to the release of endothelium-derived hyperpolarizing factor (EDHF). The NO causes relaxation by activating the formation of cyclic guanosine monophosphate cGMP from guanosine triphosphate (GTP) by soluble guanylate cyclase (GC). The EDHF causes hyperpolarization and relaxation by opening $K^+$ channels. Prostacyclin ($PGI_2$) causes relaxation by activating adenylate cyclase (AC) leading to the formation of of cyclic adenosine monophosphate (cAMP). Any increase in cytosolic calcium (including that induced by the calcium ionophore A23187) causes the release of relaxing factors. When agonists activate the endothelial cells, an increase in inositol phosphate ($IP_3$) may contribute to the increase in cytoplasmic $Ca^{2+}$ by releasing it from the sarcoplasmic reticulum. In certain arteries endogenous cannabinoids may act as EDHF (upper right). At the microcirculatory level cell-to-cell conduction may underly endothelium-dependent hyperpolarizations (lower right). Abbreviations: ACh, acetylcholine; BK, bradykinin; $B_2$, kinin receptor; $CB_1$, cannabinoid receptor; EET, epoxyeicosatrienoic acid; M, muscarinic receptor; SP, substance P; TEA, tetraethylammonium; NK, neurokinin receptor.

associated with inhibition of the contractile apparatus. The production of NO is a major contributor to endothelium-dependent relaxations in large isolated arteries including coronary, systemic, mesenteric, pulmonary, and cerebral arteries. Its significance in vivo is suggested by the observations that inhibitors of NOS cause vasoconstriction in most vascular beds and an increase in systemic arterial pressure both in animals and in humans.[13]

The endothelial cell releases NO not only toward the underlying vascular smooth muscle cells but also in the lumen of the blood vessel. Thus, NO inhibits the adhesion of platelets and leukocytes to the endothelium. It acts (synergistically with prostacyclin) to inhibit platelet aggregation.[3,4,10,13] It also inhibits the growth of the vascular smooth muscle cells and prevents the production of adhesion molecules and endothelin (ET) (Figure 2).[14]

The release of NO is modulated by physical and humoral stimuli. Among the physical stimuli, the shear stress exerted by the blood on the arterial wall is one of the main factors regulating the local release of NO. Indeed, flow-induced vasodilatation is endothelium-dependent in vivo.[15] Several neurohumoral mediators cause the release of NO through activation of specific endothelial receptors (Figure 3). The endogenous substances stimulating this release are either circulating hormones (eg, catecholamines and vasopressin), autacoids generated within the vascular wall (eg, bradykinin and histamine), or mediators released by platelets [serotonin, adenosine diphosphate (ADP)] or formed during coagulation (thrombin). The receptors for these substances are connected to the produc-

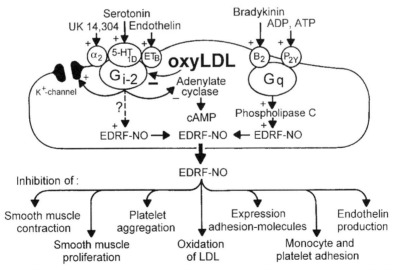

**Figure 2.** Postulated signal transduction processes in a normal endothelial cell. Activation of the cell causes the release of EDRF-NO, which has important protective effects in the vascular wall. Abbreviations: α, alpha-adrenergic; 5-HT, serotonin receptor; ET, endothelin receptors; B, bradykinin receptor; P, purinoceptor; G, coupling proteins; cAMP, cyclic adenosine monophosphate; NO, nitric oxide; LDL, low-density lipoproteins.

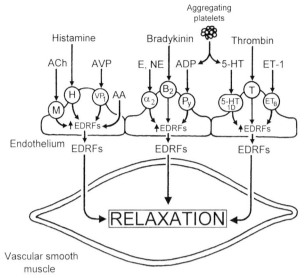

**Figure 3.** Some of the neurohumoral mediators which cause the release of endothelium-derived relaxing factor (EDRF) through activation of specific endothelial receptors (circles). Abbreviations: A, adrenaline (epinephrine); AA, arachidonic acid; ACh, acetylcholine; ADP, adenosine diphosphate; $\alpha$, alpha adrenergic receptor; AVP, arginine vasopressin; B, kinin receptor; ET, endothelin, endothelin receptor; H, histaminergic receptor; 5-HT, serotonin (5-hydroxytryptamine), serotoninergic receptor; M, muscarinic receptor; NA, noradrenaline (norepinephrine); P, purinergic receptor; T, thrombin receptor; VP, vasopressinergic receptor.

tion of NO by different coupling proteins (Figure 2). For example, in porcine endothelial cells, $\alpha_2$ adrenergic receptors, serotonin receptors, and thrombin receptors are coupled to pertussis toxin–sensitive Gi proteins, whereas for ADP or bradykinin receptors mediate the production of NO by activation of pertussis toxin–insensitive Gq proteins.[16] The substances produced during platelet aggregation also are important releasers of NO. This conclusion is based on the findings that in various species, including humans, aggregating platelets induce endothelium-dependent relaxations and that the presence of endothelial cells substantially inhibits the vasoconstriction induced by thromboxane A2 and platelet-derived serotonin. There are two major mediators of the endothelial response to platelets: serotonin and ADP, which act on 5-HT1D serotonin and P2y purinergic receptors, respectively (Figure 2). The endothelial action of thrombin and platelet products is crucial for the protective role played by the normal endothelium against unwanted coagulation (Figure 4). Thus, local platelet aggregation, with the release of serotonin and ADP, as well as the production of thrombin (because of the local activation of the coagulation cascade), leads to massive local release of NO, which diffuses toward the underlying vascular smooth muscle, induces its relaxation and thus dilatation of the artery. This reaction helps to eliminate the microaggregate. The release of NO toward the blood vessel lumen also inhibits platelet adhesion at the endothelium-blood

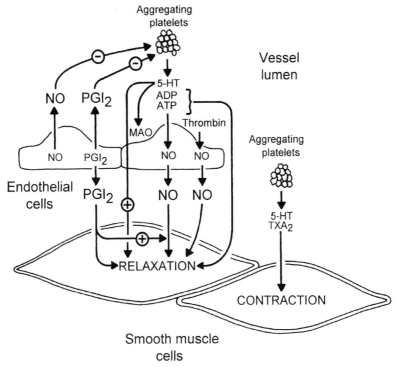

**Figure 4.** Interaction between platelet products, thrombin, and endothelium. If the endothelium is intact, several of the substances released from the platelets [in particular, the adenine nucleotides [ adenosine diphosphate (ADP) and adenosine triphosphate (ATP)] and serotonin (5-HT)] cause the release of EDRF and prostacyclin ($PGI_2$). The same is true for any thrombin formed. The released EDRF will relax the underlying vascular smooth muscle, opening up the blood vessel, and thus flushing the microaggregate away; it also will be released toward the lumen of the blood vessel to brake platelet adhesion to the endothelium and, synergistically with prostacyclin, inhibit platelet aggregation. In addition, monoamine oxidase (MAO) and other enzymes will break down the vasoconstrictor serotonin, limiting the amount of the monoamine that can diffuse toward the smooth muscle. Finally, the endothelium acts as a physical barrier that prevents the access to the smooth muscle of the vasoconstrictor platelet products serotonin and thromboxane $A_2$ ($TXA_2$). These different functions of the endothelium play a key role in preventing unwanted coagulation and vasospastic episodes in blood vessels with a normal intima. If the endothelial cells are removed (eg, by trauma), the protective role of the endothelium is lost locally, platelets can adhere and aggregate, and vasoconstriction follows; this contributes to the vascular phase of hemostasis (+, activation; −, inhibition).

interface and, in synergy with prostacyclin, eliminates the imminent danger of vascular occlusion. Conversely, if the endothelial barrier has been removed, there is a breakdown in the feedback control of platelet aggregation by NO (and prostacyclin). Aggregation proceeds with the continuous release of serotonin and thromboxane $A_2$, both of which have unrestricted access to smooth muscle cells, thereby constricting the blood vessel to constitute the vascular phase of hemostasis (Figure 5).[3,9,10]

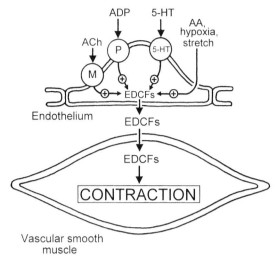

**Figure 5.** A number of physicochemical stimuli, neurohumoral mediators can evoke endothelium-dependent contractions in certain blood vessels, presumably because they evoke the release of endothelium-derived constricting factors (EDCFs). Abbreviations: AA, arachidonic acid; ACh, acetylcholine; ADP, adenosine diphosphate; 5-HT, serotonin and serotonin receptor; M, muscarinin receptor; P, P receptor.

## Prostacyclin

Prostacyclin, a product of cyclooxygenase, is formed primarily in endothelial cells, in response to shear stress, hypoxia, and several mediators that also release NO. Prostacyclin causes relaxation of certain vascular smooth muscle cells by activating adenylate cyclase and increasing the production of cyclic $3',5'$-adenosine monophosphate (cAMP). In most blood vessels the contribution of prostacyclin to endothelium-dependent relaxation is negligible, and its effect essentially is additive to that of NO. However, the two substances act synergistically to inhibit platelet aggregation (Figure 4).[17]

## Endothelium-Dependent Hyperpolarizing Factor

Electrophysiological studies in various arteries, including the human coronary artery, demonstrate that ACh, and other endothelium-dependent dilators, cause endothelium-dependent hyperpolarizations and relaxations, which are caused by a diffusible endothelium-derived hyperpolarizing factor (EDHF) different from NO and prostacyclin, although the latter two can hyperpolarize certain vascular smooth muscle cells. The chemical nature of EDHF remains speculative. In some blood vessels, epoxyeicosatrienoic acids (EETs), formed from arachidonic acid by the action of cytochrome P450, may correspond to EDHF (Figure 1).[18-21] The hyperpolarization of smooth muscle cells induced by EDHF is mediated by an increased movement of potassium ions. The type of potassium channels involved is not established definitively but more likely seems to be calcium-dependent rather than adenosine triphosphate (ATP)-dependent potassium channels (Figure 1).[18–21]

The contribution of hyperpolarization to endothelium-dependent relaxations varies as a function of the size of the arteries[22] and is prominent in resistance vessels. In large arteries, both mediators can contribute to endothelium-dependent relaxations, but the role of NO predominates under normal circumstances. However, in these arteries, EDHF can mediate near normal endothelium-dependent relaxations when the synthesis of NO is inhibited.[18–21] In certain cases, NO exerts an inhibitory effect on endothelium-dependent hyperpolarizations.[23]

## Chronic Modulation

Several chronic modulatory influences can up-regulate the releasse of relaxing factors by endothelial cells. These include estrogens,[24] increases in blood flow,[25] exercise training[26] and intake of $\omega_2$-unsaturated fatty acids.[27,28]

# Endothelium-Dependent Contractions

Endothelial cells also can initiate contraction of the underlying smooth muscle cells by releasing constricting substances. The EDCFs include the peptide ET, vasoconstrictor prostanoids such as thromboxane $A_2$, and prostaglandin $H_2$ as well as superoxide anions and components of the renin–angiotensin system.[2,3,29–31]

## Contractions Blocked by Inhibitors of Cyclooxygenase

A group of EDCFs is generated by the metabolism of arachidonic acid involving cyclooxygenase. In peripheral veins, but also in the cerebral circulation and in some arteries from hypertensive animals, endothelium-dependent contractions are mediated by thromboxane $A_2$ or prostaglandin $H_2$, which activate the same thromboxane-endoperoxide receptor.[32–35] Among the stimuli that cause endothelium-dependent contractions sensitive to inhibitors of cyclooxygenase, an important physiological response probably is that to stretch. The endothelium-dependent contraction of a cerebral artery in response to stretch closely resembles the autoregulatory response. A possible explanation for autoregulation of the cerebral circulation initiated by a sudden stretch of the vessel wall in response to an increase in blood pressure is the release of EDCFs, which would activate the underlying smooth muscle cells to restore a normal flow rate.

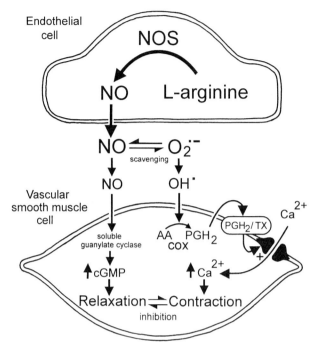

**Figure 6.** Interactions between NO and superoxide anions ($O_2^-$). Superoxide anions cause contraction of vascular smooth muscle by scavenging endothelium-derived NO and by activating the production of vasoconstrictor prostaglandins in the vascular smooth muscle cells. Abbreviations: AA, arachidonic acid; COX, cyclooxygenase; cGMP, cyclic guanosine monophosphate; NOS, nitric oxide synthase; $PGH_2$, endoperoxides, TX, thromboxane.

In addition, cyclooxygenase is a source of superoxide anions, which can cause contraction directly[36] or indirectly by inactivating EDRF-NO[37] (Figure 6).

## Hypoxia-Induced Contractions

Coronary, cerebral, and pulmonary arteries rapidly contract when exposed to sudden hypoxia. This endothelium-dependent contraction is caused by the transfer of a diffusible substance that remains unknown. It is not dependent on cyclooxygenase and is exacerbated by a reduced release of NO.[38,39]

## Endothelin-1

Endothelial cells produce endothelin-1 (ET-1). Translation of mRNA generates preproendothelin, which is converted to big ET; its conversion to the mature peptide ET-1 by ET-converting enzymes is necessary for the

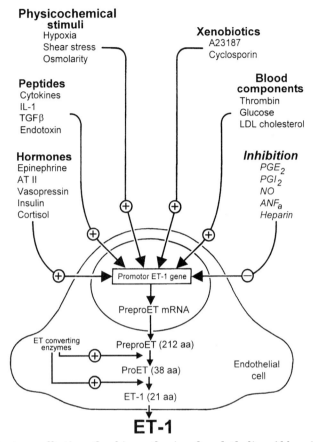

**Figure 7.** Factors affecting the biosynthesis of endothelin. Abbreviations: ANF$_a$, atrial natriuretic factor; AT II, angiotensin II; IL-1, interleukin 1; LDL, low-density lipoproteins; PF, prostaglandins; TGF$_\beta$, tumor growth factor $\beta$.

development of its vascular activity.[40–42] The expression of messenger RNA and the release of the peptide from cultured endothelial cells are stimulated by thrombin (Figure 7),[43] transforming growth factor b$_1$, interleukin-1 (IL-1), epinephrine, angiotensin II (Ang II), arginine vasopressin, calcium ionophore, and phorbol ester and are inhibited by NO.[35,41] ET-1 causes vasodilatation at a lower concentration by activating endothelial ET$_B$ receptors coupled to the release of NO, prostacyclin, and EDHF. At higher concentrations, it causes marked and sustained contractions by activation of ET$_A$ receptors and in some blood vessels of ET$_B$ receptors on vascular smooth muscle cells (Figure 8).[44,45] The circulating levels of ET-1 are low suggesting either a discrete endogenous production under physiological conditions, the presence of potent inhibitory mechanisms (such as the negative control induced by NO[46]), or a preferential abluminal release of the peptide toward vascular smooth muscle cells.

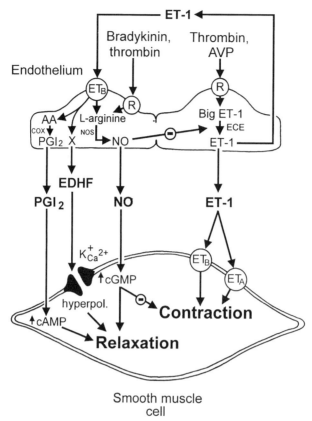

**Figure 8.**   Interaction between endothelin-1 and EDRFs. Abbreviations: AA, arachidonic acid; cAMP, cyclic adenosine monophosphate; cGMP, cyclic guaonsine monophosphate; COX, cyclooxygenase; ECE, endothelium-converting enzyme; EDHF, endothelium-derived hyperpolarizing factor; ET, endothelin, endothelin receptor; hyperpol., hyperpolarization; $K_{Ca^{2+}}^{+}$, calcium-dependent potassium channel; NO, nitric oxide; NOS, nitric oxide synthase; $PGI_2$, prostacyclin; R, receptor; $X$, unknown precursor.

# Endothelial Dysfunction

In several types of vascular disease and hypertension, the endothelial cells become dysfunctional.[3,4,8,10–12] Usually, this dysfunction expresses itself as an impairment in endothelium-dependent relaxations, mainly caused by a reduced release (or action) of EDRFs although production of endothelium-derived vasoconstrictor substances may contribute.[3–30,47]

## Regenerated Endothelium

Even the normal aging process induces a turnover and regeneration of endothelial cells resulting in an abnormal function. Regenerated endothelial cells lose some of their ability to release EDRF, in particular in response to platelet aggregation and thrombin.[48,49] Indeed, regenerated endothelium responds poorly to serotonin and other substances using the pertussis toxin–sensitive pathway controlling the release of EDRF (Figure 2). In regenerated endothelial cells, pertussis toxin–sensitive Gi proteins are expressed normally but have a reduced activity.[50] The loss of pertussis toxin–sensitive response is selective and does not apply to endothelium-dependent responses induced by ADP or bradykinin. It may be caused by the greater accumulation of low-density lipoprotein (LDL) by the regenerated endothelial cells (Figure 2).[51] The area of regenerated endothelium becomes a site of predilection for triggering exaggerated vasoconstriction in response to serotonin or ergonovine.[52]

## Hypercholesterolemia and Atherosclerosis

In experimental animals, hypercholesterolemia induced by high-fat and/or high-cholesterol diets impairs endothelium-dependent relaxations.[53,54] By contrast, endothelium-independent relaxations to nitroglycerin, sodium nitroprusside, or adenosine are normal or only slightly impaired.

In the early stage of the atherosclerotic process, the endothelial dysfunction appears to be limited to the pertussis toxin–sensitive Gi protein–dependent pathway, which leads to NO formation (Figure 2). Thus, the ability of regenerated endothelial cells, chronically exposed to high-cholesterol levels, to ADP-ribosylate pertussis toxin is reduced.[55] Consequently, in coronary arteries from hypercholesterolemic pigs, endothelium-dependent relaxations evoked by agents that activate the pertussis toxin–sensitive Gi protein (eg, serotonin, $\alpha_2$ adrenergic agonists, aggregating platelets, and thrombin) are depressed while those induced by ADP, bradykinin, or the $Ca^{2+}$-ionophore A23187 are preserved.[16,48,49,54,55] Oxidized LDLs, which are considered to be more atherogenic than native LDL, induce, in vitro, a similar selective endothelial dysfunction for stimuli activating the pertussis-sensitive Gi protein pathway, while at higher concentrations they also inhibit endothelium-dependent responses evoked by receptor-independent stimuli (Figure 2).[55,56]

The most important mechanism in the reduction in endothelium-dependent responses is a lesser release of NO. Nevertheless, as the disease progresses and the artery thickens and stiffens, it becomes increasingly difficult for NO to reach smooth muscle cells that are still able to relax. Endothelial dysfunction is probably a fundamental initial step in the progression of atherosclerosis. This hypothesis argues that aging and prolonged exposure to shear stress, coupled with risk factors such as hypertension, smoking, and stress, accelerate endothelial aging and hence the process of endothelial regeneration. As a result, larger and larger sections of the endothelium become unable to resist platelet adhesion and aggregation and respond less well to thrombin formation. The feedback effect of NO (together with prostacyclin) on platelet aggregation decreases steadily, while vasoconstrictor factors (serotonin and thromboxane $A_2$) are released in increasingly greater amounts, together with growth factors [ such as platelet-derived growth factor (PDGF)], which probably are responsible for initiating the characteristic morphological changes in atherosclerosis (Figure 9).[3,7,9,10,16]

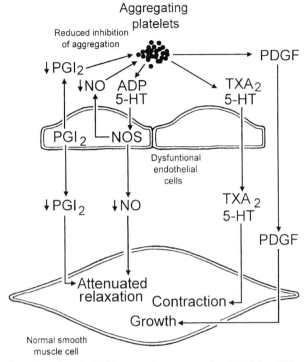

**Figure 9.** Dysfunctional endothelium and response to platelets. Abbreviations: 5-HT, 5-hydroxytryptamine; ADP, adenosine diphosphate, NO, nitric oxide; NOS, nitric oxide synthase; PDGF, platelet-derived growth factor; PGI$_2$, prostacyclin; TXA$_2$, thromboxane A$_2$; $\downarrow$, reduced production.

# Therapeutic Implications: Inhibition of Converting Enzyme

Although endothelial dysfunction can be improved by dietary measures, the most efficient way to up-regulate the failing release of NO and EDHF is to inhibit the converting enzyme. Indeed, angiotensin-converting enzyme (ACE) is located mainly at the cell membrane of the endothelial cells. It converts the less active peptide Ang I into the powerful vasoconstrictor Ang II, which acts both as direct activator of vascular smooth muscle, and as an amplifier of the sympathetic nervous system. Hence, it is not surprising that inhibitors of the enzyme can cause peripheral vasodilatation by reducing the local and circulating levels of Ang II, particularly in patients with high renin. The ACE also is the main pathway for the breakdown of bradykinin into inactive peptides; thus, the vasodilator effects of converting enzyme inhibitors are caused by in part by their protective effect against the breakdown of locally produced bradykinin.[57–61]

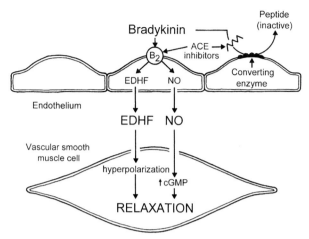

**Figure 10.** Converting enzyme (ACE) and endothelium-derived vasodilator mediators. Converting enzyme, which is expressed abundantly at the surface of endothelial cells, catalyzes the generation of the vasoconstrictor AT II (not shown) and the degradation of the endothelium-dependent vasodilator bradykinin. Bradykinin, through activation of endothelial $B_2$ kinin receptors, induces the release of EDHF and/or NO. Inhibitors of converting enzyme potentiate both actions. They also may interact directly with the $B_2$ kinin receptor.

## Exogenous Bradykinin

The ACE inhibitors cause a shift to the left of the concentration-relaxation curve to bradykinin in isolated blood vessels with endothelium, without affecting the lack of response in the absence of endothelial cells. If rings of isolated arteries with endothelium are exposed under control conditions to increasing concentrations of an ACE inhibitor, no changes in tension are observed. However, if the preparations are studied in the presence of a subthreshold concentration of bradykinin,[57] or even hours after a previous exposure to the peptide,[62] ACE inhibitors cause a marked relaxation. The potentiating effect of ACE inhibitors on the endothelium-dependent relaxation to bradykinin is accompanied by an increased production of cGMP, illustrating the greater release of NO.[63] Likewise, ACE inhibitors augment the endothelium-dependent hyperpolarizing effect of the kinin.[64] Both components are inhibited equally by $B_2$ kinin receptor antagonists either in the absence or during ACE inhibition. These experiments demonstrate that both the greater release of NO and the larger endothelium-dependent hyperpolarization contribute to the augmented endothelium-dependent relaxations to bradykinin caused by ACE inhibition. In addition, the inhibitors of the enzyme probably interact directly with the $B_2$ kinin receptors of the endothelial cells (Figure 10).

## Endogenous Bradykinin

Plasma and tissue kallikreins are the main enzymes involved in the formation of kinins from kininogens. Kininogens can cause endothelium-dependent relaxations.[65] Rings of isolated arteries with (but not those without) endothelium relax to kallikrein, a response that is potentiated by the ACE inhibitor perindoprilat. Both the response to kallikrein and its augmentation by perindoprilat are prevented by an inhibitor of kallikrein.[66] These studies indicate that the arterial wall contains a precursor of kinins and that the local activation of the kallikrein-bradykinin system can yield enough kinins to activate the endothelial cells to release relaxing factors, particularly when ACE is inhibited by perindoprilat.

Increases in shear stress augment the release of EDRFs (see above). When the ACE inhibitor perindoprilat is given into perfused isolated arteries with (but not in those without) endothelium, it causes marked relaxation, which can be attributed to the release of endothelial factors.[67] The relaxations are reversed by a selective $B_2$ kinin antagonist but are not affected by losartan, a selective antagonist of Ang I receptors. Actually, even the basal release of EDRFs is inhibited in part by the $B_2$ kinin receptor antagonist. These experiments strongly suggest that shear stress activates the local kallikrein-kinin system in the arterial wall, and that this system contributes to the increased release of EDRFs, which underlies flow-induced vasodilatation. A similar conclusion has been reached in the human coronary circulation.[68]

## Significance

Although in the face of an increased production of renin a major pharmacological target for ACE inhibitors remains the reduced production of Ang II, augmented endothelium-dependent relaxations to bradykinin produced locally may help to explain the acute vasodilator properties of these compounds, particularly in hypertensive patients with low levels of renin. Although ACE inhibitors are not considered as antianginal drugs, they may be useful in the treatment of ischemic heart disease and acute myocardial infarction. The beneficial effect of ACE inhibitors may be caused by, in part, the augmentation of coronary diameter by preventing the degradation of bradykinin generated by shear stress and therefore increasing the formation of endothelium-derived NO and EDHF.

Because NO not only is involved in the regulation of vascular tone but also inhibits the adhesion and aggregation of platelets as well as the growth of vascular smooth muscle (Figure 2), the potentiated release of endothelium-derived NO may contribute to the vascular protective effect of ACE inhibitors.

*Acknowledgments:* The author thanks M Palumbo for outstanding editorial assistance.

# References

1. Furchgott RF, Zawadzki JV. The obligatory role of the endothelial cells in relaxation of arterial smooth muscle by acetylcholine. *Nature* 1980;288:373–376.
2. Furchgott RF, Vanhoutte PM. Endothelium-derived relaxing and contracting factors. *FASEB J* 1989;3:2007–2018.

3. Lüscher TF, Vanhoutte PM. *The Endothelium:Modulator of Cardiovascular Function*. Boca Raton, FL: CRC Press; 1990:1–228.
4. Vanhoutte PM. The endothelium:modulator of vascular smooth-muscle tone. *New Engl J Med* 1988;319:512–513.
5. Vanhoutte PM. The other endothelium-derived vasoactive factors. *Circulation* 1993;87(suppl):V9–V17.
6. Vanhoutte PM, Boulanger CM. Endothelium-dependent responses in hypertension. *Hypertens Res* 1995;18:87–98.
7. Vanhoutte PM, Shimokawa H. Endothelium-derived relaxing factor(s) and coronary vasospasm. *Circulation* 1989;80:1–9.
8. Vanhoutte PM, Gräser T, Lüscher TF. Endothelium-derived contracting factors. In: Rubanyi G, ed. *Endothelin*. Oxford: Oxford University Press; 1992:3–16.
9. Vanhoutte PM. Hypercholesterolaemia, atherosclerosis and release of endothelium-derived relaxing factor by aggregating platelets. *Eur Heart J* 1991;12(suppl E):25–32.
10. Vanhoutte PM. State of the art lecture: Endothelium and control of vascular function. *Hypertension* 1989;13(pt 2):658–667.
11. Vanhoutte PM, Boulanger CM, Mombouli JV. Endothelium-derived relaxing factors and converting enzyme inhibition. *Am J Cardiol* 1995;76:3E–12E.
12. Vanhoutte PM. Endothelial dysfunction and inhibition of converting enzyme. *Eur Heart J* 1998;19:J7–J156.
13. Moncada S, Palmer RMJ, Higgs EA. Nitric oxide: physiology, pathophysiology, and pharmacology. *Pharmacol Rev* 1991;43:109–142.
14. Scott-Burden T, Vanhoutte PM. The endothelium as a regulator of vascular smooth muscle proliferation. *Circulation* 1993;87(suppl):V51–V55.
15. Bassenge E, Heuch G. Endothelial and neuro-humoral control of coronary blood flow in health and disease. *Rev Physiol Biochem Pharmacol* 1990;116:79–163.
16. Flavahan NA, Vanhoutte PM. Endothelial cell signaling and endothelial dysfunction. *Am J Hypertens* 1995;8:28S–41S.
17. Moncada S, Vane JR. Pharmacology and endogenous roles of prostaglandin endoperoxides, thromboxane A2 and prostacyclin. *Pharmacol Rev* 1979;30:293–331.
18. Komozi K, Vanhoutte PM. Endothelium-derived hyperpolarizing factor. *Blood Vessels* 1990;27:238–245.
19. Vanhoutte PM. *Endothelium-Derived Hyperpolarizing Factor*. The Netherlands: Harwood Academic Publishers;1996:1–338.
20. Mombouli JV, Vanhoutte PM. Endothelium-derived hyperpolarizing factor(s). Updating the unknown. *Trends Physiol* 1997;18:252–256.
21. Campbell WB, Gebremedhin D, Pratt PF, et al. Identification of epoxyeicosatrienoic acids as endothelium-derived hyperpolarizing. *Circ Res* 1996;78:415–423.
22. Nagao T, Illiano S, Vanhoutte PM. Heterogeneous distribution of endothelium-dependent relaxations resistant to nitro-L-arginine in the arterial tree of the rat. *Am J Physiol* 1992;263:90–94.
23. Olmos L, Mombouli JV, Illiano S, et al. cGMP mediates the desensitization to bradykinin in isolated canine coronary arteries. *Am J Physiol* 1995;268:H865–H870.
24. Gisclard V, Miller V, Vanhoutte PM. Effect of 17β-estradiol on endothelium-dependent responses in the rabbit. *J Pharmacol Exp Ther* 1988;244:19–22.
25. Miller VM, Aarhus LL, Vanhoutte PM. Modulation of endothelium-dependent responses by chronic alterations of blood flow. *Am J Physiol* 1986;251:H520–H527.
26. Mombouli JV, Nakashima M, Hamra M, et al. Endothelium-dependent relaxation and hyperpolarization evoked by bradykinin in canine coronary arteries: Enhancement by exercise-training. *Br J Pharmacol* 1996;117:413–418.
27. Shimokawa H, Lam JY, Chesebro T, et al. Effects of dietary supplementation with cod-liver oil on endothelium-dependent responses in porcine coronary arteries. *Circulation* 1987;76:898–905.

28. Nagao T, Nakashima M, Smart FW, et al. Potentiation of endothelium-dependent hyperpolarization to serotonin by dietary intake of NC 020, a defined fish oil, in the porcine coronary artery. *J Cardiovasc Pharmacol* 1995;26:679–681.
29. De Mey JG, Vanhoutte PM. Heterogeneous behavior of the canine arterial and venous wall: Importance of the endothelium. *Circ Res* 1982;5:439–447.
30. Lüscher TF, Vanhoutte PM. Dysfunction of the release of endothelium-derived relaxing factor. In: Simionescu N, Simionescu M. eds. *Endothelial Cell Dysfunction.* New York: Plenum Press; 1992:65–102.
31. Vanhoutte PM, Rubanyi GM, Miller VM, et al. Modulation of vascular smooth muscle contraction by the endothelium. *Annu Rev Physiol* 1986;48:307–320.
32. Katusic Z, Shepherd JT, Vanhoutte PM. Endothelium-dependent contraction to stretch in canine basilar arteries. *Am J Physiol* 1987;21:H671–H673.
33. Lüscher TF, Vanhoutte PM. Endothelium-dependent contractions to acetylcholine in the aorta of the spontaneously hypertensive rat. *Hypertension* 1986;8:344–348.
34. Auch-Schwelk W, Katusic ZS, Vanhoutte PM. Thromboxane A2 receptor antagonists inhibit endothelium-dependent contractions. *Hypertension* 1990;15:699–703.
35. Ge T, Hughes H, Junquero DC, et al. Endothelium-dependent contractions are associated with both augmented expression of prostaglandin H synthase-1 and hypersensitivity to prostaglandin H2 in the SHR aorta. *Circ Res* 1995;76:1003–1010.
36. Auch-Schwelk W, Katusic ZS, Vanhoutte PM. Contractions to oxygen-derived free radicals are augmented in aorta of the spontaneously hypertensive rat. *Hypertension* 1989;13:859–864.
37. Rubanyi GM, Vanhoutte PM. Superoxide anions and hyperoxia inactivate endothelium-derived relaxing factor(s). *Am J Physiol* 1986;250:H822–H827.
38. Rubanyi GM, Vanhoutte PM. Hypoxia releases a vasoconstrictor substance from the canine vascular endothelium. *J Physiol.* 1985;364:45–56.
39. Gräser T, Vanhoutte PM. Hypoxic contraction of canine coronary arteries: Role of endothelium and cGMP. *Am J Physiol* 1991;261:H1769–H1777.
40. Yanagisawa M, Kurihara H, Kimura S, et al. A novel potent vasoconstrictor peptide produced by vascular endothelial cells. *Nature* 1988;332:411–415.
41. Masaki T, Yanagisawa M, Goto K. Physiology and pharmacology of endothelins. *Med Res Rev* 1992;12:391–421.
42. Schini VB, Vanhoutte PM. Endothelin-1: A potent vasoactive peptide. *Pharmacol Toxicol* 1991;69:1–7.
43. Schini VB, Hendrickson H, Heublein DM, et al. Thrombin enhances the release of endothelin from cultured porcine aortic endothelial cells. *Eur J Pharmacol* 1989; 165:333–334.
44. Schini VB, Kim ND, Vanhoutte PM. The basal and stimulated release of EDRF inhibits the contractions evoked by endothelin-1 and endothelin-3 in aortae of normotensive and spontaneously hypertensive rats. *J Cardiovasc Pharmacol* 1991; 17:S266–S270.
45. Nakashima M, Vanhoutte PM. Endothelin-1 and endothelin-3 cause endothelium-dependent hyperpolarization in the rat mesenteric artery. *Am J Physiol* 1993;265: H2137–H2141.
46. Miller VM, Komori K, Burnett JC Jr, et al. Differential sensitivity to endothelin in canine arteries and veins. *Am J Physiol* 257: 1989:H1127–H1131.
47. Vanhoutte PM. Is endothelin involved in the pathogenesis of hypertension ? *Hypertension* 1993;21:747–751.
48. Shimokawa H, Aarhus LL, Vanhoutte PM. Porcine coronary arteries with regenerated endothelium have a reduced endothelium-dependent responsiveness to aggregating platelets and serotonin. *Circ Res* 1987;61:256–270.
49. Shimokawa H, Flavahan NA, Vanhoutte PM. Natural course of the impairment of endothelium-dependent relaxations after balloon endothelial removal in porcine coronary arteries. Possible dysfunction of a pertussis toxin-sensitive G protein. *Circ Res* 1989;65:740–753.

50. Borg-Capra C, Fournet-Bourguignon MP, Janiak P, et al. Morphological heterogeneity with normal expression but altered function of Gi proteins in cultured regenerated porcine coronary endothelial cells. *Br J Pharmacol* 1997;122:999–1008.
51. Castedo-Delrieu M, Fournet-Bourguignon MP, Bidouard JP, et al. Phenotypic, and functional characterization of regenerated endothelial cells after balloon injury in the pig. *J Vasc Res* 1997;34(suppl 1):10.
52. Shimokawa H, Vanhoutte PM. Angiographic demonstration of hyperconstriction induced by serotonin and aggregating platelets in porcine coronary arteries with regenerated endothelium. *J Am Coll Cardiol* 1991;17:1197–1202.
53. Shimokawa H, Vanhoutte PM. Impaired endothelium-dependent relaxation to aggregating platelets and related vasoactive substances in porcine coronary arteries in hypercholesterolemia and atherosclerosis. *Circ Res* 1989;64:900–914.
54. Shimokawa H, Flavahan NA, Vanhoutte PM. Loss of endothelial pertussis toxin-sensitive G protein function in atherosclerotic porcine coronry arteries. *Circulation* 1991;83:652–660.
55. Shibano T, Codina J, Birnbaumer L. Pertussis toxin-sensitive G-proteins in regenerated endothelial cells after balloon denudation of porcine coronary artery. *Am J Physiol* 1994;267:H979–H981.
56. Cox DA, Cohen ML. Effects of oxidized low-density lipoprotein on vascular contraction and relaxation: Clinical and pharmacological implications in atherosclerosis. *Pharmacol Rev* 1996;48:3–19.
57. Vanhoutte PM, Auch-Schwelk W, Biondi ML, et al Why are converting enzyme inhibitors vasodilators ? *Br J Clin Pharmacol* 1989;28:95S–104S.
58. Vanhoutte PM, Boulanger CM, Illiano SC, et al. Endothelium-dependent effects of converting-enzyme inhibitors. *J Cardiovasc Pharmacol* 1993;22(suppl. 5):S10–S16.
59. Vanhoutte PM, Boulanger CM, Vidal M, et al. Endothelium-derived mediators and the renin-angiotensin system. In: Robertson JIS, Nicholls MG, eds. *The Renin Angiotensin System*. London: Gower Publishers; 1993;29:1–29.
60. Mombouli JV, Vanhoutte PM. Kinins and the vascular actions of converting enzyme inhibitors. *Nephrol Hypertens* 1994;3:481–484.
61. Vanhoutte PM. Endothelium-dependent responses and inhibition of angiotensin-converting enzyme [in Russian]. *Kardiologiya* 1996;36:71–79.
62. Desta B, Vanhoutte PM, Boulanger CM. Inhibition of the angiotensin converting enzyme by perindoprilat and release of nitric oxide. *Am J Hypertens* 1995;8:15–65.
63. Mombouli JV, Illiano S, Nagao T, et al. The potentiation of endothelium-dependent relaxations to bradykinin by angiotensin-converting enzyme inhibitors in canine coronary artery involves both endothelium-derived relaxing and contracting factors. *Circ Res* 1992;71:137–144.
64. Nakashima M, Mombouli JV, Taylor AA, et al. Endothelium dependent hyperpolarization caused by bradykinin in human coronary arteries. *J Clin Invest* 1993;92:2867–2871.
65. Mombouli JV, Illiano S, Vanhoutte PM. Endothelium dependant hyperpolarization caused by bradykinin in human coronary arteries. *J Clin Invest* 1993;92:2867–2871.
66. Mombouli JV, Vanhoutte PM. Kinins mediate kallikrein-induced endothelium-dependent relaxations in isolated canine coronary arteries. *Biomed Biophys Res Commun* 1992;185:693–697.
67. Mombouli JV, Vanhoutte PM. Kinins and endothelium-dependent relaxations to converting enzyme inhibitors in perfused canine arteries. *J Cardiovasc Pharmacol* 1991;18:926–927.
68. Groves P, Kurz S, Hanjörg J, et al. Role of endogenous bradykinin in human coronary vasomotor control. *Circulation*. 1995;92:3424–3430.

# Endothelium-Derived Constricting Factors and Endothelial Dysfunction

*Frank T. Ruschitzka, MD,Georg Noll, MD, and Thomas F. Lüscher, MD*

## Introduction

In addition to endothelial vasodilators, the endothelium releases contracting factors that induce sustained vasoconstriction, platelet aggregation, cell adhesion, and vascular smooth muscle proliferation. Important endothelium-derived contracting factors are the vasoconstrictor prostanoids thromboxane $A_2$, prostaglandin $H_2$, free radicals such as superoxide anions, and the 21 amino acid peptide endothelin-1 (ET-1).

Particularly in veins, agonists such as arachidonic acid, acetylcholine (ACh), histamine, and serotonin can evoke endothelium-dependent contractions, which are mediated by thromboxane $A_2$ or prostaglandin $H_2$ and activate the thromboxane receptor in the vascular smooth muscle and platelets. In addition, the cyclooxygenase pathway, as well as the renin angiotensin system, is a source of free radicals such as superoxide, which are formed by univalent reduction of molecular oxygen and known to counteract the effects of nitric oxide (NO).

The most important endothelium-derived vasoconstrictors are the ETs, which represent a family of three isopeptides, ET-1, ET-2, and ET-3. The ETs are cleaved from big ET-1 (bigET-1) by ET-converting enzymes (ECEs) and exert their effects by activation of two membrane bound, G-protein–coupled receptors, termed $ET_A$ and $ET_B$. There is experimental and clinical evidence that ET-1, in particular, is activated in atherosclerosis, myocardial infarction, coronary spasm, congestive heart failure, and pulmonary hypertension. Although still controversial, ET-1 also may be involved in blood pressure regulation as well as functional and structural changes particularly in salt-sensitive hypertension. Beneficial effects of ET blockade in experimental mod-

Original research work was supported by Grant 3200–051069.97/1 of the Swiss National Research Foundation and a grant from the Swiss Heart Foundation.

From Panza JA, Cannon RO III (eds): *Endothelium, Nitric Oxide, and Atherosclerosis* ©Futura Publishing Co, Inc, Armonk, NY, 1999.

els and human disease have set the stage for large-scale clinical trials, which are already under way to prove if ET antagonism may represent a further therapeutic advance in cardiovascular medicine.

## Endothelium-Derived Contracting Factors

Soon after the discovery of endothelium-derived relaxing factors it became clear that endothelial cells also can mediate contraction, at least under certain conditions (Figure 1).[1] Endothelium-derived contracting factors include the 21 amino acid peptide ET, vasoconstrictor prostanoids such as thromboxane $A_2$ and prostaglandin $H_2$, and components of the renin angiotensin system as well as free radicals.[1–3]

Particularly in veins, but also in the cerebral and ophthalmic circulation, agonists such as arachidonic acid, ACh, histamine, and serotonin can evoke endothelium-dependent contractions, which are mediated by thromboxane $A_2$ or prostaglandin $H_2$ (Figure 1).[4,5] Thromboxane $A_2$ and prostaglandin $H_2$

# Endothelium-Derived Vasoactive Substances

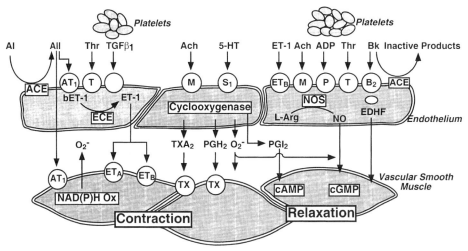

**Figure 1.** The vascular endothelin-system: schematic diagram shows that production of endothelin-1 (ET)-1 is stimulated by thrombin and other receptor-operated agonists (open circles). Released ET-1 can activate receptors on vascular smooth muscle mediating contraction ($ET_A$ receptors) and on endothelial cells releasing nitric oxide (NO) and prostacyclin ($PGI_2$) ($ET_B$ receptors). Increases in cyclic guanosine monophosphate (cGMP) and cyclic adenosine monophosphate (cAMP) in endothelial cells evoked by the latter inhibit the production of ET-1. At the level of vascular smooth muscle, both NO and $PGI_2$ blunt or prevent ET-1–induced contraction. Abbreviations: A, angiotensin; ACE, angiotensin-converting enzyme; ECE, endothelin-converting enzyme; $O_2^-$, superoxide; $PGH_2$, prostaglandin $H_2$; $TGFb_1$, transforming growth factor $b_1$; Thr, thrombin; $TXA_2$, thromboxane $A_2$; circles represent receptors (AT, angiotensinergic; M, muscarinic; P, purinergic; T, thrombin receptor).

activate the thromboxane receptor in vascular smooth muscle and platelets and hence counteract the effects of NO and prostacyclin in both cells.[5] In addition, the cyclooxygenase pathway and the renin angiotensin system are a source of free radicals such as superoxide (Figure 1). Superoxide anion is an oxygen-derived free radical formed by univalent reduction of molecular oxygen that is known to interact with NO and reduce its ability to act as a vasodilator.[2,5,6] Furthermore, the interaction of superoxide anions with NO results in the production of the cell-damaging prooxidant peroxynitrite.[7,8] As endothelial cells are constantly being subjected to oxidative stress, alterations in endogenous free-radical production under conditions of oxidative stress may play an important role in modulating spontaneous and agonist-stimulated NO production and thus alter vascular function.

Moreover, the endothelium regulates the activity of the renin angiotensin system; the angiotensin-converting enzyme (ACE), which activates angiotensin I (Ang I) into Ang II, is expressed on the endothelial cell membrane (Figure 1).[9] The ACE is identical to kinase II, which breaks down bradykinin. However, whether or not other components of the renin angiotensin system are produced in endothelial cells is still controversial. Ang II can activate endothelial angiotensin receptors, which in turn stimulate ET production[10] and possibly that of other mediators such as plasminogen activator inhibitor (PAI-1).[11]

## Regulation of Endothelin Production

ETs have been implicated in the pathogenesis of several, mainly cardiovascular disorders in view of their powerful vasoconstrictor and growth-promoting properties.[12] The three members of the family—ET-1, ET-2, and ET-3—are 21 amino acid residue peptides that are produced in a variety of tissues, where they act as modulators of vasomotor tone, cell proliferation, and hormone production (Figure 1).[13] Because of degradation by endopeptidases in the plasma, lung, and kidney, circulating ET-1 has a short half-life, of approximately 4–7 minutes.[14] Correspondingly, the mRNA half-life of preproendothelin is approximately 15 minutes indicating that vascular cells can rapidly adjust ET production as required for the regulation of vasomotor tone.[15] The ET-2 is produced predominantly within the kidney and the intestine, but the cells of origin are still not clear. The ET-3 is associated with neuronal cells and has been found in high concentrations in the brain.[16]

Stimuli for the release of ETs include hypoxia and shear stress, as well as endotoxin, adrenaline, angiotensin II, vasopressin, insulin, thrombin, transforming growth factor $\beta$, and interleukin-1 $\beta$.[13] Prostacyclin and NO inhibit ET production via a cyclic guanosine monophosphate (cGMP)-dependent mechanism.[17] Atrial natriuretic peptide also inhibits both basal production of ET-1 as well as basal production stimulated by Ang II and thrombin.[18]

Under most conditions, the production of ET appears to require de novo protein synthesis.[17] After expression of the ET gene, a transcript of 6836 base pair is formed, which leads to the production of preproendothelin, a peptide with 203 amino acids.[12,15,19] Posttranslational cleavage yields the 39 amino acid peptide bigET-1 that undergoes an additional cleavage between the non-dibasic bond of $Trp^{21}$ $Val^{22}$ to form mature ET-1.[15] The ET-1 synthesis is catalyzed by at least two ECEs, ie, ECE-1 and ECE-2.[20,21] Cloning of ECE-1 was first reported in bovine adrenal cortex,[21] but ECE-1 mRNA expression also was demonstrated in various other organs, including the heart, lung, and kidney.[22,23] Interestingly, the pH optimum of ECE-1 is 6.8, whereas that of ECE-2 is in the acidic range (pH 5.5).[20] The ECE-2 is the predominant form in neuronal tissue,[20] but expression has not been shown yet in humans. Both ECEs are membrane-bound proteinases that show structural similarity with a cytoplasmatic N terminus, a single transmembrane domain and a large extracellular C terminus, containing the catalytic domain. The ECE-1 is a zinc metalloprotease displaying 40% similarity to neutral endopeptidase 24.11[21,22] that is present at the cell surface and on intracellular vesicles.[24,25] Two subtypes of ECE-1 have been identified, ECE-1a and ECE-1b.[26] Both are encoded by the same gene by alternative splicing and differ only by their N termini.

## Endothelin Receptors

ETs exert their biological effects via activation of specific receptors (Figure 1). These membrane-bound receptors consist of seven transmembrane domains and are coupled to G-proteins. Two types of ET receptors have been cloned ($ET_A$ and $ET_B$) in mammalian tissues.[27,28] The existence and role of an $ET_C$ receptor from amphibian tissue still remains elusive.[29] The ET-1, the primary product of endothelial cells, is secreted predominantly abluminally toward the vascular smooth muscle, where it binds to $ET_A$ receptors and causes vasoconstriction with a potency 100 times that of norepinephrine on a molar basis.[28] The $ET_B$ receptors on smooth muscle cells that partly contribute to these effects exert no isoform specificity, while the putative $ET_C$ receptor preferentially binds ET-3. Endothelial cells express only $ET_B$ receptors linked to NO and prostacyclin formation.[27] The order of affinity of ETs for the $ET_A$-receptor is ET-1 $\geq$ ET-2 $\gg$ ET-3 (ET-1 affinity is approximately 100 times that of ET-3).[30,31] The $ET_B$ receptors have equipotent affinity for all three isoforms.[32]

The regulation of the production of the receptors often parallels that of the ETs. Epidermal growth factor, basic fibroblast growth factor, cyclic adenosine monophosphate (cAMP), and estrogen up-regulate $ET_A$ receptors, whereas the latter is down-regulated by the ETs, Ang II, platelet-derived growth factor 3. The $ET_A$ receptors have a 10-fold higher binding affinity to ET-1 than to ET-3. The C-type natriuretic hormone and angiotensin II and, although controversial, basic fibroblast growth up-regulate cAMP and catecholamines down-regulate $ET_B$ receptors (for review see Lüscher et al[13] and Levin[33]).

After binding to its receptors, ET-1 activates phospholipase C and in turn leads to the formation of inositol triphosphate ($IP_3$) and diacylglycerol.[34,35] The increase in $IP_3$ is more pronounced and lasts longer than with other vasoconstrictor hormones. The ET-1 also evokes a rapid and transient increase in cytosolic $Ca^{2+}$, which is associated with a rapid efflux of $Ca^{2+}$, while the influx of the cation remains unaffected.[36] Thus, the rise in cytosolic $Ca^{2+}$ induced by the peptide is derived mainly from intracellular stores due to the formation of $IP_3$. In line with this interpretation, in the human internal mammary artery, removal of extracellular $Ca^{2+}$ only slightly reduces ET-induced contractions, while removal of intracellular calcium markedly depresses the response.[37] In certain vascular smooth muscle such as the porcine coronary artery, the peptide indirectly—via a G-protein—activates voltage-operated $Ca^{2+}$ channels and in turn evokes the influx of extracellular $Ca^{2+}$.[38] Similar mechanisms might be operative in the human forearm circulation where the contraction induced by ET-1 is prevented by calcium antagonists.[39]

The ET-1 affects the membrane potential of vascular smooth muscle cells, particularly in veins.[40] Activation of $Ca^{2+}$-sensitive potassium ($K^+$) channels by the peptide provokes a transient hyperpolarization followed by a sustained depolarization caused by the opening of nonspecific cation channels permeable to $Ca^{2+}$ and magnesium ($Mg^{2+}$).[41] The depolarization leads to an activation of L-type $Ca^{2+}$ channels, which may explain why $Ca^{2+}$ antagonists are more effective in reversing than in preventing ET-induced contractions.[37,41]

ET-1 is a potent vasoconstrictor both in vitro and in vivo.[1,12,42,43] In healthy subjects, ET-1 infusion decreases and receptor antagonism increases forearm blood flow indicating a role of ET-1 in the regulation of vascular tone.[39,44–46] Moreover, the vasoconstrictor response to ET is enhanced in the human hand vein circulation of patients with essential hypertension.[47] In isolated blood vessels, the contractions induced by ET-1 are long-lasting and difficult to wash out presumably because the peptide binds very tightly to its receptor. In perfused arteries, the vasoconstrictor effects of ET-1 are more pronounced with extraluminal than with intraluminal application of the peptide.[48,49] Low and threshold concentrations of ET-1, which by themselves exert no significant contraction can potentiate the effects of other vasoconstrictor hormones, such as norepinephrine in the human internal mammary artery and serotonin in the mammary and coronary arteries.[50] The potentiating effects of low concentrations of ET-1 are sensitive to $Ca^{2+}$ antagonists and may be related to an increased influx of extracellular $Ca^{2+}$ through voltage-operated calcium channels and/or an increased sensitivity to extracellular $Ca^{2+}$.[51]

Endothelin can stimulate the release and action of NO and prostacyclin via a distinct endothelial receptors ($ET_B$-receptors).[27,52] This explains why in intact animals and in the human forearm circulation studied in vivo ET causes a transient vasodilatation at lower concentrations, which precedes its pressor effect.[12,39,53] During intravenous infusion of ET in the intact organism and after exposure of cultured endothelial cells to the peptide, the formation of prostaglandins is stimulated.[54] Indomethacin, on the other hand, augments the pressor effects of the peptide in the rabbit.[14] In cultured human vascular smooth muscle cells, ET-1 activates phospholipase $A_2$ and in turn the metabolism of arachidonic acid.[55] In rat perfused mesenteric resistance arteries, the vasodilator effects of ET-1 are prevented by indomethacin, but not $N^G$-monomethyl-L-arginine (L-NMMA), indicating that endothelium-derived prostacyclin mediates the response.[48]

In the heart, $ET_A$ receptors are localized and produced in cardiomyocytes and fibroblasts.[56] In the coronary circulation, $ET_B$ receptors virtually are absent under physiological conditions thus indicating that ETs may act predominantly as coronary vasoconstrictors.[56] In other vascular beds, ET-1 most likely acts as a paracrine constrictor when overexpressed in disease states, while it is a vasorelaxant through its effect on endothelial $ET_B$ receptors under normal conditions.[46] However, the function of the $ET_B$ receptor may vary considerably between species. For example, the effects of ET-1 in the rat kidney are mediated largely by $ET_B$ receptors, whereas in the dog they are dependent on activation of $ET_A$ receptors.[57] In the human kidney, 70% of the ET receptors are those of the $ET_B$ receptor subtype, but effects of ET-1 are mediated predominantly by the $ET_A$ receptor.[58] These species differences indicate that data obtained in animal models cannot always be extrapolated to the situation in human physiology.

## Endothelin Receptor Antagonists

Recently, an increasing number of ET receptor antagonists have been synthesized (Figure 2). Certain compounds inhibit $ET_A$ receptors only, while others interfere with both $ET_A$ and $ET_B$ receptors. Several pharmacodynamic aspects of ET receptor blockers have to be considered in clinical medicine. Some of the ET receptor blockers becoming available for clinical use will be nonselective $ET_A/ET_B$ receptor blockers. Although the $ET_A$ receptor has been implicated in the vasoconstrictive and mitogenic effects of ET, the $ET_B$ receptor activation has been shown to either mediate vasodilation or vasoconstric-

| Drug | Receptor | Proposed Indication | Development Status |
|---|---|---|---|
| ABT 627 | $ET_A$ | Prostate cancer | phase I/II |
| BMS 193884 | $ET_A$ | CHF | phase I |
| BMS 20794 | $ET_A$ | CHF | preclinical |
| Bosentan | $ET_A$ / $ET_B$ | CHF | phase II/III |
| EMD 94246 | $ET_A$ | CHF, hypertension | preclinical |
| L 743929 | $ET_A$ | | preclinical |
| LU-135252 | $ET_A$ | CHF, hypertension | phase I/II |
| PD 142893 | $ET_A$ / $ET_B$ | CV diseases | preclinical |
| PD 145065 | $ET_A$ / $ET_B$ | | preclinical |
| PD 56707 | $ET_A$ | | preclinical |
| PD 159433 | $ET_A$ | | preclinical |
| Ro 61-1790 | $ET_A$ | SAH | preclinical (only iv) |
| S 0139 | $ET_A$ | Hypertension | preclinical |
| SB 209670 | $ET_A$ | CV diseases | phase I |
| SB 217242 | $ET_A$ / $ET_B$ | COPD | phase I |
| T 0115 | $ET_A$ | Hypertension | preclinical |
| TAK-044 | $ET_{A(/B)}$ | CAD, SAH, RTR | phase II (only iv) |
| TBC 11251 | $ET_A$ | CHF, PPH | phase I/II |
| ZD 1611 | | COPD, PPH | preclinical |

**Figure 2.** The ET receptor antagonists: a variety of nonselective, combined $ET_A/ET_B$ receptor and selective $ET_A$ receptor antagonist currently are under investigation in preclinical and clinical trials. Abbreviations: CHF, congestive heart failure; CV, cardiovascular; CAD, coronary artery disease; SAH, subarachnoidal hemorrhage; PPH, primary pulmonary hypertension; RTR, renal transplant rejection; COPD, chronic obstructive pulmonary disease.

tion. Under normal physiological conditions, the peripheral vasculature probably is not subject to important $ET_B$ receptor–mediated vasoconstriction.[59,60] However, in some organs, such as the human kidney, the $ET_B$ receptor subtype predominates over the $ET_A$ receptor.[58] Importantly, the function of the $ET_B$ receptor subtype also may vary considerably between species. In dogs ET-induced vasoconstriction appears to be mediated exclusively by the $ET_A$ receptor,[61] whereas the $ET_B$ receptor is crucial for the renal vasoconstrictive effects and stimulation of water and sodium excretion and regeneration of tubular cells in the rat.[62] Thus it is possible that blockade of this receptor subtype could be harmful under pathological conditions associated with $ET_B$ receptor up-regulation.

Gene-disruption experiments of the ET receptor subtypes also point toward an important role of these receptors in mammalian neural crest development. For example, knockout of the $ET_A$ receptor gene results in defects of the branchial arch and endocardial cushion,[63] while knockout of the $ET_B$ receptor could be linked to defects in the enteric ganglia and Hirschsprungs's disease.[64,65] Of course these knockout experiments cannot be extrapolated to side effects of receptor blockade, but they clearly indicate potential teratogenic effects of ET receptor–blocking drugs.

## Endothelium-Derived Constricting Factors and Cardiovascular Disease

The endothelium is that structure of the blood vessel wall that is most exposed to the mechanical forces of the blood and hormones and noxious substances therein. Morphological studies have demonstrated changes in endothelial cell morphology with aging and disease, in particular increased endothelial cell turnover and density, a marked heterogeneity in endothelial cell size, and bulging of the cells into the lumen. However, endothelial cell denudation does not occur except in very late stages of atherosclerosis and plaque rupture. Almost invariably associated with these changes in endothelial cell morphology are functional alterations and intimal thickening with accumulation of white blood cells, vascular smooth muscle cells and fibroblasts, and matrix deposition.

# Hypertension

Endothelial dysfunction in hypertension could contribute to the increase in peripheral vascular resistance (particularly if it occurs in resistance arteries) and to the vascular complications of the disease (if present in large- and medium-sized conduit arteries). In most models of hypertension, high blood pressure is associated with reduced endothelium-dependent relaxations.[5] This defect is more dominant in certain blood vessels and appears to occur as blood pressure rises and hence is a consequence rather than a cause of hypertension. In hypertensive subjects, ACh causes paradoxical vasoconstriction of epicardial coronary arteries. The increase in blood flow to ACh in the forearm and coronary circulation was found to be decreased in all but one study.[66-68]

The mechanism of endothelial dysfunction differs in different models of hypertension. In the spontaneously hypertensive rat (SHR), the activity of NO synthase (NOS) is increased markedly but inefficacious probably because of an increased deactivation of NO (Figure 3).[69] In addition, the endothelium of spontaneously hypertensive and ren-2 transgenic rats produces increased amounts of prostaglandin $H_2$, which offsets the effects of NO in vascular smooth muscle and platelets.[70] Whether or not this occurs in man is uncertain; however, in the forearm circulation of patients with essential hypertension infusion of a cyclooxygenase inhibitor such as indomethacin enhances the vasodilation to ACh.[71]

Because of its vasoconstrictor action and its effects on vascular hypertrophy, ET-1 also has been implicated in the pathogenesis and/or the maintenance of hypertension. However, whether or not ET production is altered in human hypertension remains elusive.[72,73] Although some studies found increased plasma levels of ET, most found no differences as compared with controls. Interestingly, patients with ET secreting hemangioendotheliomas are hypertensive.[74] Specific activation of the ETs in African-Americans who often present with severe and salt-sensitive (low-renin) hypertension, points to severity and salt sensitivity as important denominators of the activation of the ET system in hypertension.[75] However, circulating ET may not reflect local levels of the peptide, because in the blood vessel wall ET is released primarily abluminally.[76]

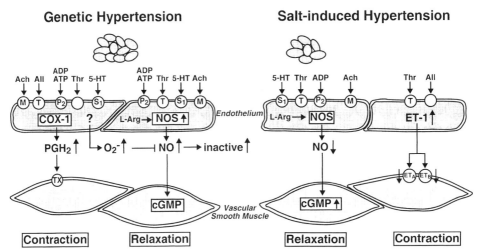

**Figure 3.** Heterogeneity of endothelium dysfunction in hypertension: In spontaneously hypertensive rats (SHR; left) NO synthase (NOS) activity is increased, but the biological activity of NO is reduced, possibly because of inactivation. In addition, the production of thromboxane $A_2$ (TXA$_2$) and prostaglandin $H_2$ (PGH$_2$) via cyclooxygenase (COX-1) is increased. In contrast, in salt-related hypertension(Dahl rats, Sabra rat, deoxycorticosterone acetate (DOCA) salt hypertension), NO production is reduced but no TXA$_2$ or PGH$_2$ is produced. ET-1 production is augmented in DOCA-salt hypertension but reduced in SHR. (See Figure 1 for more abbreviations.)

Infusion of ET-1 increases blood pressure in experimental animals and in man.[77] In essential hypertensives, ET-1 induces a rise in blood pressure and systemic vascular resistance, while cardiac index and natriuresis are reduced.[45] Interestingly, normotensive offsprings of hypertensive parents exhibit enhanced plasma ET responses to mental stress indicating that genetically determined activation of the ET system is already present at this early stage of disease.[78] Furthermore, ET-1 gene expression is enhanced in small arteries of patients with moderate to severe hypertension, whereas expression is similar in control subjects and untreated mild hypertensives.[79]

Experimental findings suggest that ET may be involved differently in different forms of hypertension (Figure 3). In fact, in some animal models of hypertension, such as the deoxycorticosterone acetate (DOCA) salt hypertensive rat, ET receptor blockade causes marked reductions in blood pressure, which also is associated with regression of vascular hypertrophy.[80,81] In keeping with that, ET-1 secretion is augmented in cultured endothelial cells from DOCA-salt hypertensive rats.[82] Accordingly, ET antagonists lower blood pressure in salt-depleted monkeys.[83] However, the effects of ET antagonism in other experimental models of hypertension, notably the SHR, are less clear. In SHR, both circulating and vascular ET as well as ET tissue content of the renal medulla are reduced.[84,85] In contrast, in the stroke-prone SHR the ET axis is activated and ET antagonism significantly reduces blood pressure and prevents cardiac and vascular hypertrophy.[86,87] In addition, in Dahl salt-sensitive rats, ET levels are increased and ET antagonists lower blood pressure indicating that the ET system is activated particularly in severe, salt-sensitive (low-renin) hypertension (Figure 3).[88] Similarly, the circulating and tissue ET-1 system is increased in one-kidney, one-clip (low-renin) hypertension[89] and two-kidney, two-clip acute renal failure.[90] At variance, the ET expression is augmented only in the late phase of two-kidney, one-clip Goldblatt (high-renin) hypertension resembling true renovascular hypertension and activation of the renin-angiotensin system in man.[91] In contrast, 2 weeks administration of Ang II increases the production of ET in the blood vessel wall of the rat.[10,92] Most interestingly, selective $ET_A$ receptor antagonism reduced blood pressure, vascular hypertrophy,[10] and endothelial dysfunction[92] under these experimental conditions. These data strongly suggest that ET antagonists may be of particular value in conditions of increased activity of the renin-angiotensin system. This is consistent with additional hypotensive effects of ET-1 receptor antagonism in hypertensive dogs already treated with ACE inhibitor.[93] However, the discrepancy between the beneficial effects of selective $ET_A$ receptor blockade in Ang II induced hypertension and the lack of effects in two-kidney, one-clip model is difficult to reconcile, but may be caused by a lesser extent of activation of the tissue (rather than circulating) renin-angiotensin and ET system or activation of vasodilatory systems preventing increased ET production.

In NO-deficient hypertension induced by L-NMMA or nitro-L- arginine methylester (NAME), ET production is enhanced, but the peptide only is involved in the increase of blood pressure under acute but not chronic conditions.[94,95] Recently, a role of ET also was suggested in fructose-fed hypertensive rats exhibiting hyperinsulinemia and insulin resistance, as chronic combined ET blockade reduces blood pressure in this experimental model of hypertension.[96] Interestingly, hepatic overexpression of preproendothelin-1 in rats also resulted in elevation of blood pressure that was reduced by an $ET_A$ antagonist.[97]

To further elucidate the role of ET, transgenic and gene knockout rats have been developed. The ET-2 transgenic rats exhibit elevated ET-1 plasma levels, but do not develop hypertension (possibly because of the activation of compensatory vasodilator mechanisms).[98] Surprisingly, ET-1 gene knockout mice are actually hypertensive.[99] It is likely that the small increase in blood pressure in ET knockout mice is related to hypoxia and disturbances in the central regulation of respiration that in turn may activate the sympathetic nervous system. The finding that ET knockout rats have profound malformations of the throat indicates that the peptide may be involved importantly in the development of these organs.[63]

Thus, there is mounting evidence from animal and human studies that ET-1 is involved in the pathogenesis and/or maintenance of hypertension, at least in salt-sensitive and severe forms of the disease. The first clinical trial evidence now is available demonstrating that combined $ET_A/ET_B$ receptor antagonism effectively lowers blood pressure in patients with mild to moderate hypertension; indeed, the antihypertensive effects of bosentan were comparable with that of the ACE inhibitor enalapril (Figure 4).[100] However, so far, experimental data do not provide evidence in favor of combined $ET_A/ET_B$ versus $ET_A$ receptor blockade in hypertension, except as to the surrogate parameter endothelial dysfunction that only is ameliorated by selective $ET_A$ receptor blockade.[92] Thus, head-to-head comparative, large-scale studies with combined $ET_A/ET_B$ and selective $ET_A$ receptor antagonist are needed to further delineate the best approach of pharmacologically blocking the ET axis in human hypertension.

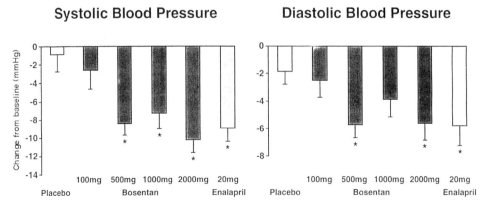

**Figure 4.** Effects of ET antagonism in patients with essential hypertension: $ET_A/ET_B$ receptor antagonist bosentan lowers blood pressure in patients with essential hypertension as compared with the ACE inhibitor enalapril. Reproduced with permission from Reference 100.

# Pulmonary Hypertension

In contrast to systemic hypertension, primary and secondary pulmonary hypertension clearly is associated with an activation of the ET system.[101] In young patients with pulmonary hypertension and congenital heart disease, elevated plasma ET levels were reduced after surgical correction.[102] In addition, ET levels are correlated positively with the degree of pulmonary hypertension and negatively with prognosis.[103] There also is a strong association between the intensity of ET-1-like immunoreactivity and pulmonary vascular resistance in the patients with plexogenic pulmonary arteriopathy.[104] Furthermore, ET-1 also appears to be an important local mediator in acute pulmonary hypertension associated with hypoxia, as plasma ET levels are increased twofold and inversely correlated to arterial $P_{O_2}$ in high-altitude pulmonary hypertension.[105]

In addition, experimental data strongly provide evidence for a pathogenetic role for ET-1 in pulmonary hypertension. Indeed, the circulating and tissue ET system is increased in the fawn-hooded rat that develops idiopathic pulmonary hypertension.[106] Moreover, ET-1 exerts proinflammatory effects[107] and collagen remodeling in the lung.[108] Overexpression of ET-1 contributes to the enhanced growth of pulmonary artery smooth muscle cells via an $ET_A$-dependent mechanism. Indeed, selective $ET_A$ antagonism reversed hypoxia-induced pulmonary hypertension in rats.[109] Correspondingly, pulmonary hypertension caused by congestive heart failure also is ameliorated by long-term application of an $ET_A$ receptor antagonist in the rat.[110] At variance, in beagles with dehydromonocrotaline-induced pulmonary hypertension, ET-1 decreased pulmonary artery pressure via an $ET_B$ receptor–dependent mechanism.[111] Interestingly, $ET_B$-mediated vasoconstriction also has been demonstrated in pulmonary arteries from humans and rats.[112]

Thus, the most effective profile, that is, $ET_A$ and/or $ET_B$ receptor antagonism, in pulmonary hypertension remains to be defined. Because the $ET_B$ receptor is involved predominantly in the clearance of ET-1 from the pulmonary circulation, selective blockade of the $ET_A$ receptor appears to be more favorable. In view of the lack of any therapy that retards deterioration (with the exception of intravenously applied prostacyclin), the rationale of blocking the ET axis appears to be particularly exciting in patients with primary or secondary pulmonary hypertension.

# Congestive Heart Failure

In patients with heart failure, plasma ET-1 and bigET-1 levels are increased, are related to the degree of hemodynamic compromise, and predict clinical outcome.[103,113–115] In addition, experimental data strongly suggest that the ET system is activated and plays a contributory role in exacerbating left ventricular dysfunction and symptoms associated with congestive heart failure.[103,114,116,117] In particular, activation of the $ET_A$ receptor has direct effects on myocyte contractile function, protein expression, and electrophysiology.[118–124] In a rat model of myocardial infarction, up-regulation of the myocardial ET system contributes to the progression of chronic heart failure, as selective $ET_A$ receptor antagonism decreased the rate and force of contraction of the failing heart suggesting a direct inotropic action of ET-1.[110] In addition, long-term administration improved survival by approximately 50% in these animals.[125] The favorable effects of $ET_A$ receptor antagonism were attributed to the inhibition of the cytotoxic actions of ET-1 on cardiac cells, regression of maladaptive cellular hypertrophy, reduction of myocardial contractility, and inhibition of ET-induced arrhythmias. However, therapy was started 10 days after myocardial infarction in this experimental model leaving the question unanswered whether up-regulation of the ET system could or should be blocked instantly after infarction or at a later stage of the disease, particularly in view of the impact of the ETs on wound healing and ventricular remodeling.

Interestingly, combined $ET_A/ET_B$ receptor antagonist with bosentan also improved ventricular performance and vascular resistance in dogs with heart failure.[126] In patients with severe congestive heart failure, bosentan lowers arterial and pulmonary pressures.[127] Selective $ET_A$ receptor antagonism and ECE inhibition produced a significant reduction in forearm vascular resistance in patients with heart failure already treated with conventional therapy including ACE inhibitors.[128] In line with that, the postischemic effects of ACE inhibitors in rat hearts in large part are caused by suppression of ET-1 secretion and action.[129]

Hence, inhibition of the ET axis may represent a further therapeutic advance in the treatment of congestive heart failure. However, as both $ET_A$ and $ET_B$ receptors mediate vasoconstriction in congestive heart failure, the ideal compound would block both receptors but preserve endothelial $ET_B$ receptor–mediated vasodilation and clearance of ET-1.

# Atherosclerosis

Endothelium-dependent relaxations are reduced in hyperlipidemia and atherosclerosis,[130,131] most likely because of the action of low-density lipoproteins (LDL).[132] Indeed, incubation of isolated coronary arteries with oxidized but not native LDLs (ox-LDLs) selectively inhibits endothelium-dependent relaxations to serotonin, aggregating platelets and thrombin, while the response to bradykinin is unaffected.[132] In more advanced stages of atherosclerosis, a more generalized endothelial dysfunction occurs and endothelium-derived vasoconstrictors come into play. Indeed, experiments in the hypercholesteremic rabbit aorta suggest that the overall production of NO is not reduced but markedly augmented; however, NO is inactivated by superoxide radicals produced within the endothelium (Figure 5).[133]

In contrast to native LDLs, ox-LDLs, which are present in human atherosclerotic plaque,[134] induce the expression of preproendothelin mRNA and an increase in ET-1 release (Figure 5).[135]

The ET-1 is a strong chemoattractant for monocytes and macrophages that are major cellular components of human atherogenic lesions.[136] Enhanced

# Pathogenesis of Atherosclerosis

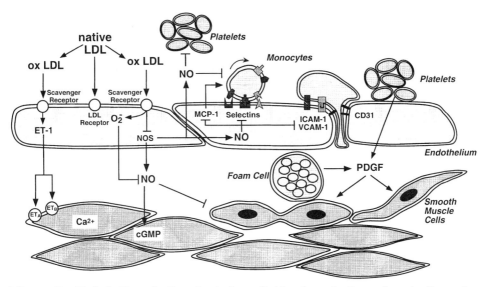

**Figure 5.** Endothelium dysfunction in hyperlipidemia and atherosclerosis: the major components are oxidized low-density lipoproteins (ox-LDLs), which by activating scavenger receptors impair the activity of the L-arginine NO pathway. The mechanism may involve inactivation of G-proteins ($G_i$), decreased intracellular availibility of L-arginine (L-Arg) and increased breakdown of NO by superoxide ($O_2^-$). ox-LDLs further activate ET gene expression and production via protein kinase C (PKC). (See Figure 1 for more abbreviations.)

expression of ET-1 in smooth muscle cells migrating into the intima of arteries in atherosclerosis thus may contribute to the enhanced vasoconstrictor responses of atherosclerotic blood vessels as well as—through their proliferative effects on vascular smooth muscle (see reviews byYanagisawa and Masaki[19] and Simonson et al[34])—to the development of the atherosclerotic plaque. It remains uncertain, at this point, whether the enhanced production of the peptide occurring in the presence of modified LDL and atherosclerosis is sufficient to alter vascular function. As even threshold concentrations of ET-1 potentiate contractile responses to other agonists such as norepinephrine and serotonin[50], locally increased ET levels may increase vascular reactivity in atherosclerosis.

In patients with hyperlipidemia and atherosclerosis, the circulating levels of ET are increased and correlate with the anatomical extent of the disease.[137] In addition, increased ET-1 immunoreactivity in atherosclerotic lesions is associated with acute coronary syndromes.[138]

In hypercholesterolemic pigs, the vasoconstrictive effect on the coronary circulation in response to intracoronary ET-1 administered exogenously are enhanced.[139] However, no changes in ET receptor density or binding affinity occurs, whereas endothelial NOS (eNOS) immunoreactivity decreases. In addition to exaggerated vasoconstriction, ET-1 within atherosclerotic lesions may be involved in smooth muscle cell proliferation[140] and neovascularization.[141] In smooth muscle cells of human coronary arteries $ET_A$ receptors dominate, while $ET_B$ receptors are up-regulated in atherosclerotic coronaries.[142]

Most interestingly, selective $ET_A$ receptor blockade decreases number and size of macrophage-foam cells in hamsters fed a high-cholesterol diet.[143] Correspondingly, selective $ET_A$ receptor blockade significantly inhibited the development of atherosclerotic lesions and normalized endothelial dysfunction in apolipoprotein-E (apoE)-deficient mice.[144]

## Coronary Artery Disease

In patients with variant angina (coronary vasospasm), plasma and coronary sinus ET levels are elevated.[145] During spasm the levels decrease in the coronary sinus, possibly because of decreased local clearance of the peptide from the ischemic areas of the heart.

Patients with acute myocardial infarction exhibit elevated plasma ET levels very early in the course of the disease.[146] Stimuli for the increased ET levels might be hypoxia and ischemia, and the enhanced release of secretagogues for ET-1, such as thrombin. Interestingly, the plasma levels of ET are important predictors of clinical outcome.[147] Indeed, patients with plasma ET 6.5 pg/mL at 3 hours after onset of myocardial infarction have a much poorer survival than those with lower values. This may be related to the fact that the patients with poor outcome have a lower ejection fraction and hence on average higher pulmonary pressures.

In vitro and animal studies of the role of ET-1 in the pathogenesis of coronary artery disease are still inconsistent. Mixed $ET_A/ET_B$ receptor antagonism with TAK-044 or bosentan either decreased or did not affect infarct size, respectively.[148,149] $ET_A$ receptor antagonism with PD 156707, following coronary artery occlusion and reperfusion in pigs, did not reduce infarct size either.[150] In contrast, when given during rather than after occlusion, $ET_A$ receptor antagonist FR 139317 significantly decreased infarct size in rabbits.[151]

Moreover, increased plasma immunoreactivity of ET-1 was demonstrated after percutaneous transluminal coronary angioplasty.[152,153] After carotid artery balloon angioplasty preproendothelin-1 mRNA was up-regulated and ET-1 immunoreactivity was localized particularly in neointima cells.[154] Indeed, combined $ET_A/ET_B$ receptor antagonism and ECE inhibition reduced neointimal formation[155,156] suggesting that ET-1 may contribute to intimal proliferation in restenosis after coronary angioplasty. Furthermore, selective $ET_A$ receptor antagonism also acts favorably on proliferating vascular smooth muscle cells to reduce vessel reocclusion following angioplasty.[157]

## Conclusions

In cardiovascular disease, endothelium-derived contracting factors, such as vasoconstrictor prostanoids and the ETs, counteract the effects of NO and thus induce sustained vasoconstriction, platelet aggregation, and vascular smooth muscle proliferation.

In particular, there is experimental and clinical evidence that the circulating and tissue ET system is activated in atherosclerosis, myocardial infarction, coronary spasm, congestive heart failure, and pulmonary hypertension. Although still controversial, ET also may be involved in blood pressure regulation as well as functional and structural changes, particularly in salt-sensitive hypertension. Whereas short-term activation of the ETs may be beneficial under physiological conditions to provide hemodynamic support; sustained activation of the ETs may induce enhanced vasoconstriction and proliferation of vascular smooth muscle cells, all events known to occur in cardiovascular disease. The first clinical trial evidence is available proving beneficial effects of ET antagonism in patients with essential hypertension. Further clinical trials with ET receptor antagonists are already under way, which will provide deeper insights in the pathophysiological role of this endothelium-dependent vasoconstrictor and prove if blocking the ETs offers a new therapeutical approach for the benefit of patients with cardiovascular disease.

# References

1. Lüscher TF, Yang Z, Tschudi M, et al. Interaction between endothelin-1 and endothelium-derived relaxing factor in human arteries and veins. *Circ Res* 1990; 66:1088–1094.
2. Rubanyi GM, Vanhoutte PM. Superoxide anions and hyperoxia inactivate endothelium-derived relaxing factor. *Am J Physiol* 1986;250:H822–H827.
3. Katusic ZS, Vanhoutte PM. Superoxide anion is an endothelium derived contracting factor. *Am J Physiol* 1989;257:H33–H37.
4. Moncada S, Vane VR. Pharmacology and endogenous roles of prostaglandin endoperoxides, thromboxane A2 and prostacyclin. *Pharmacol Rev* 1979;30:293–331.
5. Lüscher TF, Vanhoutte PM. *The Endothelium: Modulator of Cardiovascular Function*. Boca Raton, FL: CRC Press; 1990:1–215.
6. Gryglewski RJ, Palmer RM, Moncada S. Superoxide anion is involved in the breakdown of endothelium-derived vascular relaxing factor. *Nature* 1986;320: 454–456.
7. Moro MA, Darley-Usmar VM, Goodwin DA, et al. Paradoxical fate and biological action of peroxynitrite on human platelets. *Proc Natl Acad Sci U S A* 1994;91: 6702–6706.
8. White CR, Brock TA, Chang LY, et al. Superoxide and peroxynitrite in atherosclerosis. *Proc Natl Acad Sci U S A* 1994;91:1044–1048.
9. Rajagopalan S, Kurz S, Münzel T, et al. Angiotensin II mediated hypertension in the rat increases vascular superoxide production via membrane NADH/NADPH oxidase activation: Contributions to alterations of vasomotor tone. *J Clin Invest* 1996;97:1916–1923.
10. Moreau P, d'Uscio LV, Shaw S, et al. Angiotensin II increases tissue endothelin and induces vascular hypertrophy. *Circulation* 1997;96:1593–1597.
11. Kerins DM, Hao Q, Vaughan DE. Angiotensin induction of PAI-1 expression in endothelial cells is mediated by the hexapeptide angiotensin IV. *J Clin Invest* 1996;96:2515–2520.
12. Yanagisawa M, Kurihara H, Kimura S, et al. A novel potent vasoconstrictor peptide produced by vascular endothelial cells. *Nature* 1988;332:411–415.
13. Lüscher TF, Boulanger CM, Dohi Y, et al. Endothelium-derived contracting factors. *Hypertension* 1992;19:117–130.

14. de Nucci G, Thomas R, D'Orleans JP, et al. Pressor effects of circulating endothelin are limited by its removal in the pulmonary circulation and the release of prostacyclin and endothelium-derived relaxing factor. *Proc Natl Acad Sci U S A* 1988;85:9797–9800.

15. Inoue A, Yanigasawa M, Takuwa Y, et al. The human preproendothelin-1 gene. *J Biol Chem* 1989;264:14954–14959.

16. Shinmi O, Kimura S, Sawamura T, et al. Endothelin-3 is a novel neuropeptide: Isolation and sequence determination of endothelin-1 and endothelin-3 in porcine brain. *Biochem Biophys Res Commun* 1989;164:587–593.

17. Boulanger C, Lüscher TF. Release of endothelin from the porcine aorta. Inhibition by endothelium-derived nitric oxide. *J Clin Invest* 1990;85:587–590.

18. Hu RM, Levin ER, Pedram A, et al. Atrial natriuretic peptide inhibits the production and secretion of endothelin-1from cultured endothelial cells: Mediation through the C receptor. *J Biol Chem* 1992;267:17384–17389.

19. Yanagisawa M, Masaki T. Molecular biology and biochemistry of the endothelins. *Trends Pharmacol Sci* 1989;10:374–378.

20. Emoto N, Yanagisawa M. Endothelin-converting enzyme-2 is a membrane-bound, phosphoramidon-sensitive metalloprotease with acidic pH optimum. *J Biol Chem* 1995;270:15262–15268.

21. Xu D, Emoto N, Giaid A, et al. ECE-1: A membrane-bound metalloprotease that catalyzes the proteolytic activation of big endothelin-1. *Cell* 1994;78:473–485.

22. Shimada K, Takahashi M, Tanzawa K. Cloning and functional expression of endothelin-converting enzyme from rat endothelial cells. *J Biol Chem* 1994;269: 18275–18278.

23. Shimada K, Matsushita Y, Wakabayashi K, et al. Cloning and functional expression of human endothelin-converting enzyme cDNA. *Biochem Biophys Res Commun* 1995;207:807–812.

24. Takahashi M, Fukuda K, Shimada K, et al. Localization of rat endothelin converting enzyme to vascular endothelial cells and some secretory cells. *Biochem J* 1995;311:657–665.

25. Barnes K, Brown C, Turner AJ. Endothelin-converting enzyme. Ultrastructural localization and its recycling from the cell surface. *Hypertension* 1998;31(pt 1):3–9.

26. Valdenaire O, Rohrbacher E, Mattei MG. Organization of the gene encoding the human endothelin converting enzyme (ECE-1). *J Biol Chem* 1995;270:29794–29798.

27. Sakurai T, Yanagisawa M, Takuwa Y, et al. Cloning of a cDNA encoding a non-isopeptide-selective subtype of the endothelin receptor. *Nature* 1990;348:732–735. Comments.

28. Arai H, Hori S, Aramori I, et al. Cloning and expression of a cDNA encoding an endothelin receptor. *Nature* 1990;348:730–732. Comments.

29. Karne S, Jayawickreme CK, Lerner MR. Cloning and characterization of an endothelin-3 specific receptor (ETC receptor) from Xenopus laevis dermal melanophores. *J Biol Chem* 1993;268:19126–19133.

30. Hosoda K, Nakao K, Hiroshi A, et al. Cloning and expression of human endothelin-1 receptor cDNA. *FEBS Lett* 1991;287:23–26.

31. Lin HY, Kaji EH, Winkel G, et al. Cloning and functional expression of a vascular smooth muscle endothelin 1 receptor. *Proc Natl Acad Sci U S A* 1991;88:3185–3189.

32. Sakamoto A, Yanagisawa M, Sakurai T, et al. Cloning and functional expression of human cDNA for the ETB endothelin receptor. *Biochem Biophys Res Commun* 1991;178:656–663.

33. Levin ER. Endothelins. *N Engl J Med* 1995;333:356–363.

34. Simonson MS, Wann S, Mene P. Endothelin stimulates phospholipase C, Na+/H+ exchange, c-fos expression, and mitogenesis in rat mesangial cells. *J Clin Invest* 1989;83:708–712.

35. Resink TJ, Scott-Burden T, Bühler FR. Endothelin stimulates phospholipase C in cultured vascular smooth muscle cells. *Biochem Biophys Res Commun* 1988;157: 1360–1368.

36. Wallnöfer A, Weir S, Rüegg U, et al. The mechanism of action of endothelin-1 as compared with other agonists in vascular smooth muscle. *J Cardiovasc Pharmacol* 1989;13(suppl 5):23–31.

37. Yang Z, Bauer E, von Segesser L, et al. Different mobilization of calcium in endothelin-1-induced contractions in human arteries and veins: Effects of calcium antagonists. *J Cardiovasc Pharmacol* 1990;16:654–660.

38. Goto K, Kasuya Y, Matsuki N, et al. Endothelin activates the dihydropyridine sensitive, voltage-dependent Ca(2+) channel in vascular smooth muscle. *Proc Natl Acad Sci U S A* 1989;86:3915–3918.

39. Kiowski W, Lüscher TF, Linder L. Endothelin-1-induced vasoconstriction in humans. Reversal by calcium channel blockade but not by nitrovasodilators or endothelium-derived relaxing factor. *Circulation* 1991;83:469–475.

40. Miller VM, Komori K, Burnett JC Jr, et al. Differential sensitivity to endothelin in canine arteries and veins. *Am J Physiol* 1989;257:H1127–H1131.

41. Van Renterghem C, Vigne P, Barhanin J, et al. Molecular mechanism of action of the vasoconstrictor peptide endothelin. *Biochem Biophys Res Commun* 1988;157: 977–985.

42. Miller WL, Redfield MM, Burnett JJ. Integrated cardiac, renal, and endocrine actions of endothelin. *J Clin Invest* 1989;83:317–320.

43. Goetz KL, Wang BC, Madwed JB, et al. Cardiovascular, renal, and endocrine responses to intravenous endothelin in conscious dogs. *Am J Physiol* 1988;255: R1064–R1068.

44. Haynes WG, Webb DJ. Contribution of endogenous generation of endothelin-1 to basal vascular tone. *Lancet* 1994;344:852–854.

45. Kaasjager KA, Koomans HA, Rabelink TJ. Endothelin-1-induced vasopressor responses in essential hypertension. *Hypertension* 1997;30(pt 1):15–21.

46. Verhaar MC, Strachan FE, Newby DE, et al. Endothelin-A receptor antagonist-mediated vasodilation is attenuated by inhibition of nitric oxide synthesis and by endothelin-B receptor blockade. *Circulation* 1998;97:752–756.

47. Haynes WG, Moffat S, Webb DJ. An investigation into the direct and indirect venoconstrictor effects of endothelin-1 and big endothelin-1 in man. *Br J Pharmacol* 1995;40:307–311.

48. Dohi Y, Lüscher TF. Endothelin in hypertensive resistance arteries. Intraluminal and extraluminal dysfunction. *Hypertension* 1991;18:543–549.

49. Pohl U, Busse R. Differential vascular sensitivity to luminally and adventitially applied endothelin-1. *J Cardiovasc Pharmacol* 1989;13(suppl 5):188–190.

50. Yang Z, Richard V, von Segesser L, et al. Threshold concentrations of endothelin-1 potentiate contractions to norepinephrine and serotonin in human arteries: A new mechanism of vasospasm? *Circulation* 1990;82:188–195.

51. Godfraind T, Mennig D, Morel N, et al. Effect of endothelin-1 on calcium channel gating by agonists in vascular smooth muscle. *J Cardiovasc Pharmacol* 1989; 13(suppl 5):112–117.

52. Mizuguchi T, Nishiyama M, Moroi K, et al. Analysis of two pharmcologically predicted endothelin B receptor subtypes by using the endothelin B receptor gene knock out mouse. *Br J Pharmacol* 1997;120:1427–1430.

53. Wright CE, Fozard JR. Regional vasodilation is a prominent feature of the haemodynamic response to endothelin in anaesthetized, spontaneously hypertensive rats. *Eur J Pharmacol* 1988;155:201–203.

54. Thiemermann C, Lidbury PS, Thomas GR, et al. Endothelin-1 releases prostacyclin and inhibits ex vivo platelet aggregation in the anesthetized rabbit. *J Cardiovasc Pharmacol* 1989;13(suppl 5):138–141.

55. Resink TJ, Scott-Burden T, Bühler FR. Activation of phospholipase A2 by endothelin in cultured vascular smooth muscle cells. *Biophys Biochem Res Commun* 1989;158:279–286.

56. Davenport AP, Kuc RE, Maguire JJ, et al. ETA receptors predominate in the human vasculature and mediate constriction. *J Cardiovasc Pharmacol* 1995;l26: S265–S267.
57. Clavell A, Stingo A, Margulies K, et al. Role of endothelin receptor subtypes in the in vivo regulation of renal function. *Am J Physiol* 1995;268:F455–F469.
58. Kaasjager KA, Shaw S, Koomans HA, et al. Role of endothelin receptor subtypes in the systemic and renal responses to endothelin-1 in humans. *J Am Soc Nephrol* 1997;8:32–39.
59. Clozel M, Fischli W, Guilly C. Specific binding of endothelin on human vascular smooth muscle cells in culture. *J Clin Invest* 1989;83:1758–1761.
60. Dashwood M, Turner M, Jacobs M. Endothelin-1: Contractile responses and autoradiographic localization of receptors in rabbit blood vessels. *J Cardiovasc Pharmacol* 1989;13(suppl 5):183–185.
61. Lee CY, Chiappinelli VA, Takasaki C, et al. Similarity of endothelin to snake venom toxin. *Nature* 1988;335:303.
62. Wellings RP, Corder R, Warner TD, et al. Evidence from receptor antagonists of an important role for ETB receptor-mediated vasoconstrictor effects of endothelin-1 in the rat kidney. *Br J Pharmacol* 1994;111:515–520.
63. Kurihara Y, Kurihara H, Suzuki H, et al. Targeted disruprion of mouse endothelin-1 gene (I): Lethality and craniofacial anomaly in homozygotes. *Circulation* 1993;88:1–182.
64. Hosoda K, Hammer R, Richardson J, et al. Targeted and natural (piebald–lethal) mutations of endothelin-b receptor gene produces megacolon associated spotted coat color in mice. *Cell* 1994;79:1267–1276.
65. Puffenberger KG, Hosoda K, Washington SS, et al. A missense mutation of the endothelin-b receptor gene in Hirschsprung disease. *Cell* 1994;79:1257–1266.
66. Linder L, Kiowski W, Bühler FR, et al. Indirect evidence for release of endothelium-derived relaxing factor in human forearm circulation in vivo. Blunted response in essential hypertension. *Circulation* 1990;811990:1762–1767.
67. Panza JA, Quyyumi AA, Brush JJ, et al. Abnormal endothelium-dependent vascular relaxation in patients with essential hypertension. *N Engl J Med* 1990;323:22–27.
68. Cockcroft JR, Chowienczyk PJ, Benjamin N, et al. Preserved endothelium-dependent vasodilatation in patients with essential hypertension. *N Engl J Med* 1994;330:1036–1040.
69. Nava E, Noll G, Lüscher TF. Increased activity of constitutive nitric oxide synthase in cardiac endothelium in spontaneous hypertension. *Circulation* 1995;91:2310–2313.
70. Küng CF, Lüscher TF. Different mechanisms of endothelial dysfunction with aging and hypertension in rat aorta. *Hypertension* 1995;25:194–200.
71. Taddei S, Virdis A, Mattei P, et al. Vasodilation to acetylcholine in primary and secondary forms of human hypertension. *Hypertension* 1993;21:929–933.
72. Lüscher TF, Seo BG, Bühler FR. Potential role of endothelin in hypertension. Controversy on endothelin in hypertension. *Hypertension* 1993;21:752–757.
73. Vanhoutte P. Other endothelium-derived vasoactive factors. *Circulation* 1993;87(suppl):V9–V17.
74. Yokokawa K, Tahara T, Kohno M, et al. Hypertension associated with endothelin-secreting malignant hemangioendothelioma. *Ann Intern Med* 1991;114:213–215.
75. Ergul S, Parish DC, Puett D, et al. Racial differences in plasma endothelin-1 concentrations in individuals with essential hypertension. *Hypertension* 1996;28:652–655.
76. Wagner OF, Christ G, Wojta J, et al. Polar secretion of endothelin-1 by cultured endothelial cells. *J Biol Chem* 1992;267:16066–16068.
77. Pernow J, Kaijser L, Lundberg JM, et al. Comparable potent coronary vasoconstrictor effects of endothelin-1 and big endothelin-1 in humans. *Circulation* 1996;94:2077–2082.

78. Noll G, Wenzel RR, Schneider M, et al. Increased activation of sympathetic nervous system and endothelin by mental stress in normotensive offspring of hypertensive parents. *Circulation* 1996;93:866–869.
79. Schiffrin EL, Deng LY, Sventek P, et al. Enhanced expression of endothelin-1 gene in endothelium of resistance arteries in severe human essential hypertension. *J Hypertens* 1997;15:57–63.
80. Li JS, Lariviere R, Schiffrin EL. Effect of a nonselective endothelin antagonist on vascular remodeling in DOCA-salt hypertensive rat: Evidence for a role of endothelin in vascular hypertrophy. *Hypertension* 1994;24:183–188.
81. Schiffrin EL, Sventek P, Li JS, et al. Anti hypertensive effect of bosentan, a mixed ETA/ETB endothel in receptor antagonist, in DOCA-salt spontaneously hypertensive rats. *Br J Pharmacol* 1995;115:1377–1381.
82. Takada K, Matsumara Y, Miyazaki Y, et al. Endothelin-1 secretion form cultured vascular endothelial cells of DOCA-salt hypertensive rats. *Life Sci* 1996;59:PL1111–PL1116.
83. Clozel M, Breu V, Burri K, et al. Pathophysiological role of endothelin revealed by the first orally active endothelin receptor antagonist. *Nature* 1993;365:759–761.
84. Li JS, Schiffrin EL. Chronic endothelin receptor antagonist treatment of young spontaneously hypertensive rats. *J Hypertens* 1995;13:647–652.
85. Kitamura K, Tanaka T, Kato J, et al. Immunoreactive endothelin in rat kidney inner medulla: marked decrease in spontaneously hypertensive rats. *Biochem Biophys Res Commun* 1989;162:38–44.
86. Stasch JP, Hirth-Dietrich C, Frobel K, et al. Prolonged endothelin blockade prevents hypertension and cardiac hypertrophy in strokeprone spontaneously hypertensive rats. *Am J Hypertens* 1995;8:1128–1134.
87. Chillon JM, Heistad DD, Baumbach GL. Effect of endothelin receptor inhibition on cerebral arterioles in hypertensive rats. *Hypertension* 1996;27:794–798.
88. d'Uscio LV, Barton M, Shaw S, et al. Structure and function of small arteries in salt-induced hypertension: effects of chronic endothelin-subtype-A-receptor blockade. *Hypertension* 1997;30:905–911.
89. Li JS, Knafo L, Turgeon A, et al. Effect of endothelin antagonism on blood pressure and vascular structure in renovascular hypertensive rats. *Am J Physiol* 1996;271:H88–H93.
90. Ruschitzka FT, Shaw S, Gygi D, et al. Endothelial dysfunction in acute renal failure. Role of circulating and tissue endothelin- 1. *J Am Soc Nephrol* 1998. In press
91. Sventek P, Turgeon A, Schiffrin EL. Vascular and cardiac overexpression of endothelin-1 gene in 1-kidney, one clip Goldblatt hypertensive rats but only in the late phase 2-kidney, one clip Goldblatt hypertension. *J Hypertens* 1996;14:57–64.
92. d'Uscio LV, Moreau P, Shaw S, et al. Effects of chronic ETA-receptor blockade in angiotension 11-induced hypertension. *Hypertension* 1996;29:435–441.
93. Donckier JE, Massart PE, Hodeige D, et al. Additional hypotensive effects of ET-1 receptor antagonism in hypertensive dogs already under ACE inhibition. *Circulation* 1997;96:1250–1256.
94. Sventek P, Turgeon A, Schiffrin EL. Vascular endothelin-1 gene expression and effect on blood pressure of chronic ETA-receptor antagonism after nitric oxide synthase inhibition with l-NMMA in normal rats. *Circulation* 1997;95:240–244.
95. Moreau P, Takase H, Kung CF, et al. Blood pressure and vascular effects of endothelin blockade in chronic nitric oxide deficient hypertension. *Hypertension* 1997;29:763–769.
96. Verma S, Bhanot S, McNeill JH. Effect of chronic endothelin blockade in hyperinsulemic hypertensive rats. *Am J Physiol* 1995;269(pt 2):H2017–H2021.
97. Niranjan V, Telemaque S, Dewit D, et al. Systemic hypertension induced by hepatic overexpression of human preproendothelin-1 in rats. *J Clin Invest* 1996;98:2364–2372.

98. Hocher B, Liefeldt L, Thone-Reineke C, et al. Characterization of the renal phenotype of transgenic rats expressing the human endothelin-2 gene. *Hypertension* 1996;28:196–201.

99. Kurihara Y, Kurihara H, Kuwaki T, et al. Targeted disruprion of mouse endothelin-1 gene (Il): Elevated blood pressure in heterozygotes. *Circulation* 1993;88:1–332.

100. Krum H, Viskoper RJ, Lacourciere Y, et al. The effect of an endothelin-receptor antagonist, bosentan, on blood pressure in patients with essenetial hypertension. *N Engl J Med* 1998;338:784–790.

101. Stewart DJ, Levy RD, Cernacek P, et al. Increased plasma endothelin-1 in pulmonary hypertension: Marker or mediator of disease? *Ann Intern Med* 1991;114:464–469.

102. Ishikawa S, Miyauchi T, Salcai S, et al. Elevated levels of plasma endothelin-1 in young patients with pulmonary hypertension caused by congenital heart disease are decreased after successful surgical repair. *J Thorac Cardiovasc Surg* 1996;110:271–273.

103. Cody RJ, Haas GJ, Binkley PF, et al. Plasma endothelin correlates with the extent of pulmonary hypertension in patients with congestive heart failure. *Circulation* 1992;85:504–509.

104. Giaid A, Yanagisawa M, Langleben D, et al. Expression of endothelin-1 in the lungs of patients with pulmonary hypertension. *N Engl J Med* 1993;328:17329.

105. Goerre S, Wenk M, Bärtsch P, et al. Endothelin-1 in pulmonary hypertension associated with high altitude. *Circulation* 1995;91:359–364.

106. Zamora MR, Stelzner TJ, Webb S, et al. Overexpression of endothelin-1 and enhanced growth of pulmonary artery smooth muscle cells from fawn-hooded rats. *Am J Physiol* 1996;270:L101–L109.

107. Filep JG, Fournier A, Foldes-Filep E. Acute pro-inflammatory actions of endothelin-1 in the guinea-pig lung: Involvement of ETA and ETB receptors. *Br J Pharamcol* 1995;115:227–236.

108. Mansoor AM, Honda M, Saida K, Iet al. Endothelin-induced remodeling in experimental pulmonary hypertension. *Biochem Biophys Res Commun* 1995;215:981–986.

109. Di Carlo VS, Chen SJ, Meng C, et al. ETA-receptor antagonist prevents and reverses chronic hypoxia-induced pulmonary hypertension in rat. *Am J Physiol* 1995;269:L690–L697.

110. Sakai S, Miyauchi T, Sakurai T, et al. Pulmonary hypertension caused by congestive heart failure is ameliorated by long-term application of an endothelin receptor antagonist. Increased expression of endothelin-1 messenger ribonucleic acid and endothelin-1-like immunoreactivity in the lung in congestive heart failure in rats. *J Am Coll Cardiol* 1996;28:1580–1588.

111. Okada M, Yamashiba C, Okada M, et al. Role of endothelin-1 in beagles with dehydromonocrotaline-induced pulmonary hypertension. *Circulation* 1995;92:114–119.

112. McCullough KM, MacLean MR. Endothelin B receptor-mediated contraction of human and rat pulmonary resistance arteries and the effect of pulmonary hypertension on endothelin responses in the rat. *J Cardiovasc Pharmacol* 1995;26(suppl 3):S169–S176.

113. Stewart DJ, Cernacek P, Costello KB, et al. Elevated endothelin-1 in heart failure and loss of normal response to postural change. *Circulation* 1992;85:510–517.

114. Wei CM, Lerman A, Rodeheffer RJ, et al. Endothelin in human congestive heart failure. *Circulation* 1994;89:1580–1586.

115. Pacher R, Stanek B, Hulsmann M, et al. Prognostic impact of big endothelin-1 plasma concentrations compared with invasive hemodynamic evaluation in severe heart failure. *J Am Coll Cardiol* 1996;27:633–641.

116. Clavell A, Stingo A, Margulies K, et al. Physiological significance of endothelin: its role in congestive heart failure. *Circulation* 1993;87(suppl 5):45–50.

117. Teerlink JR, Löffler BM, Hess P, et al. Role of endothlein in the maintenance of blood pressure in conscious rats with chronic heart failure: Acute effects of the

endothelin receptor antagonist RO 47–0203 (bosentan). *Circulation* 1994;90: 2510–2518.

118. Spinale FG, Walher JD, Mukheerjee R, et al. Concomitant endothelin receptor subtype-A blockade during the progresssion of pacing-induced congestive heart failure in rabbits. Beneficial effects on left ventricular and myocyte function. *Circulation* 1997;95:1918–1929.

119. Ono K, Tsujimoto G, Sakamoto A, et al. Endothelin-a receptor mediates cardiac inhibition by regulating calcium and potassium currents. *Nature* 1994;370:301–304.

120. Kelly RA, Eid H, Kramer BK, et al. Endothelin enhances the contractile responsiveness of adult rat ventricular myocytes to calcium by a pertussis toxin-sensitive pathway. *J Clin Invest* 1990;86:1164–1171.

121. James AF, Xie LH, Fujitani Y, et al. Inhibition of the cardiac protein kinase A-dependent chloride conductance by endothelin-1. *Nature* 1994;370:297–300.

122. Ito H, Hirata Y, Hiroe M, et al. Endothelin-1 induces hypertrophy with enhanced expression of muscle specific-genes in cultured neonatal rat cardiomyocytes. *Circ Res* 1991;69:209–215.

123. McClellan G, Weisberg A, Winegrad S. Effect of endothelin-1 on actynomyosin ATPase activity: Implications for the efficiency of contraction. *Circ Res* 1996;78: 1044–1050.

124. Kramer BK, Smith TW, Kelly RA. Endothelin and increased contractility in adult rat ventricular myocytes: Role of ontracellular alkalosis induced by activation of the protein kinase C-dependent $NA^+–H^+$ exchanger. *Circ Res* 1991;68:269–279.

125. Sakai S, Miyauchi T, Kobayashi M, et al. Inhibition of myocardial endothelin pathway improves long-term survival in heart failure. *Nature* 1996;384:353–355.

126. Shimoyama H, Sabbah HN, Borzak S, et al. Short-term hemodynamic effects of endothelin receptor blockade in dogs with chronic heart failure. *Circulation* 1996; 94:779–784.

127. Kiowski W, Sutsch G, Hunziker P, et al. Evidence for endothelin-1-mediated vasoconstriction in severe chronic heart failure. *Lancet* 1995;346:732–736.

128. Love MP, Haynes WG, Gray GA, et al. Vasodilator effects of endothelin-converting enzyme inhibition and endothelin ETA receptor blockade in chronic heart failure patients treated with ACE inhibitors. *Circulation* 1996;94:2131–2137.

129. Brunner F, Kukovetz W. Postischemic antiarrhythmetic effects of angiotensin-converting enzyme inhibitors. Role of suppression of endogenous endothelin secretion. *Circulation* 1996;94:1752–1761.

130. Harrison DG, Freiman PC, Armstrong ML, et al. Alterations of vascular reactivity in atherosclerosis. *Circ Res* 1987;61:1174–1180.

131. Creager MA, Cooke JP, Mendelsohn ME, et al. Impaired vasodilation of forearm resistance vessels in hypercholesterolemic humans. *J Clin Invest* 1990;86:228–234.

132. Tanner FC, Noll G, Boulanger CM, et al. Oxidized low density lipoproteins inhibit relaxations of porcine coronary arteries. Role of scavenger receptor and endothelium-derived nitric oxide. *Circulation* 1991;83:2012–2020.

133. Minor R Jr, Myers PR, Guerra R Jr, et al. Diet induced atherosclerosis increases the release of nitrogen oxides from rabbit aorta. *J Clin Invest* 1990;86:2109–2116.

134. Yla-Herttuala S, Palinski W, Rosenfeld ME, et al. Evidence for the presence of oxidatively modified low density lipoprotein in atherosclerotic lesions of rabbit and man. *J Clin Invest* 1989;84:1086–1095.

135. Boulanger CM, Tanner FC, Bea ML, et al. Oxidized low density lipoproteins induce mRNA expression and release of endothelin from human and porcine endothelium. *Circ Res* 1992;70:1191–1197.

136. Lüscher TF, Oemar BS, Boulanger CM, et al. Molecular and cellular biology of endothelin and its receptors–Part II. *J Hypertens* 1993;11:121–126.

137. Lerman A, Edwards BS, Hallett JW, et al. Circulating and tissue endothelin immunoreactivity in advanced atherosclerosis. *New Engl J Med* 1991;325:997–1001.

138. Zeiher AM, Ihling C, Pistorius K, et al. Increased tissue endothelin immunoreactivity in atherosclerotic lesions associated with acute coronary syndromes. *Lancet* 1994;344:1405–1406.

139. Mathew V, Cannan C, Miller VM, et al. Enhanced endothelin-mediated coronary vasoconstriction and attenuated basal nitric oxide activity in experimental hypercholesterolemia. *Circulation* 1997;96:1930–1936.

140. Haug C, Voisard R, Lenich A, et al. Increased endothelin release by cultured human smooth muscle cells from atherosclerotic coronary arteries. *Cardiovasc Res* 1996;31:807–813.

141. Timm M, Kaski JC, Dashwood MR. Endothelin-like immunoreactivity in atherosclerotic human coronary arteries. *J Cardiovasc Pharmacol* 1995;26:S442–S444.

142. Dagassan PH, Breu V, Clozel M, et al. Up-regulation of endothelin b-receptors in atherosclerotic human coronary arteries. *J Cardiovasc Pharmacol* 1996;l27:147–153.

143. Goller N, Recce R, Beyer S, et al. Selective blockade of the endothelin subtype A receptor decreases early atherosclerosis in hamsters fed cholesterol. *Am J Pathol* 1995;146:819–826.

144. Barton M, Shaw S, d'Uscio LV, et al. Endothelin ETA receptor blockade restores NO-mediated endothelial function and inhibits atherosclerosis in apolipoprotein E-deficient mice.. *Proc Natl Acad Sci U S A:* 1998;95:14367–14372.(

145. Toyo-oka T, Aizawa T, Suzuki N, et al. Increased plasma level of endothelin-1 and coronary spasm induction in patients with vasospastic angina pectoris. *Circulation* 1991;83:476–483.

146. Stewart DJ, Kubac G, Costello KB, et al. Increased plasma endothelin-1 in the early hours of acute myocardial infarction. *J Am Coll Cardiol* 1991;18:38–43.

147. Omland T, Terje Lie R, Aakvaag A, et al. Plasma endothelin determination as a prognostic indicator of 1-year mortality after acute myocardial infarction. *Circulation* 1994;89:1573–1579.

148. Richard V, Kaeffer N, Hogie M, et al. Role of endogenous endothelin in myocardial and endothelial injury after ischemia and reperfusion in rats: studies with bosentan, a mixed ETA/ETB antagonist. *Br J Pharmacol* 1994;113:869–876.

149. Watanabe T, Awane Y, Ikeda S, et al. Pharamcology of the non-selective ETA and ETB receptor antagonist TAK-044 and the inhibition of myocardial infarct size in rats. *Br J Pharmacol* 1995;114:949–954.

150. Mertz TE, McClanghan TB, Flynn MA, et al. EndothelinA receptor antagonism by PD 156707 does not reduce infarct after coronary artery occlusion/reperfusion in pigs. *J Pharmacol Exp Ther* 1996;29:87–92.

151. Burke SE, Nelson RA. Endothelin-receptor antagonist FR 139317 reduces infarct size in a rabbit model when given before, but not after, coronary artery occlusion. *J Cardiovasc Pharamcol* 1997;29:87–92.

152. Tahara A, Kohno M, Yanagi S, et al. Circulating immunoreactive endothelin in patients undergoing percutaneous transluminal coronary angioplasty. *Metabolism* 1991;40:1235–1237.

153. Hasdai D, Holmes DR, Garrat KN, et al. Mechanical pressure and stretch release endothelin-1 from human atherosclerotic coronary arteries in vivo. *Circulation* 1997;95:357–362.

154. Wang X, Douglas SA, Louden C, et al. Expression of endothelin-1, endothelin-3, endothelin-converting enzyme-1, and endothelin-A and endothelin-B receptor mRNA after angioplasty-induced neointimal formation in the rat. *Circ Res* 1996;78:322–328.

155. Douglas SA, Vickery-Clark LM, et al. Endothelin receptor subtypes in the pathogenesis of angioplasty-induced neointima formation in the rat: a comparison of selective ETA receptor antagonism and dual ETA/ETB receptor antagonism using BQ-123 and SB 209670. *J Cardiovasc Pharmacol* 1996;26(suppl 3):S186–S189.

156. Minamino T, Kurihara H, Takahashi M, et al. Endothelin-converting enzyme expression in the rat vascular injury model and human coronary atherosclerosis. *Circulation* 1997;95:221 - 230.

157. Kirchengast M, Münter K, Hergenröder M, et al. Effect of ETA receptor antagonism on coronary artery hemodynamics and remodelling. *Vasa* 1998;27:216–219.

## Chapter 10

# Endothelial Nitric Oxide and Vascular Inflammation

*James K. Liao, MD*

## Introduction

Nitric oxide (NO) is an endogenous vasodilator, which was described initially as endothelium-derived relaxing factor (EDRF).[1,2] The activity of endothelium-derived NO is not only a marker of endothelial function but also plays an important physiological role in the regulation of blood pressure and blood flow.[3,4] Therefore, it is not surprising to find that endothelial dyfunction or the lack of EDRF often is associated with cardiovascular diseases such as hypertension, atherosclerosis, and congestive heart failure. Although the mechanism by which NO mediates vasodilation occurs via activation of soluble guanylyl cyclase in vascular smooth muscle, there is growing evidence that NO may exert effects on other cell types that are independent of cyclic guanosine monophosphate (cGMP). As a result, the role of NO in the vessel wall has expanded beyond those of a vasodilator.

The NO is synthesized in many cell types from the conversion of L-arginine to L-citrulline.[4] At least three distinct NO synthases (NOSs) have been identified and found to produce various amounts of NO under different conditions. For example, both the neuronal NOS (nNOS; type I) and the endothelial NOS (eNOS; type III) isoforms are calcium-dependent and produce low levels of NO constitutively; whereas, sustained, high levels of NO are produced by macrophage or smooth muscle inducible NOS (iNOS; type II) only after induction by certain cytokines. The localization of these various NOSs in specific cell types other than vascular wall cells suggests that NO may mediate other signaling pathways in different organ systems. Such differences in the regulation and localization of these NOSs, therefore, may underlie their importance and contributions in homeostatic and inflammatory processes.

The diversity of NO-mediated processes results not only from the biological actions of NO itself, but also from the complex biochemical interactions between NO and its surrounding environment. Such environmental factors including the presence of reactive oxygen species and antioxidants can determine the ultimate biological effects and biochemical status of NO and its

From Panza JA, Cannon RO III (eds): *Endothelium, Nitric Oxide, and Atherosclerosis* ©Futura Publishing Co, Inc, Armonk, NY, 1999.

derivatives.[5,6] For example, NO can form a potent oxidant, peroxynitrite, through its interaction with superoxide anion.[7] Indeed, some of the neurotoxicity of NO in cerebral ischemia/reperfusion injury may be caused by the formation of peroxynitrite.[8] Furthermore, interaction of NO with thiol derivatives produces nitrosothiols, which can modify the activities of signaling molecules such as mitogen-activated protein (MAP) kinases and p21*ras* via S-nitrosylation.[9] Thus, NO can mediate disparate and sometimes contradictory effects in different cell types and conditions.

Recent studies from many laboratories have shown that NO modulates gene expression via its effects on multiple signaling pathways. For example, NO activates protein tyrosine phosphatases in peripheral blood mononuclear cells leading to the possiblity that NO regulates various transcription factors, which are tyrosine phosphorylated such as signal transducers and activators of transcription (STATs) and interferon regulatory factor (IRF)-1. Oxidants such as hydrogen peroxide and pervanadate stimulate protein tyrosine phosphorylation and activate transcription factors downstream of MAP kinase pathways such as p38 c-*jun* kinase (JNK) and nuclear factor–kappa B (NF-κB). Because NO can avidly scavenge superoxide anion, it can prevent superoxide anion from forming its dismutation product, hydrogen peroxide. Furthermore, under certain conditions, NO may act as an electron donor or antioxidant.[5] Indeed, antioxidants such as *N*-acetylcysteine (NAC) or pyrrolidine dithiocarbamate (PDTC) inhibit the activation of the transcription factors, AP-1 and NF-κB. Finally, S-nitrosylation of p21*ras* by nitrosothiols also may lead to the activation of NF-κB and JNK, which are involved in endothelial cell activation and proliferation.[9]

## Role of Nitric Oxide in Atherogenesis and Vascular Inflammation

An early step in atherogenesis and vascular inflammation is the activation of endothelial cells.[10] The activated endothelium expresses cell surface adhesion molecules such as vascular cell adhesion molecule (VCAM) 1, intercellular adhesion molecule (ICAM) 1, and E-selectin, which facilitate the attachment of peripheral blood leukocytes to the endothelial surface.[11] Monocyte adhesion to the vessel wall and subsequent differentiation of these cells into macrophages is required for the development of macrophage-derived–foam cells in atherosclerotic vessels. Thus, factors such as cytokines, which promote monocyte-endothelial cell interaction, may play important roles in the initiation and propagation of atherosclerosis and vascular inflammation.

Vessels affected by atherosclerosis develop endothelial dysfunction as indicated by impaired vasomotor function caused by the decreased synthesis, release, and/or activity of endothelial-derived NO.[2,4] Endothelial dysfunction, in turn, may contribute to the atherogenic process because growing evidence indicates that NO may be anti-inflammatory. For example, reduced endothelium-derived NO activity contributes to impaired vascular relaxation, enhanced platelet aggregation and increased vascular smooth muscle proliferation, and

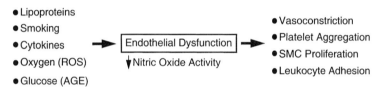

- Lipoproteins
- Smoking
- Cytokines → Endothelial Dysfunction →
- Oxygen (ROS)    ↓Nitric Oxide Activity
- Glucose (AGE)

- Vasoconstriction
- Platelet Aggregation
- SMC Proliferation
- Leukocyte Adhesion

**Figure 1.**   Factors that lead to endothelial dyfunction or decreased endothelial nitric oxide synthase (eNOS) activity. Abbreviations: ROS, reactive oxygen species; AGE, advanced glycation endproducts; SMC, smooth muscle cells; LDL, low-density lipoprotein. Reproduced with permission from Reference 31.

endothelial–leukocyte interactions (Figure 1).[12–14] Inactivation of endothelium-derived NO by $\cdot O_2^-$ generated from angiotensin II–stimulated nicotinamide-adenine dinucleotide (NADH) oxidase can lead to nitrate tolerance, vasoconstriction, and hypertension. Mutant mice lacking endothelial type III eNOS have hypertension and develop greater proliferative and inflammatory vascular response to cuff injury.

On the other hand, in vivo transfer of eNOS gene into balloon-injured vessels decreases intimal smooth muscle cell proliferation in rat carotid arteries. Enriching the diets of cholesterol-fed rabbits with L-arginine, the precursor of NO, improves endothelial-dependent relaxation, reduces leukocyte attachment to the endothelial surface, and limits the extent of atherosclerotic lesions. In fact, a single bolus treatment with a NO-generating compound, S-nitrosothiol, has been shown to inhibit intimal smooth muscle proliferation of the rabbit carotid artery following injury with a balloon-tip catheter.

## Nitric Oxide and Endothelial–Leukocyte Interaction

Although cGMP mediates many effects of NO such as vasodilation and inhibition of vascular smooth muscle proliferation and platelet aggregation, the ability of NO to attenuate leukocyte attachment to the endothelial surface is not dependent on cGMP formation.[15,16] For example, NO donors but not cGMP analogues decrease cytokine-induced expression of endothelial cell adhesion molecules and other proinflammatory mediators such as macrophage-colony stimulating factor (M-CSF or CSF-1), IL-6, and IL-8 via cGMP-independent pathways.[17]

Recent studies have shown that NO inhibits monocyte adhesion to the endothelial surface. In vivo studies demonstrate that inhibition of endogenous NO production by $N^\omega$-nitro-L-arginine methylester (L-NAME) promotes vasoconstriction and leukocyte adhesion to the endothelium during ischemia reperfusion injury in splanchnic vessels.[18] Indeed, NO inhibits monocyte adhesion to endothelium in vitro, without altering expression of CD11b/CD18, one of the cognate ligands on monocytes for certain endothelial–leukocyte adhesion molecules. In experiments superfusing a cat mesenteric preparation with inhibitors of NO production, Kubes and collaborators also showed that such inhibitors increase leukocyte (mostly neutrophil) adhesion to mesenteric venules.[19]

They also showed that increased expression of CD11b/CD18 on the leukocyte surface could not account for L-NAME's effect.

Other studies, however, have documented increased monocyte adhesion to mesenteric endothelial cells in vivo by L-NAME and reversal by cGMP analogues. These studies contrast with finding from others who found that cGMP analogues do not affect cytokine-induced expression of adhesion molecules.[19,20] Several possibilities could account for this difference. First, these in vivo studies showed induction of endothelial–leukocyte adhesion by L-NAME rather than by cytokines. Perhaps induction of VCAM-1 by L-NAME, but not by cytokines, is amenable to reversal by cGMP analogues. Second, these studies cannot separate cGMP effects on hemodynamics and/or leukocytes from direct alterations in endothelial functions. Furthermore, induction of other adhesion molecules (ie. ICAM-1 or E-selectin) by L-NAME treatment may depend partially on cGMP-dependent pathways.

Inhibition of endogenous endothelial NO production by $N^G$-monomethyl-L-arginine (L-NMMA) mildly induces VCAM-1 expression in cultured saphenous vein endothelial cells,[15,20] while exposure of cytokine-activated endothelial cells to an NO donor, S-nitrosoglutathione (GSNO), greatly diminishes leukocyte adhesion to the endothelial surface.[21] Thus, endothelial cells, therefore, serve as a potential target of NO's effect in limiting leukocyte adhesion to the vessel wall.

## Nuclear Factor-$\kappa$ B and Transcriptional Induction of Proinflammatory Genes

The genes that encode a number of cellular adhesion molecules and cytokines implicated in atherogenesis share specific DNA binding motifs in their promoters, which interact with the proinflammatory transcription factor NF-$\kappa$B (Table 1).[22,23] The NF-$\kappa$B originally was described as a heterodimeric cytosolic protein in lymphocytes, which on activation, translocates into the nucleus where it binds to specific decameric sequences in the immunoglobulin G-$\kappa$ (IgG-$\kappa$) light chain enhancer. Subsequent studies have shown that this nuclear-binding protein also can activate viral enhancer elements. All members of the mammalian NF-$\kappa$B family possess Rel homology domains, which are necessary for dimerization, nuclear translocation, and DNA binding.

The NF-$\kappa$B family can be divided further into two groups based on their structure and function. The first group consists of p65 (RelA), c-Rel, and RelB, which contain transcriptional activation domains necessary for gene induction. The second group consists of p105 and p100, which on proteolytic processing give rise to p50 (NF-$\kappa$B1) and p52 (NF-$\kappa$B2), respectively. The carboxy terminal regions of p105 and p100 share structural features with the endogenous NF-$\kappa$B inhibitor (I-$\kappa$B) and, thus functions to retain NF-$\kappa$B in the cytoplasm. However, the mature proteins p50 and p52 can form functional dimers with members of both groups. With the exception of RelB, which cannot form homodimers, members of both groups can bind in a tissue-specific manner as homo- or heterodimers to enhancer elements of target genes. In vascular

Table 1
**Genes Requiring Nuclear Factor-Kappa B (NF-κB)
for Transactivation**

Cellular adhesion molecules
  Intercellular adhesion molecule-1 (ICAM-1)
  Vascular cell adhesion molecule-1 (VCAM-1)
  Endothelial leukocyte adhesion molecule-1 (ELAM-1 or E-Selectin)

Inflammatory cytokines
  Interleukin (IL)-2, -6, and -8
  Tumor necrosis factor (TNF)-$\alpha$ and -$\beta$
  Macrophage-colony stimulating factor (M-CSF or CSF-1)
  Granulocyte-colony stimulating factor (G-CSF)
  Granulocyte/macrophage-colony stimulating factor (GM-CSF)
  Interferon-$\beta$
  Tissue factor
  Macrophage chemotactic protein-1 (MCP-1)

Immunologic mediators
  Immunoglobulin (IgG)-$\kappa$ light chain
  T-cell receptor-$\alpha$ and -$\beta$ chain
  Major histocompatability complex (MHC) class I
  MHC class II invariant chain (Ii)
  $\beta_2$-Microglobulin
  Type II inducible nitric oxide synthase (iNOS)

Viral enhancers
  Human immunodeficiency virus-1 (HIV-1)
  Cytomegalovirus (CMV)
  Adenovirus
  Simian virus 40 (SV40)

Transcription factors
  I-$\kappa$B-$\alpha$
  c-Rel
  NF-kB p105
  c-myc
  Interferon regulatory factor-1 (IRF-1)

Reproduced with permission from Reference 32.

endothelial cells, the transcriptional induction of proinflammatory genes predominantly depends on the activation of the RelA/p50 heterodimer.[23]

The NF-κB is activated under numerous conditions associated with vascular inflammation (Table 2). For example, bacterial or viral products such as lipopolysaccharide (LPS) or double-stranded RNA can trigger the activation of NF-κB.[22] In addition, the production of cytokines and growth factors at sites of inflammation also can activate NF-κB. There is growing evidence that reactive oxygen species (ROS) such as hydrogen peroxide ($H_2O_2$) and possibly peroxynitrite ($ONOO^-$) contibutes to cellular "oxidative stress" and may be a common pathway for the activation of NF-κB (Figure 2).[24] Indeed, recent studies have shown that the dismutated product of superoxide anion ($O_2^-$), $H_2O_2$ is a potent oxidant, which not only can activate NF-κB but also other transcription factors such as AP-1 and *egr*-1. These findings suggest that activation of NF-κB and endothelial cells occur, through generation of ROS

---

Table 2
**Factors That Activate NF-κB**

---

Inflammatory mediators
  TNF-α
  IL-1 and -2
  Lymphotoxin
  Leukotriene B4

Growth factors
  Platelet-derived growth factor (PGDF)
  Transformin growth factor-β1 (TGF-β1)

Viral mediators
  Viral infection (HIV, EBV, CMV, etc.)
  Double-stranded RNA
  Epstein–Barr nuclear antigen-2

Bacterial mediators
  Lipopolysaccharide (LPS)
  Muramyl proteins
  Exotoxin B

Oxidants
  Hydrogen peroxide
  Ultraviolet light

Drugs
  Phorbolesters
  Okadaic acid
  Cycloheximide
  Anisomycin
  Pervanadate

Physical stress
  Laminar shear stress
  Stretch
  Cyclic strain

---

Reproduced with permission from Reference 32.

and that antioxidants would be effective inhibitors of NF-κB and endothelial cell activation.

The activation of NF-κB involves the degradation of its cytoplasmic inhibitor I-κB and activation of bound protein kinase A (Figure 3). Presently, five distinct I-κB proteins (I-κB-α, -β, -γ, -δ, and -ε) have been described and function to retain NF-κB in the cytoplasm and render it inactive.[25] These I-κB proteins contain ankyrin repeat motifs, which mask the nuclear localization sequence of NF-κB subunits. Of the different I-κB proteins, the most well characterized is I-κB-α, a 37-kd protein. Following cytokine stimulation or oxidative stress, I-κB-α is phosphorylated by a novel ubiquitinated serine kinase NF-κB inhibitor called Iκ-B kinase (IKK).

However, the signaling pathway from cytokine interaction with cell surface receptors to phosphorylation of I-κB-α involves the recruitment of many other kinases into a large protein complex. Stimulation with tumor necrosis factor α TNF-α induces a trimerization of TNF receptor 1 and 2 (TNFR-1 and TNFR-2). The signaling domain of both receptors interacts with certain cytoplasmic proteins such as TNFR-1–associated death domain (TRADD) protein,

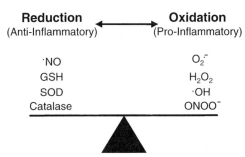

**Figure 2.** Redox balance in the vascular wall. Oxidants, especially superoxide anion ($O_2^-$) and its dismutation product hydrogen peroxide ($H_2O_2$) produced by vascular smooth muscle cells and macrophages oxidize low-density lipoprotein and activate oxidant-sensitive transcription factors such as NF-$\kappa$B leading to the transcriptional induction of proinflammatory genes. Hydroxyl radical ($\cdot$OH) is generated by catalysis of $H_2O_2$ in the presence of transitional metals while peroxynitrite ($ONOO^-$) is formed by the interaction of $O_2^-$ and NO ($\cdot$NO). The cellular antioxidant or anti-inflammatory mechanisms include $\cdot$NO, glutathione (GSH), superoxide dismutase (SOD), and catalase. Note that $\cdot$NO can participate on both sides depending on the enviromental mileiu. Reproduced with permission from Reference 31.

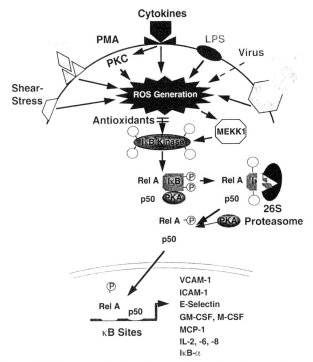

**Figure 3.** Schematic diagram of signaling pathway leading to the activation of NF-$\kappa$B. Reproduced with permission from Reference 32.

Fas-associated death domain (FADD) protein, and TNFR- associated factor 2 (TRAF-2). The TRAF-2 interacts directly with TNFR-2 and indirectly via TRADD and receptor interacting protein (RIP) with TNFR-1. The downstream target of TRAF-2 is a member of the MAP kinase kinase kinase (MAPKKK) family called the NF-κB–inducing kinase (NIK). The NIK has been shown to activate directly IKK. The NIK interacts with I-κB-associated protein (IAP) and I-κB kinases (IKK). Phosphorylation of NIK, IAP, and IKK is required for the activation of IKK.

Recently, at least two kinase subunits, IKK-1 (or CHUK) and IKK-2, have been identified. Both IKK-1 and -2 phosphorylate serine residues 32 and 36 of the I-κB-α protein. Phosphorylation of I-κB-α targets the I-κB-α for ubiquitination and rapid degradation by 26S proteasomes. The proteasomes are large multimeric assemblies of intracellular enzymes, which digest proteins marked for degradation by ubiquitination. Serine phosphorylation of p105 and p100 targets these proteins for limited proteolytic cleavage rather than complete degradation through the ubiquitin-proteasome pathway. The degradation of I-κB-α or proteolytic cleavage of p105/p100 then allows the unbound NF-κB to translocate into the nucleus where it can transactivate the κB enhancer elements in the regulator region of proinflammatory genes (Table 1).

Because the phosphorylation of I-κB-α by IKK is a key regulatory step in the activation of NF-κB, factors that influence IKK activity might modulate inflammatory processes. Indeed, recent studies indicate that salicylates and agents with antioxidant activity such as NAC or PDTC inhibit cytokine-induced NF-κB by preventing I-κB-α phosphorylation. Alternatively, stabilization of phosphorylated I-κB-α by inhibitors of 26S proteasomes such as the peptide aldehyde derivatives MG132 or lactacystin attenuates cytokine-induced VCAM-1 expression in endothelial cells. However, evidence indicates that NO and antioxidants prevent NF-κB activation by different mechanisms.[26]

Interestingly, one of the main factors that limits NF-κB activity is NF-κB itself. Depending on the species, the I-κB-α promoter contains at least three to five functional κB-binding sites. Thus, the induction of I-κB-α by NF-κB serves as an inducible autoregulatory feedback mechanism for terminating NF-κB activity.[27] However, the induction of I-κB-α is not limited to NF-κB. Recent studies have demonstrated that the glucocorticoids can modulate NF-κB stability and transcriptionally induce the expression of I-κB-α in T lymphocytes (ie, Jurkat cells).[28,29] Consequently, the induction of I-κB-α by glucocorticoids and the subsequent inhibition of NF-κB activity may underlie some of the anti-inflammatory effects of glucocorticoids.

# Nitric Oxide and Nuclear Factor-κB Activation

Vascular endothelial cells produce NO constitutively and can express the inducible isoform of NOS in response to cytokine stimulation. Thus, the net activation of NF-κB in vascular wall cells during inflammation probably de-

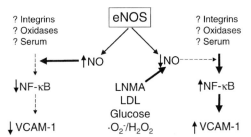

**Figure 4.** Endothelial dysfunction can lead to endothelial cell activation. Inactivation or decrease production of NO allows many factors such as integrins and oxidases to activate the proinflammatory transcription factor NF-κB. Unhindered activation of NF-κB leads to the expression of cellular adhesion molecules such as VCAM-1. Reproduced with permission from Reference 32.

pends on a complex balance between stimulatory and inhibitory factors. The finding that inhibition of endogenous eNO (eNO) production by L-NMMA could activate NF-κB, induce VCAM-1 expression, and stimulate endothelial–leukocyte adhesion suggests that constitutively produced NO may play an important physiological role in tonically inhibiting endothelial cell activation under basal conditions (Figure 4).[16,17] This inhibitory effect of NO also is supported by the finding in vivo that inhibition of endogenous NO production by L-NAME promotes endothelial–leukocyte interactions through the expression of NF-κB-dependent adhesion molecules.

Although under static conditions, cultured endothelial cells do not produce sufficient NO to inhibit cytokine-induced activation of NF-κB, higher levels of NO may be produced by endothelial cells in vivo in response to fluid shear stress, which is known to stimulate endothelial cell type III eNOS gene transcription. As eNOS expression increases with shear stress, regions of normal laminar flow may have sufficient NO production to suppress NF-κB activation. However, regions of distrubed flow, lacking the stimulus to augment NO production, may lose this potentially protective action of NO. This phenomenon could help explain why the regions of physiological shear stress tend to be less susceptible to the development of nascent atherosclerotic lesions than regions of changing or disturbed flow (ie, near brach points or flow dividers), which have increased predilection to develop these lesions (Figure 5).

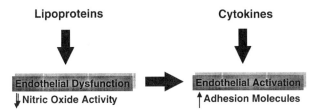

**Figure 5.** Relationship of endothelial dysfunction and endothelial cell activation. Endothelial dysfunction is defined as decreases in eNO activity whereas endothelial cell activation is defined as the expression of cellular adhesion molecules. Note that endothelial dysfunction can lead to endothelial cell activation. Reproduced with permission from Reference 32.

In addition to NO produced by eNOS, endothelial cells may encounter higher levels of NO generated by iNOS at sites of vascular inflammation. Exposure of rodent macrophages and human vascular smooth muscle cells to cytokines leads to the induction of iNOS, which produces substantially higher levels of NO compared with that of eNOS. Furthermore, compared with in vitro studies, higher NO concentrations could be achieved locally because endothelial cells are in close proximity to cells expressing iNOS in vivo. Indeed, iNOS produced by macrophages in coculture with endothelial cells inhibit the expression of endothelial cell adhesion molecules.[20,21] Thus, the amount of NO produced by iNOS can be approximated with NO donors, which have been shown to inhibit NF-κB activation.

Additionally, NO may form adducts with sulfhydryl compounds forming more stable nitrosothiols.[5,6] Such increased availability of NO may be required to suppress cytokine-activated NF-κB in endothelial cells. Interestingly, the higher levels of NO produced by activated macrophages also may provide for an endogenous feedback mechanism for limiting NO production because the induction of iNOS requires the activation of NF-κB. The regulation of NF-κB by NO, therefore, might serve as a mechanism by which NO can modulate the expression of various proinflammatory mediators during atherogenesis and vascular inflammation.

## Stabilization of Nuclear Factor-κB by Nitric Oxide

Treatment of cells with NO appears to stabilize the inactive NF-κB/I-κB-α complex following stimulation by cytokines (Figure 4).[30] By preventing the degradation of I-κB-α, the NF-κB is retained in the cytoplasm and hence cannot activate transcription of target genes within the nucleus. Several studies indicate that antioxidants such as NAC or PDTC stabilize the NF-κB/I-κB-α complex through scavenging ROS such as superoxide anion and inhibiting I-κB kinase activity. However, NO does not inhibit IKK activity or prevent the degradation of I-κB-α following cytokine stimulation.[26] Thus, NO and antioxidants exert differential effects on NF-κB activation in terms of I-κB-α phosphorylation.

In contrast, recent studies have shown that NO produces some of its effects through its interaction with thiol groups to form nitrosothiols.[5,6] Nitrosothiols such as GSNO, in turn, can modify the activity of signaling molecules via protein S-nitrosylation. For example, S-nitrosylation of the prokaryotic oxygen-sensitive transcription factor OxyR leads to its activation via S-nitrosylation of critical cysteine residues. The S-nitrosylation of p21ras, which is involved in mitogenesis and possibly NF-κB activation, induces guanosine triphosphate/guanosine diphosphate (GTP/GDP) exchange on p21ras.[9] Thus, the generation of nitrosothiols by NO may be an important pathway for activating NF-κB in unstimulated endothelial cells. However, these effects of nitrosothiols are not consistent with the net effect of NO on cytokine-stimulated endothelial cells, an inhibitor of NF-κB activation.

# Enhanced Nuclear Translocation of Nuclear Factor-κB by Nitric Oxide

Of particular interest is the ability of I-κB-α to inhibit NF-κB–mediated signaling events in the nucleus.[21] Recent studies have demonstrated that I-κB-α can translocate into the nucleus and displace NF-κB subunits from their cognate DNA sequences. It is somewhat surprising though that I-κB-α can enter the nucleus because the carboxyterminus of I-κB-α contains multiple ankyrin repeat motifs, which may inhibit its entry into the cell nucleus. Nevertheless, the nuclear translocation of I-κB-α has been documented by several investigators and appears to constitute an effective mechanism that can terminate rapidly NF-κB–mediated transactivation of proinflammatory genes.

However, it is not known for certain whether enhanced nuclear translocation of I-κB-α results from an active I-κB-α nuclear transporter or if it is the result of passive diffusion of increased amounts of newly synthesized I-κB-α. For example, nuclear translocation of I-κB-α occurs following stimulation with TNF-α, which also induces I-κB-α synthesis indirectly via activation of NF-κB. Thus, the process of nuclear translocation of I-κB-α may not be restricted to the actions of NO, but rather occurs through a more general mechanism for terminating NF-κB transactivation.

# Induction of Nuclear Factor-κB Inhibitor-α by Nitric Oxide

A particularly novel effect of NO is its ability to induce the expression of I-κB-α (Figure 6).[21,30] Exposure to NO does not affect the expression of NF-κB subunits RelA and p50, or cause the activation of NF-κB in human endothelial cells. However, several recent studies noted an increase in NF-κB activation by NO-generating compounds in peripheral blood mononuclear cells. Perhaps differences in the intracellular redox regulation of thiols in different cell types could account for the observed differences between endothelial cells and peripheral blood mononuclear cells. Furthermore, the actions of NO may be quite different depending on whether or not the cells have been activated by cytokines.

Transfection studies using the I-κB-α promoter linked to the chloramphenicol acetyltransferase reporter gene suggests that the induction of I-κB-α by NO occurs at the transcriptional level.[26,30] Previous analyses of the human, porcine, and murine I-κB-α promoters have revealed multiple functional κB sites necessary for transcriptional induction by NF-κB. All of these sites are located within -350 bp of the transcriptional start site and provide for an inducible autoregulatory pathway for terminating the activation of NF-κB.[27] However, NO's effects on I-κB-α gene transcription probably is not mediated by NF-κB because NO inhibits NF-κB and alone does not induce VCAM-1 gene transcription. Further analyses of the upstream I-κB-α promoter will be

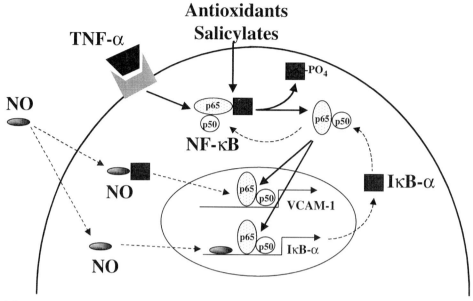

**Figure 6.** Schematic diagram showing the potential mechanisms by which NO inhibits NF-κB activity. Note that NO induces the transcription and enhances the nuclear translocation of the NF-κB inhibitor I-κB-α while antioxidants and salicylates prevent I-κB-α phosphorylation and degradation. Reproduced with permission from Reference 32.

necessary to determine which DNA-binding domain(s) constitute the NO-responsive *cis*-regulatory element(s) in the I-κB-α promoter.

The induction of I-κB-α gene transcription also occurs following treatment with corticosteroids in Jurkat or T cells.[28,29] However, we have observed that the induction of I-κB-α by glucocorticoids in vascular endothelial cells is modest at best, producing only about a twofold increase in I-κB-α steady-state mRNA levels compared with greater than 10-fold with NO (unpublished observations). It is possible that NO and glucocorticoids may share similar or identical pathways for transactivating the I-κB-α gene. It remains to be determined whether NO production in endothelial cells mediates the induction of I-κB-α by glucocorticoids.

## Summary

The role of NO in biological processes continues to expand. This discussion has described how this endogenous mediator can affect vascular inflammation via regulation of NF-κB. Elucidation of the further molecular mechanisms by which NO or its derivatives regulate I-κB-α stability and gene transcription remains to be determined. Thus, what started as a mysterious and evanescent vasodilator in the pharmacology laboratory and as a nefarious pollutant by atmospheric chemists has now emerged as a novel regulator of vascular inflammation. Further investigation into NO's effects will undoubtly furnish further surprises in the future.

# References

1. Furchgott RF, Zawadzki JV. The obligatory role of endothelial cells in the relaxation of arterial smooth muscle muscle by acetylcholine. *Nature* 1980;288:373–376.
2. Ignarro LJ, Buga GM, Wood KS, et al. Endothelium-derived relaxing factor produced and released from artery and vein is nitric oxide. *Proc Natl Acad Sci U S A* 1987;84:9265–9269.
3. Palmer RMJ, Ferrige AG, Moncada S. Nitric oxide release accounts for the biological activity of endothelium-derived relaxing factor. *Nature* 1987;327:524–526.
4. Moncada S, Palmer RMJ, Higgs EA. Nitric oxide: Physiology, pathophysiology and pharmacology. *Pharmacol Rev* 1991;43:109–140.
5. Stamler JS, Singel DJ, Loscalzo J. Biochemistry of nitric oxide and its redox-activated forms. *Science* 1992;258:1898–1902.
6. Stamler JS. Redox signaling: nitrosylation and related target interactions of nitric oxide. *Cell* 1994;78:931–936.
7. Beckman JS, Beckman TW, Chen J, et al. Apparent hydroxyl radical production by peroxynitrite: implications for endothelial injury from nitric oxide and superoxide. *Proc Natl Acad Sci U S A* 1990;87:1620–1624.
8. Huang Z, Huang P, Panahian N, et al. Effects of cerebral ischemia in mice deficient in neuronal nitric oxide synthase. *Science* 1994;265:1883–1885.
9. Lander HM, Jacovina AT, Davis RJ, et al. Differential activation of mitogen-activated protein kinases by nitric oxide-related species. *J Biol Chem* 1996;271:19705–19709.
10. Ross R. The pathogenesis of atherosclerosis: A perspective for the 1990s. *Nature* 1993; 362:801–809.
11. Cybulsky MI, Gimbrone MA Jr. Endothelial expression of a mononuclear leukocyte adhesion molecule during atherogenesis. *Science* 1991;251:788–791.
12. Radomski MW, Palmer RM, Moncada S. An L-arginine/nitric oxide pathway present in human platelets regulates aggregation. *Proc Natl Acad Sci U S A* 1990;87:5193–5197.
13. Cayatte AJ, Palacino JJ, Horten K, et al. Chronic inhibition of nitric oxide production accelerates neointima formation and impairs endothelial function in hypercholesterolemic rabbits. *Arterioscler Thromb* 1994;14:753–759.
14. Cooke JP, Singer AH, Tsao P, et al. Antiatherogenic effects of L-arginine in the hypercholesterolemic rabbit. *J Clin Invest* 1992;90:1168–1172.
15. De Caterina R, Libby P, Peng HB, et al. Nitric oxide decreases cytokine-induced endothelial activation. Nitric oxide selectively reduces endothelial expression of adhesion molecules and proinflammatory cytokines. *J Clin Invest* 1995;96:60–68.
16. Khan BV, Harrison DG, Olbrych MT, et al. Nitric oxide regulates vascular cell adhesion molecule 1 gene expression and redox-sensitive transcriptional events in human vascular endothelial cells. *Proc Natl Acad Sci U S A* 1996;93:9114–9119.
17. Peng HB, Rajavashisth TB, Libby P, et al. Nitric oxide inhibits macrophage-colony stimulating factor gene transcription in vascular endothelial cells. *J Biol Chem* 1995;270:17050–17055.
18. Gauthier TW, Davenpeck KL, Lefer AM. Nitric oxide attenuates leukocyte-endothelial interaction via P-selectin in splanchnic ischemia-reperfusion. *Am J Physiol* 1994;267:G562–G568.
19. Kubes P, Suzuki M, Granger DN. Nitric oxide: an endogenous modulator of leukocyte adhesion. *Proc Natl Acad Sci U S A* 1991;88:4651–4655.
20. Peng HB, Spiecker M, Liao JK. Inducible nitric oxide: an autoregulatory feedback inhibitor of vascular inflammation. *J Immunol* 1998;161:1970–1976.

21. Spiecker M, Peng HB, Liao JK. Inhibition of endothelial vascular cell adhesion molecule-1 expression by nitric oxide involves the induction and nuclear translocation of I-$\kappa$B-$\alpha$. *J Biol Chem* 1997;272:30969–30974.

22. Baeuerle PA, Henkel T. Function and activation of NF-$\kappa$B in the immune system. *Annu Rev Immunol* 1994;12:141–179.

23. Collins T. Endothelial nuclear factor-$\kappa$B and the initiation of the atherosclerotic lesion. *Lab Invest* 1993;68:499–508.

24. Marui N, Offermann MK, Swerlick R, et al. Vascular cell adhesion molecule-1 (VCAM-1) gene transcription and expression are regulated through an antioxidant-sensitive mechanism in human vascular endothelial cells. *J Clin Invest* 1993;92: 1866–1872.

25. Baeuerle PA, Baltimore D. NF-$\kappa$B: Ten years after. *Cell* 1996;87:13–20.

26. Spiecker M, Darius H, Kaboth K, et al. Differential regulation of endothelial cell adhesion molecule expression by nitric oxide donors and antioxidants. *J Leukoc Biol* 1998;63:732–739.

27. Sun SC, Ganchi PA, Ballard DW, et al. NF-$\kappa$B controls expression of inhibitor I-$\kappa$B-$\alpha$-Evidence for an inducible autoregulatory pathway. *Science* 1993;259:1912–1915.

28. Scheinman RI, Cogswell PC, Lofquist AK, et al. Role of transcriptional activation of I-$\kappa$B-$\alpha$ in mediation of immunosuppression by glucocorticoids. *Science* 1995;270: 283–286.

29. Auphan N, DiDonato JA, Rosette C, et al. Immunosuppression by glucocorticoids: Inhibition of NF-$\kappa$B activity through induction of I-$\kappa$B synthesis. *Science* 1995;270: 286–290.

30. Peng HB, Libby P, Liao JK. Induction and stabilization of I-$\kappa$B-$\alpha$ by nitric oxide mediate inhibition of NF-$\kappa$B. *J Biol Chem* 1995;270:14214–14219.

31. Liao JKE. Endothelium and acute coronary syndromes. *Clin Chem.* 1998;44 (pt 2):1799–1808.

32. Liao JK, Libby P. Nitric oxide and gene transcription. In Rubanyi GM, ed. *The Pathophysiology and Clinical Applications of Nitric Oxide.* Armonk, NY: Futura Publishing; 1998:99–120.

## Chapter 11

# Vascular Oxidant Stress and Nitric Oxide Bioactivity

*A. Maziar Zafari, MD, PhD, David G. Harrison, MD, and Kathy K. Griendling, PhD*

## Introduction

During the past decade, a growing body of evidence has accumulated in regard to the role of different oxygen species in disease states such as atherosclerosis and hypertension. Recently, it has become apparent that the renin-angiotensin system, with angiotensin II (Ang II) as its effector, and the vascular L-arginine/nitric oxide synthase (NOS) system with NO as its main agonist have effects on vascular tone and endothelial function that are interrelated closely and interdependent. One major integrating factor is oxidant stress, which affects both Ang II signaling and the integrity of NO. It appears that there is a tenuous balance in the vessel wall between the steady-state levels of NO and superoxide anion ($O_2^-$), and that imbalances between these two systems predispose to alterations of vascular regulation in the setting of such diverse disease conditions such as hypertension, hypercholesterolemia, diabetes mellitus, and heart failure. The mechanisms responsible for alterations of endothelial function are varied and multifactorial. This chapter will highlight the role of oxidant stress generated in vascular smooth muscle (VSM) on the bioactivity of NO as one such mechanism in physiological and pathophysiological conditions.

## Destruction of Nitric Oxide by Reactive Oxygen Species

Endothelial and smooth muscle cells produce $O_2^-$ and hydrogen peroxide ($H_2O_2$) and are exposed to free oxygen radicals generated and released by circulating blood cells and macrophages.[1] Even before the identification of

From Panza JA, Cannon RO III (eds): *Endothelium, Nitric Oxide, and Atherosclerosis* ©Futura Publishing Co, Inc, Armonk, NY, 1999.

endothelium-derived relaxing factor (EDRF) as NO, it was shown that its biological activity is compromised by oxygen-derived free radicals.[2] In fact, if the antioxidant defense systems are inhibited, endothelium-dependent relaxations to acetylcholine (ACh) are impaired.[3] Apparently, this is not caused by a decrease in the amount of NO released, but rather by the functional destruction of NO by $O_2^-$.[2–4] (Figure 1). Because $O_2^-$ and NO are both radicals and contain unpaired electrons in their outer orbitals, they undergo an exteremely rapid, diffusion-limited radical/radical reaction, which occurs at a rate estimated to be $6.7 \times 10^9$ mol/L per second.[5] This rate is approximately 10 000 times faster than the reaction between $O_2^-$ and the common antioxidant vitamins, such as vitamins A, C, and E, and three times faster than the reaction of $O_2^-$ with the manganese or copper–zinc superoxide dismutases (SODs). Combined with the fact that orally administered vitamins produce small alterations in tissue vitamin concentrations, it is unlikely that vitamin therapy will impact on the interaction between $O_2^-$ and NO. In compartments where both NO and SOD exist, there is the potential for $O_2^-$ to react predominantly with NO, depending on the relative concentrations of NO and SOD present. The reaction with $O_2^-$ markedly alters the biological activity of NO.[6]

A major product of this reaction is peroxynitrite anion ($OONO^-$)[7] (Figure 1). The $OONO^-$ is a powerful oxidant but is sufficiently stable to diffuse through a cell to react with a target. It is a weak vasodilator compared with NO, and thus conversion of NO to $OONO^-$ markedly impairs the vasodilator capacity of NO. Likewise, many of the other beneficial effects of NO [inhibition of platelet aggregation and smooth muscle cell growth, inhibition of vascular cell adhesion molecule-1 (VCAM-1) expression, etc.] are lost. As a strong oxidant, $OONO^-$ likely is involved in numerous pathophysiological processes. It is particularly efficient at oxidizing iron-sulfur clusters, zinc-fingers, and protein thiols, and these reactions contribute to cellular energy depletion.[8] Additionally, in the presence of peroxynitrite, SOD catalyzes the 3-nitration of protein tyrosine residues, particularly those in cytoskeletal proteins.[8] At phys-

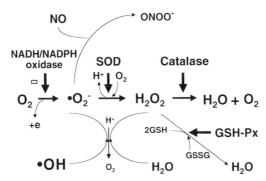

**Figure 1.** Metabolism of reactive oxygen species in the vasculature. As described in the text, the vascular nicotinamide-adenine dinucleotide/nicotinamide-adenine-dinucleotide phosphate (NADH/NADPH) oxidase converts molecular oxygen to superoxide. Superoxide is then converted to hydrogen peroxide by superoxide dismutase (SOD), and hydrogen peroxide is metabolized to water by catalase or glutathione peroxide (GSH-Px). The interaction of superoxide with NO produces peroxynitrite ($ONOO^-$). Reproduced with permission from Reference 28.

iological pH, OONO$^-$ is protonated to form peroxynitrous acid, which can yield nitrogen dioxide and a hydroxyl-like radical, both of which are highly reactive. In the vessel wall, OONO$^-$ and peroxynitrous acid may contribute to lipid peroxidation and membrane damage.[9] In the past, it was unclear how scavenging of O$_2^-$ by SOD could be beneficial in biological systems, because the product of this reaction is H$_2$O$_2$, a more potent oxidant than O$_2^-$. One currently accepted explanation for this paradox is that SOD prevents the formation of OONO$^-$, which is a much stronger oxidizing agent than H$_2$O$_2$.

The rapid rate of the reactions between O$_2^-$ and NO and O$_2^-$ and SODs suggests that in compartments where these three entities coexist, there may be interactions such that alterations in the amounts of either O$_2^-$ or SOD markedly could change levels of NO. In the normal vessel, the balance between NO and O$_2^-$ favors the net production of NO and produces basal vasodilation and maintenance of normal blood pressure. Notably, this is altered in several vascular diseases, including hypertension, atherosclerosis, diabetes mellitus, and conditions such as aging and cigarette smoking.[10] All of these conditions are associated with an increase in oxidative stress,[1] suggesting that impaired endothelial reactivity is a function of the increase in free oxygen radicals. This has been demonstrated most clearly for hypercholesterolemia. Vessels from hypercholesterolemic animals produce excess quantities of O$_2^-$, leading to destruction of NO and impaired endothelium-dependent vascular relaxation, which can be corrected by administration of polyethylene-glycolated SOD.[11] Likewise, infusion of ascorbic acid markedly improves endothelium-dependent vasodilation of forearm vessels in human subjects with diabetes mellitus and in cigarette smokers.[12]

## Sources of Oxidant Stress in Vascular Cells

Potential sources of reactive oxygen species encompass components of mitochondrial electron transport, xanthine oxidase, cyclooxygenase, lipoxygenase, heme oxygenase, NOS, and nicotinamide-adenine dinucleotide/nicotinamide-adenine-dinucleotide phosphate (NADH/NADPH) oxidase. Superoxide generation in vascular cells was identified initially as an endothelium-dependent phenomenon resulting from activation of xanthine oxidase.[13] Vascular O production in cholesterol-fed rabbits appeared to be from xanthine oxidase, because oxypurinol inhibited its production. More recently, White et al[14] have shown that levels of circulating xanthine oxidase are increased in the plasma of cholesterol-fed rabbits, and when it binds to heparin-binding sites on the vessel, it produces excess O$_2^-$. Subsequently, several groups observed that vascular O$_2^-$ is derived from both endothelial and nonendothelial sources. Pagano et al[15] noted ACh-insensitive O$_2^-$ generation from rabbit aorta and concluded that vascular O$_2^-$ is derived mainly from a nonendothelial source. Mohazzab and Wolin[16] described an O$_2^-$-generating NADH oxidase in pulmonary arteries that is modulated by hypoxia and is based on a cytochrome b558 electron transport system. Concomitantly, they demonstrated that other sources of free oxygen radicals, such as xanthine oxidase or cyclooxygenase, play a minor role in the vessel wall.[17] Consistent with these observations our laboratory defined NADH- and NADPH-dependent $O_2^-$ production in VSM cells (VSMCs). This activity was increased markedly by both Ang II and tumor necrosis factor $\alpha$ (TNF-$\alpha$), two agonists with demonstrable roles in oxidant stress-related vascular diseases.[18,19] Long-term (2–6 hours) treatment of cultured VSMCs with nanomolar levels of Ang II markedly increased NADH/NADPH oxidase activity, and caused subsequent generation of $O_2^-$ and $H_2O_2$.[18,20] The TNF-$\alpha$ caused a slightly more rapid (30 min to 2 hours) but equally robust activation of this enzyme.[19] This activity is membrane associated and is inhibited by diphenylene iodonium (DPI), an inhibitor of flavin-containing enzymes.[18] The VSMC-associated reactive oxygen species appear to derive mainly from this oxidase.

The importance of the NADH/NADPH oxidase in intact animals was demonstrated by Rajagopalan et al,[21] who used osmotic minipumps to infuse Ang II or norepinephrine into rats and measured $O_2^-$ production in aortas after the development of hypertension. Importantly, Ang II infusion but not norepinephrine infusion increased $O_2^-$ production in the vessel wall, suggesting that hypertension alone is not responsible for the oxidase activation. This conclusion was confirmed by additional experiments in which low concentrations of Ang II were infused, resulting in a small increase in blood pressure. In these animals, a perturbation of vascular $O_2^-$ production was observed, similar to that found in rats made overtly hypertensive by Ang II infusion. In experiments in which the endothelium was removed intentionally, the increase in $O_2$ production between vessels from Ang II–treated and sham-operated animals persisted, indicating that the source of the increase in $O_2^-$ likely is the VSM. Subsequent studies indicated that the oxidase involved in the increase in $O_2^-$ production was indeed the NADH/NADPH oxidase.[22] In concordance with the data of Mohazzab and Wolin,[16,17] this oxidase accounted for 90% of vascular $O_2^-$. An NADPH-dependent $O_2^-$ -generating system in the media or adventitia also was reported recently by Pagano et al.[23] Additionally, transient pulmonary vasorelaxation occurring during posthypoxic reoxygenation and photorelaxation of deendothelialized pulmonary arteries has been shown to be a consequence of $H_2O_2$ derived from n NADH oxidase.[24] Taken together, these data strongly indicate that a nonendothelial NADH/NADPH oxidase is the major source of $O_2^-$ in the vessel wall.

# Molecular Structure of the Vascular Nicotinamide-Adenine Dinucleotide/ Nicotinamide-Adenine-Dinucleotide Phosphate Oxidase

The vascular NADH/NADPH oxidase is a membrane-associated enzyme that generates $O_2^-$ from NADH or NADPH. The complete molecular structure has not been identified; however, it shares some similarity with the phagocytic NADPH oxidase that is responsible for the respiratory burst in neutrophils (Table 1). The neutrophil enzyme is a multicomponent oxidase: a plasma

Table 1
**Characteristics of Phagocytic and Nonphagocytic Oxidases**

|  | Phagocytic | Nonphagocytic |
|---|---|---|
| Substrate preference | NADPH | NADH |
| Kinetics of activation | Seconds | Minutes |
| Capacity (nmol/min per milligrams) | 130 | 40 |
| Fate of release $O_2^-$ | Extracellular | Intracellular |
| Cellular location | Plasma membrane | Nonmitochondrial membrane association |
| Activators | f-met-leu-phe | Angiotensin II |
|  | Cytokines | Cytokines |
|  | Arachidonate | Arachidonate |
|  | PMA |  |
| Inhibitors | DPI | DPI |
|  | Apocynin | Quinacrine |

Reproduced with permission from Reference 45.

membrane–associated cytochrome $b_{558}$ composed of two subunits, p22phox and gp91phox; two cytosolic components, p47phox and p67phox; and a small molecular weight G-protein, either rac-1 or rac-2. On activation, the cytosolic subunits translocate to the membrane and associate with cytochrome $b_{558}$, creating the active enzyme. The cytochrome harbors the full electron transfer activity of the phagocytic NADPH oxidase. Furthermore, the $SH_3$ domain of p47phox interacts directly with the proline-rich region of p22phox, making the p22phox subunit central to the normal functioning of the oxidase, because it is responsible for electron transfer and serves a docking function for the cytosolic factors. Many of the neutrophil components seem to be absent in SMCs, although all have been found in the endothelium and in the adventitia.[25,26] One component p22phox has been cloned in VSMCs and is relatively abundant at the mRNA level.[27] Functionally, p22phox appears to be critical for the activity of the oxidase, because stable transfection of VSMCs with a full-length p22phox antisense transgene results in a marked decrease in the capacity of these cells to produce $O_2^-$ and $H_2O_2$ in response to Ang II.[28]

Many of the characteristics of the neutrophil NADPH oxidase are shared by the vascular oxidase, including possession of flavin-binding and heme-binding regions, stimulation by phosphatidic acid and arachidonic acids, and association with the membrane. The vascular oxidase differs, however, from that of phagocytes because (1) the time course of stimulation of vascular oxidase occurs over a period of hours, unlike the "burst" activity of neutrophil oxidase; (2) the output of the vascular oxidase is much lower than that of neutrophil oxidase; (3) unlike the neutrophil oxidase, the vascular oxidase utilizes NADH for electron transfer to a greater extent than NADPH; (4) in contrast to the neutrophil oxidase, the vascular oxidase is stimulated by Ang II; and (5) the physiologic function of the $O_2^-$ accumulation is quite different from that of phagocytic cells, serving a signaling function for vascular tone or growth.

# Nitric Oxide and Vascular Smooth Muscle Growth

Like other mammalian cell types, VSM growth is redox sensitive. Recently, we have shown a sequential link between Ang II-induced NADH/NADPH oxidase activity, an increase in intracellular $H_2O_2$ leading to p38 mitogen-activated protein kinase (MAPK) activity and VSMC hypertrophy[18,28,29] (Figure 2). Pollman et al[30] have suggested that NO and Ang II serve opposing roles to maintain a balance between VSM proliferation and apoptosis. The NO has been shown to exert an antiproliferative effect on VSMC by abrogating Ang II-induced smooth muscle migration via a cyclic guanosine monophosphate (cGMP)-dependent mechanism. Thus, one function of the increase in reactive oxygen species produced by Ang II may be to inactivate NO and thus permit prohypertrophic pathways to function without their normal checks. Although many recent studies support the pro–proliferative effects of reactive oxygen species on VSMCs, some conflicting results have been reported.[31] It appears that although a certain level of oxidant stress is growth promoting, more severe stress may lead to cell death. One explanation for these apparently disparate results may be the magnitude of alterations in redox state. It is intriguing that atherosclerosis, restenosis after angioplasty, and hypertension are characterized by decreased bioactivity of NO and/or increased generation of Ang II. Further studies clearly are required to delineate the regulatory mechanisms that control the bioactivity of NO and its interactions with Ang II under a given oxidant stress.

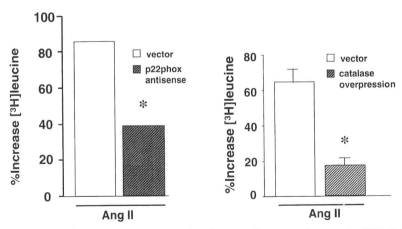

**Figure 2.** Role of reactive oxygen species in vascular smooth muscle (VSM) hypertrophy. As assessed by [³H]leucine incorporation, angiotensin II (Ang II; 100 nmol/L, 24 hours) causes hypertrophy of VSM cells (VSMCs) (open bars). Transfection of antisense p22phox to disrupt functioning of the NADH/NADPH oxidase inhibits Ang II-induced [³H]leucine incorporation (hatched bar, **left panel**). Furthermore, overexpression of catalase to decrease intracellular hydrogen peroxide levels also decreases hypertrophy (hatched bar, **right panel**). Modified from References 20 and 28.

# Hemodynamic Stress and the Integrity of Nitric Oxide

The integrity and production of NO also is influenced by different types of hemodynamic stresses to which the vessel wall is exposed. Over a decade ago, it was demonstrated that prolonged elevations of flow in vivo increase endothelial production of EDRF and enhance endothelium-dependent vascular relaxation.[32] More recently, it has been shown that expression of endothelial NOS and copper–zinc SOD is regulated in response to shear stress.[33,34] Because copper–zinc SOD plays an important role in modulating the release of bioactive NO,[3] alterations of its expression or $O_2^-$-scavenging activity potentially may alter the vasorelaxant capacity of endothelium-derived NO. Preservation of the half-life of NO may have antiatherogenic properties, such as inhibition of platelet and neutrophil adhesion and inhibition of VSM growth. Additionally, Howard et al[35] showed that cyclic strain causes an early (2 hours), transient increase in NADH/NADPH oxidase activity and a sustained increase in extracellular $H_2O_2$ in cultured porcine aortic endothelial cells. The increase in oxidative stress is reflected in an increase in lipid peroxidation products released from the cells. Chappell et al[36] showed that oscillatory shear stress induces the expression of the adhesion molecules VCAM-1 and intercellular adhesion molecule 1 (ICAM-1) in an oxidant-sensitive manner. It also has been observed that laminar shear induces the expression of SOD, thus increasing the antioxidant defenses of the cell.[34] In contrast, oscillatory shear apparently causes a sustained activation of the NADH/NADPH oxidase without increasing SOD expression.[37] These latter data suggest that oscillatory shear creates a more prooxidant environment than laminar shear stress, probably reducing the steady-state level of NO and providing a potential explanation for the fact that atherosclerotic lesions are more prone to develop in areas of low, oscillatory shear stress. These observations are of utmost relevance in the pathogenesis of hypertension and its association with atherosclerosis, because it has become increasingly clear that vasoactive substances such as NO and Ang II also have the capacity to induce long-term changes in vessel structure in addition to acute effects on vessel tone.

# Oxidant Stress and Hypertension

Nakazano and coworkers[38] showed that a form of SOD, modified to bind to heparin sulfates in the vessel extracellular matrix, acutely lowered blood pressure in spontaneously hypertensive rats, while having no effect on blood pressure in normal rats. Furthermore, we have shown that the increase in VSMC $O_2^-$ production caused by Ang II in vivo is associated with a marked impairment in endothelium-dependent vascular relaxation, probably by inactivation of NO[21] (Figure 3). We demonstrated that this elevated enzymatic activity was accompanied by an increase in the expression of p22phox mRNA, suggesting that the amount of oxidase present in the vessel wall is upregulated in this model of hypertension.[22] Both oxidase activity and p22phox

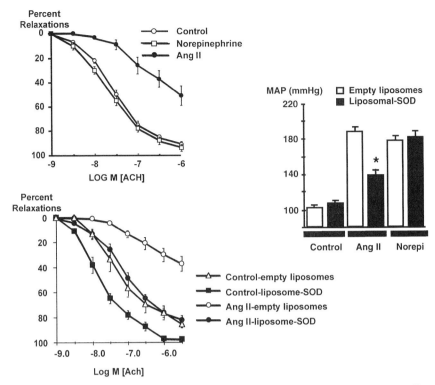

**Figure 3.**   Role of reactive oxygen species in Ang II–induced hypertension. For the experiments depicted in this graph, rats were infused with Ang II (0.7 mg/kg per day) or norephinephrine (2.8 mg/kg per day) for 5 days. **Upper left,** endothelium-dependent relaxations to acetylcholine in aortas from sham-operated (control), Ang II-infused or norepinephrine-infused animals. The Ang II infusion caused a selective impairment of endothelium-dependent vasodilation. **Lower left,** the impaired response to Ang II can be corrected by coadministration of liposomal SOD. Empty liposomes were used as a control. **Right,** treatment of these animals with liposomal SOD also partially corrected the increase in blood pressure caused by Ang II but not norepinephrine. These studies indicate that reactive oxygen species play a role in mediating relaxation and blood pressure elevation to Ang II but not norepinephrine. Reproduced with permission from References 21 and 39.

expression are blocked by the antihypertensive agent hydralazine, which also has antioxidant properties, and by the angiotensin $AT_1$ receptor antagonist losartan, raising the possibility that oxidant stress may play a role in blood pressure regulation. In fact, daily administration of liposome-entrapped SOD beginning 3 days before Ang II infusion normalizes endothelium-dependent vascular relaxation and relaxations to nitroglycerin.[39] This reduction in endogenous steady-state levels of vascular $O_2^-$ attenuates the subsequent rise in blood pressure significantly, providing direct evidence for the contribution of oxidative stress to blood pressure regulation[39] (Figure 3). These studies focused on the role of $O_2^-$ as a modulator of NO's biological activity. Another mechanism involved in Ang II-induced hypertension is the observation that Ang II can enhance endothelin-1 (ET-1) gene expression in the vessel wall.[40] We and others have shown that ET-1 antagonists can prevent hypertension caused by Ang II.[41,42] The mechanisms whereby increased oxidative stress, loss of NO bioactivity, and Ang II interplay to enhance ET-1 production in vivo are unclear but are likely to be quite important in the pathogenesis of hypertension and probably other vascular diseases.

## Polymorphisms of the p22phox Gene and Coronary Heart Disease

Recently, in the first clinical cardiovascular investigation of the NADH/NADPH oxidase, a specific polymorphism of the p22phox gene was found to be more prevalent in healthy Japanese patients compared with patients with established coronary heart disease (CHD).[43] The T-allele frequencies of the C242T polymorphism of the p22phox gene in control patients was significantly higher than in patients with CHD, and the prevalence of the TC+TT genotype was more frequent in control subjects than in case patients. The odds ratio of the TC+TT versus the CC genotype of the C242T polymorphism between case patients and control subjects was 0.49 [95% confidence interval (CI), 0.28–0.87] ($P = 0.015$). The association of this polymorphism with CHD was statistically significant and independent of the A640G polymorphism and other coronary risk factors when subjected to logistic regression analysis. The C242T polymorphism, which substitutes histidine-72 for tyrosine, is located in the heme-binding site of the NADPH oxidase. This polymorphism in the p22phox gene may modulate the activity and regulation of the oxidase, potentially decreasing oxygen radical production in the vessel wall and reducing the oxidative stress required to maintain the progression of the atherosclerotic process.

This finding raises the possibility that carriers of the mutant enzyme may have reduced NADH/NADPH oxidase activity and subsequently generate less superoxide and other oxygen-derived free radicals. A reduced level of oxidative stress would prevent the degradation of NO and maintain its physiological bioactivity, which could prevent the development of or protect the vasculature against oxidant-mediated pathophysiological conditions such as hypertension and atherosclerosis. It is known that small changes in the structure of the p22phox subunit of the phagocytic oxidase lead to instability, reduced activity, and/or loss of function of this enzyme, causing the autosomal recessive form of chronic granulomatous disease (CGD).[44] Detection of polymorphisms involving the enzymatic activity of the p22phox-based oxidase may indeed provide important information to further expand our understanding of the role of oxidative stress in the pathogenesis of atherosclerosis and its association with hypertension and open new avenues to study the role of NO and its biological properties and its interactions with Ang II in these conditions.

## Future Directions

Interventions to modify vascular p22phox expression and/or function could prove to be very helpful in modulating production of reactive oxygen species and assess the impact on the bioactivity of endothelium-derived NO.

Oxidative stress is intertwined with the functional effects of both Ang II and NO. As more is learned about Ang II and NO, it becomes apparent that their vascular effects are inextricable, and future research should take into account interactions between the two. Likewise, studies examining other sources of reactive oxygen species in vascular tissues and how they are modulated will be helpful in understanding regulation of NO bioactivity. Finally, studies of regulation of the major antioxidant defense systems (ie, the SODs, catalase, cellular thiols, and antioxidant vitamins) likely will provide additional insight into how various diseases affect the NOS system.

# References

1. Alexander RW. Hypertension and the pathogenesis of atherosclerosis. Oxidative stress and the mediation of arterial inflammatory response: A new perspective. *Hypertension* 1995;25:155–161.
2. Rubanyi GM, Vanhoutte PM. Superoxide anion and hyperoxia inactivate endothelium-derived relaxing factor. *Am J Physiol* 1986;250:H822–H827.
3. Mügge A, Elwell JH, Peterson TE, et al. Release of intact endothelium-derived relaxing factor depends on endothelial superoxide dismutase activity. *Am J Physiol* 1991;260:C219–C225.
4. Rubanyi GM, Vanhoutte PM. Oxygen-derived free radicals, endothelium, and the responsiveness of vascular smooth muscle. *Am J Physiol* 1986;250:H815–H821.
5. Thomson L, Trujillo M, Telleri R, et al. Kinetics of cytochrome c2+ oxidation by peroxynitrite: Implications for superoxide measurements in nitric oxide-producing biological systems. *Arch Biochem Biophys* 1995;319:419–497.
6. Harrison DG. Perspective series: Nitric oxide and nitric oxide synthases. Cellular and molecular mechanisms of endothelial cell dysfunction. *J Clin Invest* 1997;100: 2153–2157.
7. Beckman JS, Beckman TW, Chen J, et al. Apparent hydroxyl radical production by peroxynitrite: Implications for endothelial injury from nitric oxide and superoxide. *Proc Natl Acad Sci U S A* 1990;87:1620–1624.
8. Christopherson KS, Bredt DS. Perspective series: Nitric oxide and nitric oxide synthases. Nitric oxide in excitable tissues: Physiological roles and disease. *J Clin Invest* 1997;100:2424–2429.
9. Radl R, Beckman JW, Bush KM, et al. Peroxynitrite induced membrane lipid peroxidation: The cytotoxic potential of superoxide and nitric oxide. *Arch Biochem Biophys* 1991;288:481–487.
10. Harrison DG. Endothelial function and oxidant stress. *Clin Cardiol* 1997;20:II11–II17.
11. Mügge A, Elwell JH, Peterson TE, et al. Chronic treatment with polyethylene-glycolated superoxide dismutase partially restores endothelium-dependent vascular relaxations in cholesterol-fed rabbits. *Circ Res* 1991;69:1293–1300.
12. Ting HH, Timimi FK, Boles K, et al. Vitamin C acutely improves endothelium-dependent vasodilation in patients with non-insulin-dependent diabetes mellitus. *Circulation* 1995;92(suppl 1):1747. Abstract.
13. Ohara Y, Peterson TE, Harrison DG. Hypercholesterolemia increases endothelial superoxide anion production. *J Clin Invest* 1993;91:2546–2551.
14. White CR, Darley-Usmar V, Berrington WR, et al. Circulating plasma xanthine oxidase contributes to vascular dysfunction in hypercholesterolemic rabbits. *Proc Natl Acad Sci U S A* 1996;93:8745–8749.
15. Pagano PJ, Tornheim K, Cohen RA. Superoxide anion production by rabbit thoracic aorta: Effect of endothelium-derived nitric oxide. *Am J Physiol* 1993;265:H707–H712.

16. Mohazzab-H KM, Wolin MS. Properties of a superoxide anion-generating microsomal NADH oxidoreductase, a potential pulmonary artery PO$_2$ sensor. *Am J Physiol* 1994;267:L823–L831.

17. Mohazzab-H KM, Wolin MS. Sites of superoxide anion production detected by lucigenin in calf pulmonary artery smooth muscle. *Am J Physiol* 1994;267:L815–L822.

18. Griendling KK, Minieri CA, Ollerenshaw JD, et al. Angiotensin II stimulates NADH and NADPH oxidase activity in cultured vascular smooth muscle cells. *Circ Res* 1994;74:1141–1148.

19. DeKeulenaer GW, Alexander RW, Ushio-Fukai M, et al. Tumor necrosis factor-$\alpha$ activates a p22phox-based NADH oxidase in vascular smooth muscle cells. *Biochem J* 1998;329:653–657.

20. Zafari AM, Ushio-Fukai M, Akers M, et al. Role of NADH/NADPH oxidase-derived H$_2$O$_2$ in angiotensin II-induced vascular hypertrophy. *Hypertension* 1998;32:488–495.

21. Rajagopalan S, Kurz S, Münzel T, et al. Angiotensin II mediated hypertension in the rat increases vascular superoxide production via membrane NADH/NADPH oxidase activation: Contribution to alterations of vasomotor tone. *J Clin Invest* 1996;97:1916–1923.

22. Fukui T, Ishizaka N, Rajagopalan S, et al. p22phox mRNA expression and NADPH oxidase activity are increased in aortas from hypertensive rats. *Circ Res* 1997;80:45–51.

23. Pagano PJ, Ito Y, Tornheim K, et al. An NADPH oxidase superoxide-generating system in the rabbit aorta. *Am J Physiol* 1995;268:H2274–H2280.

24. Mohazzab-H KM, Kaminski PM, Fayngersh RP, et al. Oxygen-elicted responses in calf coronary arteries: Role of H$_2$O$_2$ production via NADH-derived superoxide. *Am J Physiol* 1996;270:H1044–H1053.

25. Pagano PJ, Clark JK, Cifuentes-Pagano ME, et al. Localization of a constitutively active, phagocyte-like NADPH oxidase in rabbit aortic adventitia: Enhancement by angiotensin II. *Proc Natl Acad Sci U S A* 1997;94:14438–14488.

26. Jones SA, O'Donnell VB, Wood JD, et al. Expression of phagocyte NADPH oxidase components in human endothelial cells. *Am J Physiol* 1996;271:H1626–H1634.

27. Fukui T, Lass gue B, Kai H, et al. cDNA cloning and mRNA expression of cytochrome b$_{558}$ a-subunit in rat vascular smooth muscle cells. *Biochim Biophys Acta* 1995;1231:215–219.

28. Ushio-Fukai M, Zafari AM, Fukui T, et al. p22phox is a critical component of the superoxide-generating NADH/NADPH oxidase system and regulates angiotensin II-induced hypertrophy in vascular smooth muscle cells. *J Biol Chem* 1996;271:23317–23321.

29. Ushio-Fukai M, Alexander RW, Akers M, et al. p38MAP kinase is a critical component of the redox-sensitive signaling pathways by angiotensin II: Role in vascular smooth muscle cell hypertrophy. *J Biol Chem* 1998;273:15022–15029.

30. Pollman MJ, Yamada T, Horiuchi M, et al. Vasoactive substances regulate vascular smooth muscle cell apoptosis. Countervailing influences of nitric oxide and angiotensin II. *Circ Res* 1996;79:748–756.

31. Fiorani M, Cantoni O, Tasinato A, et al. Hydrogen peroxide- and fetal bovine serum-induced DNA synthesis in vascular smooth muscle cells: Positive and negative regulation by protein kinase C isoforms. *Biochim Biophys Acta* 1995;1269:98–104.

32. Miller VM, Aarhus LL, Vanhoutte PM. Modulation of endothelium-dependent responses by chronic alterations of blood flow. *Am J Physiol* 1986;251:H520–H527.

33. Uematsu M, Ohara Y, Navas JP, et al. Regulation of endothelial cell nitric oxide synthase mRNA expression by shear stress. *Am J Physiol*. 1995;269:C1371–C1378.

34. Inoue N, Ramaswamy S, Fukai R, et al. Shear stress modulates expression of Cu/Zn superoxide dismutase in human aortic endothelial cells. *Circ Res* 1996;79:32–37.

35. Howard AB, Alexander RW, Nerem RM, et al. Cyclic strain induces an oxidative stress in endothelial cells. *Am J Physiol* 1997;272:C421–C427.

36. Chappell DC, Varner SE, Nerem RM, et al. Oscillatory shear stimulates adhesion molecule expression in cultured human endothelium. *Circ Res* 1998;82:532–539.
37. DeKeulenaer GW, Chappell DC, Ishizaka N, et al. Oscillatory and steady laminar shear stress differentially affect human endothelial redox state. *Circ Res* 1998;82:1094–1101.
38. Nakazono K, Watanabe N, Matsuno K, et al. Does superoxide underlie the pathogenesis of hypertension? *Proc Natl Acad Sci U S A* 1991;88:10045–10048.
39. Bech-Laursen J, Rajagopalan S, Galis Z, et al. Role of superoxide in angiotensin II-induced but not catecholamine-induced hypertension. *Circulation* 1997;95:588–593.
40. Imai T, Hirata Y, Emori T, et al. Induction of endothelin-1 gene by angiotensin and vasopressin in endothelial cells. *Hypertension* 1992;19:753–757.
41. d'Uscio LV, Moreau P, Shaw S, et al. Effects of chronic $ET_A$-receptor blockade in angiotensin II-induced hypertension. *Hypertension* 1997;29:435–441.
42. Rajagopalan S, Bech-Laursen J, Borthayre A, et al. A role for endothelin-1 in angiotensin II mediated hypertension. *Hypertension* 1997;30:29–34.
43. Inoue N, Kawashima S, Kanazawa K, et al. Polymorphism of the NADH/NADPH oxidase p22phox gene in patients with coronary artery disease. *Circulation* 1998;97:135–137.
44. Dinauer MC, Pierce EA, Bruns GAP, et al. Human neutrophil: Cytochrome b light chain (p22-phox) gene structure, chromosomal location, and mutations in cytochrome negative autosomal recessive chronic granulomatous disease. *J Clin Invest* 1990;86:1729–1737.
45. Griendling KK, Ushio-Fukai M. Redox control of vascular smooth muscle proliferation. *Lab Clin Med* 1998;132:9–15. Review.

# Part III

# Clinical Studies of Endothelial Function and Dysfunction

## Chapter 12

# Endothelium, Nitric Oxide, and Hypertension

*Julio A. Panza, MD*

## Introduction

Elevated blood pressure is a common cardiovascular condition that may lead to well-defined complications including stroke, congestive heart failure, and chronic renal failure. In addition, hypertension is a well-known risk factor for the development of atherosclerosis. This condition has a tremendous impact on health care cost; for example, currently, it is estimated that 50 million Americans have elevated blood pressure or are taking antihypertensive medications, and drug treatment alone has been estimated as more than $8 billion per year. Despite the reports that antihypertensive therapy has reduced considerably the incidence of stroke, successful treatment of high blood pressure has not led to a similar reduction in the rate of development of atherosclerosis. This epidemiological observation may have a pathophysiological basis: the association between hypertension and atherosclerosis may not be linked to the elevated blood pressure per se but, instead, it might be a reflection of a mechanistic abnormality common to both conditions.

The vast majority (more than 90%—95%) of hypertensive patients have no apparent cause for their elevated blood pressure. Although this condition, commonly referred to as essential hypertension, often can be controlled easily with one or more antihypertensive drugs, there is a need to identify pathophysiological mechanisms that may participate either in the genesis or the perpetuation of the hypertensive process. In this regard, several different processes have been identified as potentially responsible for or at least related to this condition. These different mechanisms may act separately (ie, different mechanisms in different patients) or in combination. They may initiate, precipitate, or perpetuate the elevated blood pressure. Because of the obvious hereditary transmission of essential hypertension, it is tempting to speculate that a single gene mutation is the abnormality underlying the clinical presentation of high blood pressure. However, no genetic background has been discovered yet for essential hypertension and, given its widespread distribu-

From Panza JA, Cannon RO III (eds): *Endothelium, Nitric Oxide, and Atherosclerosis* ©Futura Publishing Co, Inc, Armonk, NY, 1999.

tion in populations with very different racial, socioeconomic, and geographical backgrounds, there probably is more than one genotype that can predispose to the development of hypertension.

Independently of the precise mechanisms involved in the hypertensive process, it is clear that hypertension is a disease of small resistance vessels. Further, at least in the initial phase of the disease, it is a problem of arteriolar vascular tone. Several previous reports have identified morphological changes in the microvessels of hypertensive patients, usually in the form of increased wall:lumen ratio. Although this vascular hypertrophy can be a cause or a consequence of the hypertensive process, it cannot in itself explain all the abnormalities characteristic of this disease. Thus, even considering the structural vascular changes that may be present in hypertensive patients, a dynamic phenomenon (ie, increased vascular tone) also must be involved to explain the impaired degree of vasodilation usually observed in hypertensive arteries.

## Endothelial Dysfunction in Hypertension

The concept of endothelial regulation of vascular tone emerged with the seminal observations of Robert Furchgott,[1] described in detail in another chapter, that the vascular responses to acetylcholine (ACh) and other agonists were dependent on the presence of an intact endothelium. This discovery led the way to an ever-increasing body of work devoted to the study of the role of the endothelium in blood vessel physiology. Because of the thus demonstrated critical role of the endothelium in the modulation of vascular tone, it was logical to postulate that an abnormality of endothelial function might be involved in the pathophysiology of essential hypertension.

The initial studies that addressed the possibility of impaired endothelial regulation of vascular tone in hypertension were conducted in the early 1980s. These investigations showed that endothelium-dependent vasodilator responses of the thoracic aorta from spontaneously hypertensive rats (SHR) were depressed compared with normotensive control animals.[2,3] Shortly thereafter, these observations were extended to the small resistance mesenteric arteries[4] in the same animal model of hypertension. Subsequent studies extended these findings to other forms of arterial hypertension, not related to a particular genotype. For example, Lockette et al demonstrated that endothelium-dependent relaxation in the thoracic aorta of rats with three different models of hypertension were impaired.[5] Thus, rats with deoxycorticosterone and salt-sensitive hypertension, one-kidney, one-clip renovascular hypertension, and aortic coarctation hypertension all had impaired responses to ACh. Interestingly, endothelium-dependent vasodilation improved after the reversal of hypertension, thus leading the authors to postulate that the impaired endothelium-dependent vasodilation was secondary to the elevated blood pressure.[5] These observations were confirmed by Miller et al[6] who showed that vascular preparations from rabbits undergoing coarctation-induced hypertension had impaired responses to ACh with preserved responses to sodium nitroprusside. Importantly, the extent of the responses to ACh in these animal models was correlated with the arterial pressure, indicating that the impairment of endothelium-dependent relaxation is related proportionally to the degree of blood pressure elevation. It is important to note that early studies designed to determine the mechanism underlying this decreased endothelial vasodilator function showed that, in the SHR model, the impaired responses to ACh were not related necessarily to a diminished release of endothelium-derived relaxing factor but, instead, to enhanced activity of endothelium-derived contracting substances.[7] The same authors also demonstrated that, in rats with salt-induced hypertension, antihypertensive therapy significantly improved the impaired endothelium-dependent vasodilation to ACh in aortic rings from these animals.[8] In summary, the demonstration of the critical role of the endothelium in the vascular tone was followed quickly by the publication of several reports indicating that different animal models of hypertension were associated with impaired endothelium-dependent vascular responses to ACh. Independently of the mechanism of hypertension involved in the models, it appeared that antihypertensive therapy was able to improve the diminished vascular responses.

The demonstration of impaired endothelium-dependent responses to ACh in patients with essential hypertension was first reported in preliminary form in 1988.[9] Since then, several studies from independent investigators have demonstrated that patients with hypertension have decreased vascular responses to ACh with preserved endothelium-independent responses to nitrovasodilators.[10-17] Importantly, these abnormal responses have been observed in different vascular territories including the forearm and coronary circulations and blood vessels isolated from subcutaneous biopsies. However, some investigators have not been able to confirm these findings.[18,19] It has been suggested that this discrepancy may be related to differences in the plasma cholesterol levels of the hypertensive patients included in the different studies (see Chapter 16). According to this observation, hypertensive patients included in a previous study demonstrating impaired endothelium-dependent vasodilation had slightly higher plasma cholesterol levels than control subjects,[10] while in a study reporting preserved endothelium-dependent vasodilation in hypertensive patients,[18] the normotensive and hypertensive subjects were better matched with regard to cholesterol values. However, careful analysis of plasma cholesterol levels of normotensive and hypertensive individuals reported in several previous investigations does not support this conclusion (Table 1). Instead, this analysis reveals that the plasma cholesterol levels of the normotensive subjects used as controls in those studies reporting preserved endothelium-dependent vasodilation in hypertension was significantly higher (by approximately 50 mg/dL) than the cholesterol levels of both normotensive and hypertensive individuals included in studies reporting impaired endothelium-dependent vasodilation in patients with this condition (Table 1). Given the previously reported correlation between plasma cholesterol levels and endothelium-dependent vasodilation, it is possible that the normotensive subjects included in the studies by Cockroft et al[18] and Bruning et al[19] had impaired responses to ACh because of a higher cholesterol level, which, in turn, may have masked an impaired response in the hypertensive individuals.

Table 1

**Total Plasma Cholesterol Values (in mg/dL) in Studies Investigating Endothelial Vasodilator Function in Patients with Essential Hypertension**

| Reference | Total Plasma Cholesterol Values (mg/dL) | |
| | Normotensives | Hypertensives |
| --- | --- | --- |
| Panza et al[10] * | 180 ± 18 | 191 ± 28 |
| Taddei et al[14] * | 188 ± 17 | 183 ± 15 |
| Panza et al[38] * | 170 ± 34 | 177 ± 46 |
| Panza et al[47] * | 165 ± 35 | 168 ± 43 |
| Panza et al[49] * | 168 ± 28 | 178 ± 25 |
| Taddei et al[39] * | 189 ± 12 | 193 ± 13 |
| Cardillo et al[57] * | 176 ± 28 | 179 ± 27 |
| Rizzoni et al[17] * | 186 ± 27 | 186 ± 39 |
| Cardillo et al[53] * | 184 ± 29 | 188 ± 24 |
| Taddei et al[58] * | 184 ± 17 | 189 ± 15 |
| **Corrected average†** | **180** | **185** |
| Cockroft et al[18] § | 232 ± 3.8 | 228 ± 3.8‡ |
| Bruning et al[19] § | 232 ± 8.9 | 234 ± 20 |

* Studies reporting impaired endothelium-dependent vasodilation in hypertension.

† Average values for the 10 studies referenced above corrected for the number of patients included in each study.

‡ Values reported in previously treated hypertensive patients.

§ Studies reporting preserved endothelium-dependent vasodilation in hypertension.

Thus, based on this analysis, it appears reasonable to conclude that at plasma cholesterol levels below 200 mg/dL, the presence of hypertension is associated with abnormal endothelium-dependent vasodilation. In contrast, at higher plasma cholesterol levels (approximately 230 mg/dL), hypertension may not further impair the vasodilator response to endothelial agonists.

An important pathophysiological aspect of endothelial dysfunction in hypertension is whether this phenomenon constitutes a primary or a secondary abnormality. Taddei et al[20] reported that normotensive offsprings of hypertensive parents had a reduced vasodilator response to ACh compared with normotensive offsprings of normotensive parents. More recently, the same investigators reported studies suggesting that the bioactivity of nitric oxide (NO) may be reduced in normotensive individuals with a family history of hypertension and therefore at risk of developing high blood pressure.[21] These observations seem to indicate that endothelial dysfunction (and more specifically) a decreased bioactivity of NO, may be involved partly in the genesis of the hypertensive process. Further, the finding of lack of improvement in endothelium-dependent vascular responses with clinically effective antihypertensive therapy (discussed in the following text) also appears to support the concept that endothelial dysfunction might be a primary phenomenon in patients with essential hypertension. On the other hand, previous studies in certain animal models of hypertension clearly indicate that an impaired vasodilator response to ACh may be a consequence of elevated blood pressure. Thus, as discussed previously, animals with hypertension induced by coarctation of the aorta or by clipping of the renal artery in a single-kidney model demonstrated impaired endothelium-dependent vascular responses.[5,6] Further, studies have shown that this form of endothelial dysfunction persists for several hours or even days, but eventually may be reversible.[22] Consistent with these findings, Taddei et al[20,21] also have shown that patients with secondary forms of hypertension have impaired vascular responses to ACh. Therefore, these observations would favor the hypothesis that endothelial dysfunction is a consequence rather than the cause of the elevated blood pressure. Although this dilemma has not been resolved, it is possible that endothelial dysfunction may act both as a causative mechanism and as a consequence of high blood pressure. More specifically, because essential hypertension likely is a multifactorial process and probably represents a different disease entity in different patients, it is reasonable to postulate that endothelial dysfunction may be primary in only a subset of essential hypertensive patients and secondary (ie, induced by the elevated blood pressure) in the rest of the hypertensive population. In any case, a primary role of endothelial dysfunction for the development of hypertension clearly needs to be confirmed in larger studies. This may have very important implications because, if endothelial dysfunction is at the core of the genesis of hypertension, then one could postulate screening normotensive offsprings with measurements of endothelial vasodilator function to determine the risk of each individual to develop essential hypertension. Obviously, this postulate needs to be demonstrated in prospective studies performed with appropriate controls.

The observation that induction of hypertension in animal models resulted in impaired endothelium-dependent vasodilation[6] suggested that effective antihypertensive therapy may normalize or at least improve endothelial vasodilator function.[8] Further, in SHRs, treatment with an angiotensin-converting enzyme (ACE) inhibitor or a calcium channel blocker reduced blood pressure and improved endothelial dysfunction in resistance vessels.[23] Long-term, but not short-term, treatment with an ACE inhibitor or a calcium channel blocker improved endothelial dysfunction in a rat model of NO-deficient hypertension.[24] These studies gave support to the concept that antihypertensive treatment may have a beneficial effect on endothelial function. Human studies related to the effects of antihypertensive treatment, including investigations specifically addressing the use of ACE inhibitors, have yielded negative results.[16,25,26] However, one study did demonstrate an acute improvement in endothelium-dependent forearm vasodilation with ACE inhibitor treatment,[27] although it must be pointed out that in this study vasodilator responses to ACh and sodium nitroprusside were measured only 1 hour after oral administration of captopril, which may explain the discrepancy with the aforementioned studies using chronic ACE inhibitor therapy. It is possible that ACE inhibition may improve endothelial dysfunction regardless of its antihypertensive effect, as suggested in the Trial on Reversing Endothelial Dysfunction (TREND) study.[28] On the other hand, studies addressing the issue of lowering blood pressure regardless of the particular pharmacologic agent used for control of hypertension have shown that clinically effective antihypertensive therapy does not modify the vascular response to ACh, suggesting that this form of endothelial dysfunction is either a primary phenomenon or it becomes irreversible once the hypertensive process has become established.[25]

## Nitric Oxide and the Regulation of Vascular Tone

Principal among the substances released by the endothelium to regulate vascular tone is NO, which is formed by the enzyme NO synthase (NOS) from the amino acid L-arginine.[29,30] The endothelial constitutive form of NOS, in the presence of nicotinamide-adenine-dinucleotide phosphate (NADPH), $Ca^{2+}$/calmodulin, and tetrahydrobiopterin, oxidizes L-arginine for the formation of NO and L-citrulline.[31] Importantly, this activity of NOS to synthesize NO can be inhibited by endogenous analogues of L-arginine such as asymmetric dimethylarginine (ADMA).[32] NO stimulates soluble guanylate cyclase in the underlying smooth muscle leading to elevation of intracellular levels of cyclic guanosine monophosphate (cGMP) with consequent vascular relaxation. The critical nature of the physiological role of NO in the regulation of vascular tone has been shown in different investigational settings. For example, mice with a knockout for the endothelial NOS (eNOS) gene have increased vascular resistance with elevated systemic blood pressure.[33] Similarly, animals treated with $N^{G}$-monomethyl-L-arginine (L-NMMA), an exogenous competitive inhibitor of NOS, also have elevated blood pressure.[34] In humans, it was first demonstrated by Vallance et al[35] that administration of L-NMMA into the forearm circulation causes an increase in vascular resistance with consequent reduction in forearm blood flow. This observation indicates that, under normal circumstances, there is basal release of NO that is critical for the normal maintenance of vascular tone. Furthermore, L-NMMA also significantly blunts the response to ACh but not to nitrovasodilators in normal subjects,[35] indicating that the vasodilator effect of ACh is mediated at least partly by the stimulated release of NO. In addition to its important role for the modulation of the smooth muscle tone, it is known that NO has other very important functions for regulation of vascular homeostasis.[36] For example, NO reduces monocyte and leukocyte adhesion to endothelial cells, and is an important inhibitor of platelet aggregability and platelet-vessel wall interaction. NO decreases endothelial permeability and thus diminishes the transport of lipoproteins into the vessel wall and suppresses vascular smooth muscle proliferation and migration both in vitro and in vivo. Because all these processes are important for the development of atherosclerosis, their inhibition by NO have led to the postulation of this molecule as one of the principal endogenous antiatherosclerotic substances produced by the cardiovascular system.

## Nitric Oxide and Hypertension

Because the regulation of vascular tone involves many substances and a complex interplay among numerous cellular mechanisms, an impaired vasodilator response to ACh with preserved response to nitrovasodilators suggests the presence but does not identify the nature of endothelial dysfunction. Given the importance of endothelium-derived NO in the regulation of basal arteriolar tone in normal humans, studies were conducted to determine whether a specific defect in the NO system might explain the reduced endothelial vasodilator function in hypertensive patients. To this end, the vascular effects of L-NMMA were assessed under baseline conditions and during endothelium-dependent and -independent vasodilation. Compared with normal controls, L-NMMA produces much less vasoconstriction under basal conditions in hypertensive patients,[37,38] and does not significantly modify their response to ACh.[38,39] These reduced vascular effects of L-NMMA in hypertensive patients demonstrate impaired production of NO by hypertensive arteries, both during baseline conditions and during stimulation with endothelium-dependent agents. Importantly, the decreased response to L-NMMA of hypertensive patients cannot be ascribed to the structural changes (ie, increased wall:lumen ratio) characteristic of the hypertensive process because those changes predispose the vessels to a more pronounced response to any given vasoconstrictor agent.

The observations that the bioactivity of NO is reduced in the small resistance vessels of patients with essential hypertension has important implications. First, this abnormality provides a mechanistic insight into the nature of endothelial dysfunction in these patients. Second, because of the antiatherogenic effects of NO, the diminished vascular activity of this molecule may provide a pathophysiological link between essential hypertension and atherosclerosis, which, in turn, may explain why the former is a risk factor for the latter. As mentioned previously, NO is synthesized using the amino acid L-arginine as a precursor in response to a variety of physiological and pharmacologic stimuli and is broken down primarily by superoxide anions originated both intracellularly and extracellularly.[40] Thus, a reduced activity of NO may be the consequence of an abnormality in one or several steps in the process of NO synthesis, release, breakdown, or action on the smooth muscle cells. Understanding of the precise mechanisms of impaired bioavailability of NO may provide the basis for the development of novel therapies. Over the last few years, a series of investigations have been performed with the aim of identifying abnormalities that may account for the reduced activity of NO in human hypertension.

## Mechanisms That May Explain Reduced Synthesis of Nitric Oxide

Because L-arginine is the necessary substrate for the production of NO, reduced intracellular availability of the amino acid potentially could lead to reduced NO synthesis. If this were the case, then NO synthesis might be increased by means of augmenting the intracellular levels of L-arginine. Indeed, previous investigations in animal and human models of hypercholesteremia and atherosclerosis have indicated that administration of L-arginine may improve the impaired endothelium-dependent vascular relaxation characteristic of these conditions.[41–43] These observations not only have pathophysio-logical implications, but also may prove to be of therapeutic benefit. Thus, if increasing the availability of L-arginine ameliorates endothelial dysfunction, administration of the amino acid may become a novel therapy for atheroscle-rosis or its risk factors. However, studies conducted in patients with essential hypertension have shown that intra-arterial infusion of L-arginine does not modify significantly endothelium-dependent vascular responses to ACh.[39,44] These findings therefore demonstrate that the diminished activity of NO resulting in impaired endothelial vasodilator function of hypertensive patients is not related to decreased intracellular availability of L-arginine.

The synthesis of NO by constitutive eNOS is regulated by complex intra-cellular pathways. Most physiological and pharmacologic stimuli that result in increased production and release of NO act on cell surface receptors that are coupled to membrane-bound G-proteins. Activation of specific G-proteins, in turn, leads to the initiation of a chain of events that results in stimulation of eNOS. A defect in the process that leads to activation of eNOS could be responsible for the decreased activity of NO. For example, a defect in specific cell surface receptors may explain the impaired response to ACh in athero-sclerotic coronary arteries. Previous studies have shown that coronary arteries with constricting responses to ACh may indeed show endothelium-dependent vasodilation in response to substance P.[45,46] Because substance P is an endo-thelial agonist that stimulates the production of NO by acting on specific tachykinin receptors, the finding of differential responses to ACh (a muscarinic agonist) and substance P in patients with endothelial dysfunction suggests the possibility that the reduced activity of NO might be the result of a specific cell surface receptor defect. In the case of hypertensive patients, if this were the case, one could expect that a depressed response to ACh may coexist with preserved endothelium-dependent vasodilation to substance P. Therefore, to determine whether a selective defect at the level of the muscarinic receptor may account for the impaired vasodilator response to ACh previously reported in hypertensive patients, studies were performed with intra-arterial adminis-tration of ACh and substance P. This investigation showed that hypertensive patients with impaired responses to ACh also have reduced vasodilation in response to substance P. These findings therefore rule out the possibility that a specific muscarinic receptor abnormality is the mechanism for decreased activity of NO in essential hypertension.[47]

However, it is possible that a selective defect at the level of intracellular G-protein–dependent signal transduction pathways may be responsible for the reduced synthesis of NO. That this mechanism may be operative in certain models of endothelial dysfunction has been shown in previous studies of animal models of dyslipidemia. Thus, previous studies performed in animals fed a high-cholesterol diet have indicated that the nature of their endothelial dysfunction may follow different stages from a selective abnormality of specific intracellular signal transduction pathways in the early phases of the condition to a later stage of a more generalized abnormality of endothelial function.[48] Recent studies have addressed the possibility that hypertensive patients may show this form of endothelial abnormality with different patterns of vasodila-tor responses to different endothelial agonists. In a study specifically designed

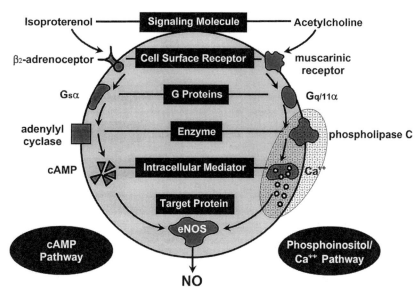

**Figure 1.** Mechanisms of stimulation of eNOS by acetylcholine (ACh) and isoproterenol. The different signaling molecules used different cell surface receptors, membrane-bound G-proteins, and intracellular signal transduction pathways to stimulate the production of nitric oxide (NO). The shaded area indicates the portion of the phosphoinositol pathway containing the defect leading to impaired NO activity in hypertensive patients, according to the results of our studies (see text for detailed explanation).

to address this issue, ACh and bradykinin were infused in patients with essential hypertension and normotensive controls. Bradykinin is an endothelial agonist, which, in contrast to ACh, acts through a pertussis toxin–insensitive G-protein–dependent pathway to activate eNOS. The results of this study showed that hypertensive patients similarly have blunted responses to ACh and bradykinin compared with normal controls.[49] Further, a significant correlation was found between the magnitude of vasodilation induced by ACh and that produced by bradykinin. In conjunction, these observations indicate that, in contrast to the animal models of dyslipidemia, the endothelial dysfunction of hypertensive patients does not appear to be localized to a single G-protein–dependent intracellular signal transduction pathway.[49] Because the patients included in this study had a long duration of hypertension, it is possible that a selective defect may be present during the early stages of the disease. Importantly, these results are different from those observed in hypercholesterolemic patients in whom a relatively preserved vasodilator response to bradykinin is observed despite the impaired responses to ACh.[50]

The results of a recent study from our laboratory appear to localize the defect in NO synthesis to a point that is distal to the activation of membrane-bound G-proteins. In this study, hypertensive patients with demonstrated impaired vasodilator response to ACh had, in contrast, a preserved response to isoproterenol, a $\beta$-adrenoceptor agonist that stimulates endothelial production of NO.[51,52] Because isoproterenol also can directly relax smooth muscle cells and induce vasodilation in an NO-independent fashion, in the same study the infusion of isoproterenol was repeated after the administration of L-NMMA. Importantly, L-NMMA blunted the response to isoproterenol to the same extent in normotensive and hypertensive individuals.[53] These findings indicate that the ability of isoproterenol to stimulate NO production is not impaired in hypertensive patients compared with normal controls. This observation has important pathophysiological implications because, for the first time, this study demonstrated normal release of NO in hypertensive arteries by means of stimulation with an endothelial agonist. The discrepancy between the results previously observed with ACh, substance P, bradykinin, and isoproterenol may be explained by the different intracellular signal transductions pathways involved in the stimulation of eNOS by these agonists (Figure 1). In particular ACh, substance P, and bradykinin act through the phosphoinositide pathway, while β-adrenoceptor stimulation with isoproterenol results in NO synthesis stimulation using cyclic adenosine monophosphate (cAMP) as a second messenger. Consequently, the findings of preserved responses to isoproterenol in subjects with previously demonstrated abnormal responses to other endothelial agonists suggest a defect in the phosphoinositide pathway as a potential mechanism responsible for endothelial dysfunction in hypertensive patients (Figure 1).[53]

## Increased Breakdown of Nitric Oxide as a Potential Mechanism of Endothelial Dysfunction

A different pathophysiological mechanism to explain the impaired activity of NO in the hypertensive vasculature may be related to increased destruction of NO after its formation (Figure 2). Thus, according to this hypothesis, the production of NO may be normal or even enhanced, but the resulting activity of this molecule would be reduced as a consequence of increased breakdown. In fact, previous studies in hypercholesterolemia and atherosclerosis have demonstrated that this mechanism may be operative in the endothelial dysfunction characteristic of these conditions.[54] This possibility may have both pathophysiological and therapeutic implications. If an enhanced breakdown of NO is responsible for the reduced vascular activity of this molecule, then interventions designed to reduce the destruction of NO may increase significantly the vascular availability of NO and therefore improve endothelial function. Because NO primarily is broken down by superoxide anions, the administration of superoxide dismutase (SOD), a scavenger of superoxide anions, may improve endothelium-dependent vascular responses. In a study designed to address this issue, the administration of copper–zinc SOD (CuZn SOD) did not result in modification of endothelium-dependent responses to ACh of either normotensive or hypertensive individuals.[55] It is important to note that CuZn SOD has very poor intracellular penetrance because of its negative charge. Therefore, administration of CuZu SOD should not be expected to curtail increased intracellular breakdown of NO. Thus, the results of these studies only indicate that the destruction of NO by extracellular superoxide anions is not increased in hypertensive patients compared with normotensive controls, but do not address the possibility of increased intracellular breakdown (Figure

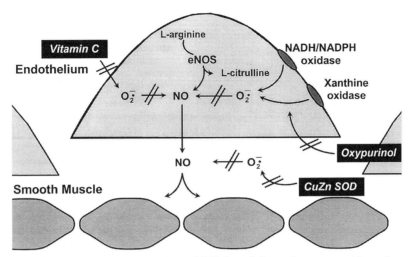

**Figure 2.** Schematic representation of NO breakdown by superoxide anions ($O_2^-$). Superoxide anions are generated both intra- and extracellularly from different enzymatic and nonenzymatic sources. The activity of superoxide anions can be modified with different pharmacologic tools. Oxypurinol inhibits xanthine oxidase; CuZn superoxide dismutase (SOD) scavenges extracellular superoxide anions; and vitamin C is a water-soluble nonspecific antioxidant with high-intracellular penetrance. These substances have been used in different studies investigating the possibility of enhanced breakdown of NO by superoxide anions in hypertensive arteries (see text for details).

2). Although other forms of SOD with increased intracellular penetrance have been shown to have a beneficial effect on animal studies[56] and potentially may have an effect on the vasodilator function of hypertensive patients, they are not available for human use.

It is important to understand that several intracellular processes may result in the production of oxygen free radicals and, in particular, superoxide anions. Among these is the xanthine oxidase system. Because xanthine oxidase can be inhibited by oxypurinol, it is possible to study the contribution of this source of superoxide anions to the endothelial dysfunction of hypertensive patients (Figure 2). Therefore, a study was designed specifically to address the possibility that an enhanced activity of the xanthine oxidase system may explain an increased breakdown of NO within the endothelial cell in hypertensive and hypercholesteremic patients. Those studies showed that oxypurinol is able to improve the response to ACh in hypercholesterolemic patients. However, the response to this endothelial agonist was not modified by oxypurinol in normal controls or hypertensive patients.[57] Importantly, the vasodilator response to sodium nitroprusside was not affected by oxypurinol in any of the three subject groups. In conjunction, these results indicate that an enhanced activity of the xanthine oxidase system may explain, at least partly, the depressed response to ACh of hypercholesterolemic patients. However, this mechanism does not seem to operate in hypertensive individuals.

A recent investigation appears to support the concept that intracellular destruction of NO by oxygen free radicals may indeed play a role in the endothelial dysfunction of hypertensive patients. Thus, Taddei et al[58] recently have demonstrated that the administration of vitamin C, a potent antioxidant with high-intracellular penetrance, can improve the impaired endothelium-dependent vasodilator response to ACh, without affecting the response to sodium nitroprusside. In the same study, the authors analyzed the effect of NO synthesis inhibition with L-NMMA on the response to ACh before and after administration of vitamin C. Prior to the infusion of the antioxidant, L-NMMA did not modify significantly the response to ACh in hypertensive patients. However, after administration of vitamin C, not only was the response to ACh enhanced, but the infusion of L-NMMA had a significant blunting effect on the increase in blood flow induced by the endothelial agonist. These findings indicate that an enhanced oxidant activity operates within the endothelial cell to reduce the availability of NO (Figure 2). It also is important to note that in the same study, the authors analyzed the effect of indomethacin (a cyclooxygenase inhibitor) on the response to ACh before and after administration of vitamin C. As reported previously,[39] indomethacin was able to augment the response to ACh in hypertensive patients, in a fashion similar to that produced by vitamin C. However, the combined administration of vitamin C and indomethacin did not enhance the response to ACh in hypertensive patients beyond the level demonstrated by vitamin C or indomethacin alone. These observations are consistent with the concept that the predominant effect by which cyclooxygenase products may impair endothelium-dependent vasodilation is related to enhanced oxidant activity that, in turn, results in diminished activity of NO.

## Endothelin, Nitric Oxide, and Hypertension

A potential mechanism that may participate in the endothelial dysfunction of hypertensive patients is related to possible interactions between NO and other endothelium-derived factors (Figure 3). Among these, endothelin (ET), a vasoconstrictor and mitogenic peptide produced by endothelial cells,[59] is a prime candidate given its complex interactions with NO. Endothelin effects on the vasculature are mediated by two subtypes of endothelial receptors: $ET_A$ and $ET_B$.[60,61] $ET_A$ receptors are located primarily on vascular smooth muscle cells and mediate the vasoconstrictor effect of the peptide. In contrast, $ET_B$ receptors are located both on smooth muscle cells and on endothelial cells and mediate different effects of ET. In smooth muscle cells, $ET_B$ receptors appear to mediate vasoconstriction. However, on endothelial cells, $ET_B$ receptors participate in stimulation of NO synthesis, which ultimately results in an indirect vasodilator effect of ET.[62-64] At the same time, NO may inhibit the production of ET. Therefore, given these interactions between ET and NO, different possible scenarios can be construed that might lead to increased vasoconstrictor tone caused by diminished activity of NO, enhanced activity of ET, or both (Figure 3). Although initial studies reported increased plasma levels of ET in hypertensive patients, more recent investigations have shown negative results.[65-68] In this regard, it is important to understand that because ET is released largely abluminally, the plasma levels of the peptide may not necessarily reflect its contribution to the regulation of vascular tone.

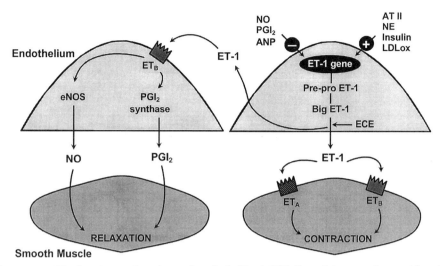

**Figure 3.**  Mechanisms of actions of endothelin-1 (ET-1) and interactions with other endothelium-derived factors. ET-1 acts on two different receptors: $ET_A$ and $ET_B$. $ET_A$ receptors are located on a smooth muscle cell surface in mediates vasoconstriction; $ET_B$ receptors are located on smooth muscle cells to induce vasoconstriction and also on endothelial cells to stimulate the production of NO and prostacyclin ($PGI_2$). In turn, these and other endothelium-derived factors regulate the production of ET-1 by endothelial cells. Abbreviations: ANP, atrial natriuretic peptide; AT II, angiotensin II; ECE, endothelin-converting enzyme; LDLox, oxidized LDL; NE, norepinephrine.

Further, it is possible that up-regulation or down-regulation of either $ET_A$ or $ET_B$ receptors could lead to enhanced or decreased vasoactive effects of ET even despite normal levels of production of the peptide. Fortunately, the development of specific $ET_A$ and $ET_B$ receptor blockers have made it possible to study the contribution of ET in the physiological and pathophysiological regulation of vascular tone. Recent studies have indicated that blockade of $ET_A$ receptors leads to substantial vasodilation in hypertensive patients with no significant response in normotensive controls.[69] These results would indicate that the vasoconstrictor effect of ET is augmented in hypertensive patients. How this abnormality is related to the previously demonstrated decreased activity of NO remains to be elucidated.

# References

1. Furchgott RF. Role of endothelium in responses of vascular smooth muscle. *Circ Res* 1983;53:557–573.
2. Konishi M, Su C. Role of endothelium in dilator responses of spontaneously hypertensive rat arteries. *Hypertension* 1983;5:881–886.
3. Winquist RJ, Bunting PB, Baskin EP, et al. Decreased endothelium-dependent relaxation in New Zealand genetic hypertensive rats. *J Hypertens* 1984;2:541–545.
4. DeMey JG, Gray SD. Endothelium-dependent reactivity in resistance vessels. *Prog Appl Microcirc* 1985;8:181–187.
5. Lockette W, Otsuka Y, Carretero O. The loss of endothelium-dependent vascular relaxation in hypertension. *Hypertension* 1986;8:II6l–II66.

6. Miller MJS, Pinto A, Mullane KM. Impaired endothelium-dependent relaxations in rabbits subjected to aortic coarctation hypertension. *Hypertension* 1987;10:164–170.

7. Luscher TF, Vanhoutte PM. Endothelium-dependent contractions to acetylcholine in the aorta of the spontaneously hypertensive rat. *Hypertension* 1986;8:344–348.

8. Luscher TF, Vanhoutte PM, Raij L. Antihypertensive treatment normalizes decreased endothelium-dependent relaxations in rats with salt-induced hypertension. *Hypertension* 1987;9:III193–III197.

9. Panza JA, Quyyumi AA, Epstein SE. Impaired endothelium-dependent vascular relaxation in hypertensive patients. *Circulation* 1988;78:II473. Abstract.

10. Panza JA, Quyyumi AA, Brush JE Jr, et al. Abnormal endothelium-dependent vascular relaxation in patients with essential hypertension. *N Engl J Med.* 1990; 323:22–27.

11. Linder L, Kiowski W, Buhler FR, et al. Indirect evidence for release of endothelium-derived relaxing factor in human forearm circulation in vivo. Blunted response in essential hypertension. *Circulation* 1990;81:1762–1767.

12. Yoshida M, Imaizumi T, Ando S, et al. Impaired forearm vasodilatation by acetylcholine in patients with hypertension. *Heart Vessels* 1991;6:218–223.

13. Brush JE Jr, Faxon DP, Salmon S, et al. Abnormal endothelium-dependent coronary vasomotion in hypertensive patients. *J Am Coll Cardiol* 1992;19:809–815.

14. Taddei S, Virdis A, Mattei P, et al. Vasodilation to acetylcholine in primary and secondary forms of human hypertension. *Hypertension* 1993;21:929–933.

15. Falloon BJ, Heagerty AM. In vitro perfusion studies of human resistance artery function in essential hypertension. *Hypertension* 1994;24:16–23.

16. Creager MA, Roddy MA. Effect of captopril and enalapril on endothelial function in hypertensive patients. *Hypertension* 1994;24:499–505.

17. Rizzoni D, Porteri E, Castellano M, et al. Endothelial dysfunction in hypertension is independent from the etiology and from vascular structure. *Circulation* 1998;31: 335–341.

18. Cockcroft JR, Chowienczyk PJ, Benjamin N, et al. Preserved endothelium-dependent vasodilatation in patients with essential hypertension. *N Engl J Med* 1994;330:1036–1040.

19. Bruning TA, Chang PC, Hendriks MGC, et al. In vivo characterization of muscarinic receptor subtypes that mediate vasodilatation in patients with essential hypertension. *Hypertension* 1995;26:70–77.

20. Taddei S, Virdis A, Mattei P, et al. Endothelium-dependent forearm vasodilation is reduced in normotensive subjects with familial history of hypertension. *J Cardiovasc Pharmacol* 1992;20(suppl):S193–S195.

21. Taddei S, Virdis A, Mattei P, et al. Defective L-arginine-nitric oxide pathway in offspring of essential hypertensive patients. *Circulation* 1996;94:1298–1303.

22. Lamping KG, Dole WP. Acute hypertension selectively potentiates constrictor responses of large coronary arteries to serotonin by altering endothelial function in vivo. *Circ Res* 1987;61:904–913.

23. Dohi Y, Criscione L, Pfeiffer K, et al. Angiotensin blockade or calcium antagonists improve endothelial dysfunction in hypertension: Studies in perfused mesenteric resistance arteries. *J Cardiovasc Pharmacol* 1994;24:372–379.

24. Takase H, Moreau P, Küng CF, et al. Antihypertensive therapy prevents endothelial dysfunction in chronic nitric oxide deficiency: Effect of verapamil and trandolapril. *Hypertension* 1996;27:25–31.

25. Panza JA, Quyyumi AA, Callahan TS, et al. Effect of antihypertensive treatment on endothelium-dependent vascular relaxation in patients with essential hypertension. *J Am Coll Cardiol* 1993;21:1145–1151.

26. Kiowski W, Linder L, Nuesch R, et al. Effects of cilazapril on vascular structure and function in essential hypertension. *Hypertension* 1996;27(pt 1):371–376.

27. Hirooka Y, Imaizumi T, Masaki H, et al. Captopril improves impaired endothelium-dependent vasodilation in hypertensive patients. *Hypertension* 1992;20:175–180.

28. Mancini GBJ, Henry GC, Macaya C, et al. Angiotensin-converting enzyme inhibition with quinapril improves endothelial vasomotor dysfunction in patients with coronary artery disease: The TREND (Trial on Reversing Endothelial Dysfunction) study. *Circulation* 1996;94:258–265.

29. Palmer RMJ, Ferrige AG, Moncada S. Nitric oxide release accounts for the biological activity of endothelium-derived relaxing factor. *Nature* 1987;327:524–526.

30. Palmer RMJ, Ashton DS, Moncada S. Vascular endothelial cells synthesize nitric oxide from L-arginine. *Nature* 1988;333:664–666.

31. Moncada S, Higgins ES. The L-arginine-nitric oxide pathway. *N Engl J Med* 1993;329:2002–2012.

32. MacAllister RJ, Fickling SA, Whitley GSJ, et al. Metabolism of methylarginines by human vasculature; implications for the regulation of nitric oxide synthesis. *Br J Pharmacol* 1994;112:43–48.

33. Huang PL, Huang Z, Mshimo H, et al. Hypertension in mice lacking the gene for endothelial nitric oxide synthase. *Nature* 1995;377:239–242.

34. Ribeiro M, Antunes E, deNucci G, et al. Chronic inhibition of nitric oxide synthesis: A new model of hypertension. *Hypertension* 1992;20:298–303.

35. Vallance P, Collier J, Moncada S. Effects of endothelium-derived nitric oxide on peripheral arteriolar tone in man. *Lancet* 1989;2:997–1000.

36. Cooke JP, Dzau VJ. Nitric oxide synthase: Role in the genesis of vascular disease. *Annu Rev Med* 1997;48:489–509.

37. Calver A, Collier J, Moncada S, et al. Effect of local intra-arterial $N^G$-monomethyl-L-arginine in patients with hypertension: The nitric oxide dilator mechanism appears abnormal. *J Hypertens* 1992;10:1025–1031.

38. Panza JA, Casino PR, Kilcoyne CM, et al. Role of endothelium-derived nitric oxide in the abnormal endothelium-dependent vascular relaxation of patients with essential hypertension. *Circulation* 1993;87:1468–1474.

39. Taddei S, Virdis A, Ghiadoni L, et al. Cyclooxygenase inhibition restores nitric oxide activity in essential hypertension. *Hypertension* 1997;29:274–279.

40. Gryglewski RJ, Palmer RM, Moncada S. Superoxide anion is involved in the breakdown of endothelium-derived vascular relaxing factor. *Nature* 1986;320:454–456.

41. Girerd XJ, Hirsch AT, Cooke JP, et al.L-arginine augments endothelium-dependent vasodilation in cholesterol-fed rabbits. *Circ Res* 1990;67:1301–1308.

42. Creager MA, Gallagher SJ, Girerd XJ, et al.L-arginine improves endothelium-dependent vasodilation in hypercholesterolemic humans. *J Clin Invest* 1992;90:1248–1253.

43. Drexler H, Zeiher AM, Meinzer K, et al. Correction of endothelial dysfunction in coronary microcirculation of hypercholesterolaemic patients by L-arginine. *Lancet* 1991;338:1546–1550.

44. Panza JA, Casino PR, Badar DM, et al. Effect of increased availability of endothelium-derived nitric oxide precursor on endothelium-dependent vascular relaxation in normal subjects and in patients with essential hypertension. *Circulation* 1993;87:1475–1481.

45. Egashira K, Inou T, Yamada A, et al. Heterogeneous effects of the endothelium-dependent vasodilators acetylcholine and substance P on the coronary circulation of patients with angiographically normal coronary arteries. *Coron Artery Dis* 1992;3:945–952.

46. Okumura K, Yasue H, Ishizaka H, et al. Endothelium-dependent dilator response to substance P in patients with coronary spastic angina. *J Am Coll Cardiol* 1992;20:838–844.

47. Panza JA, Casino PR, Kilcoyne CM, et al. Impaired endothelium-dependent vasodilation in patients with essential hypertension: Evidence that the abnormality is not at the muscarinic receptor level. *J Am Coll Cardiol* 1994;23:1610–1616.

48. Flavahan NA. Atherosclerotic or lipoprotein-induced endothelial dysfunction. Potential mechanisms underlying reduction in EDRF/nitric oxide activity. *Circulation* 1992;85:1927–1938.

49. Panza JA, Garcia CE, Kilcoyne CM, et al. Impaired endothelium-dependent vaso-dilation in patients with essential hypertension. Evidence that nitric oxide abnor-mality is not localized to a single signal transduction pathway. *Circulation* 1995; 91:1732–1738.

50. Gilligan DM, Guetta V, Panza JA, et al. Selective loss of microvascular endothelial function in human hypercholesterolemia. *Circulation* 1994;90:35–41.

51. Cardillo C, Kilcoyne CM, Quyyumi AA, et al. Decreased vasodilator response to isoproterenol during nitric oxide inhibition in humans. *Hypertension* 1997;30:918–921.

52. Daves M, Chowienczyk PJ, Ritter JM. Effects of inhibition of the L-arginine/nitric oxide pathway on vasodilation caused by β-adrenergic agonists in human forearm. *Circulation.* 1997;95:2293–2297.

53. Cardillo C, Kilcoyne CM, Quyyumi AA, et al. Selective defect in nitric oxide synthesis may explain the impaired endothelium-dependent vasodilation in pa-tients with essential hypertension. *Circulation* 1998;97:851–856.

54. Ohara Y, Peterson TE, Harrison DG. Hypercholesterolemia increases endothelial superoxide anion production. *J Clin Invest* 1993;91:2546–2551.

55. García CE, Kilcoyne CM, Cardillo C, et al. Effect of copper–zinc superoxide dis-mutase on endothelium-dependent vasodilation of patients with essential hyper-tension. *Hypertension* 1995;26:863–868.

56. White CW, Brock TA, Chang LY, et al. Superoxide and peroxynitrite in atheroscle-rosis. *Proc Natl Acad Sci U S A* 1994;91:1044–1048.

57. Cardillo C, Kilcoyne CM, Cannon RO, et al. Xanthine oxidase inhibition improves endothelium-dependent vasodilation in hypercholesterolemic but not in hyperten-sive patients. *Hypertension* 1997;30:57–63.

58. Taddei S, Virdis A, Ghiadoni L, et al. Vitamin C improves endothelium-dependent vasodilation by restoring nitric oxide activity in essential hypertension. *Circulation* 1998;97:2222–2229.

59. Yanagisawa M, Kurihara H, Kimura S, et al. A novel potent vasoconstrictor peptide produced by vascular endothelial cells. *Nature* 1988;332:411–415.

60. Arai H, Hori S, Aramori I, et al. Cloning and expression of cDNA encoding an endothelin receptor. *Nature* 1990;348:730–732.

61. Sakurai T, Yanagisawa M, Takuwa Y, et al. Cloning of a cDNA encoding a non-isopeptide-selective subtype of the endothelin receptor. *Nature* 1990;348:732–735.

62. Seo B, Oemar BS, Siebenmann R, et al. Both $ET_A$ and $ET_B$ receptors mediate contraction to endothelin-1 in human blood vessels. *Circulation* 1994;89:1203–1208.

63. Haynes WG, Strachan FE, Webb DJ. Endothelin $ET_A$ and $ET_B$ receptors cause vasoconstriction of human resistance and capacitance vessels in vivo. *Circulation* 1995;92:357–363.

64. De Nucci G, Thomas R, D'Orleans-Juste P, et al. Pressor effects of circulating endothelin are limited by its removal in the pulmonary circulation and by the release of prostacyclin and endothelium-derived relaxing factor. *Proc Natl Acad Sci U S A* 1988;85:9797–9800.

65. Kohno M, Yasumari K, Murakawa Kl, et al. Plasma immunoreactive endothelin in essential hypertension. *Am J Med* 1990;88:614–618.

66. Saito Y, Nakao K, Mukoyama M, et al. Increased plasma endothelin levels in patients with essential hypertension. *N Engl J Med* 1990;322:205. Letter.

67. Davenport AP, Ashby MJ, Easton P, et al. A sensitive radioimmunoassay measur-ing endothelin-like immunoreactivity in human plasma: Comparison of levels in patients with essential hypertension and normotensive control subjects. *Clin Sci* 1990;78:261–264.

68. Schiffrin EL, Thibault G. Plasma endothelin in human essential hypertension. *Am J Hypertens* 1991;4:303–308.

69. Cardillo C, Kilcoyne CM, Cannon RO, et al. Role of endothelin in the increased vascular tone of patients with essential hypertension. *Hypertension* 1999;33:753–758.

## Chapter 13

# Nitric Oxide Availability in Hypercholesterolemia

*Robert A. Vogel, MD*

## Introduction

Considerable data suggest a causative relationship between hypercholesterolemia and coronary heart disease.[1–9] Atherosclerosis of coronary and other arteries traditionally has been thought to result from cholesterol deposition, modification, and macrophage uptake leading to vascular smooth muscle cell proliferation and matrix formation.[10–12] Recently, hypercholesterolemia, especially in the form of oxidized low-density lipoprotein (LDL) has been shown to impair nitric oxide (NO) availability.[13–18] Lipoprotein(a), postprandial triglyceride remnants, very low-density lipoprotein (VLDL) remnants, and free fatty acids also appear to impair endothelial function. Improvements in endothelium-dependent vasoactivity have been demonstrated by several cholesterol-lowering clinical trials. Reduced NO availability leads to a proatherogenic state.[19–21] Although considerable evidence supports increased NO destruction in hypercholesterolemia by superoxide anion, other data point to decreased NO production.[22] The impaired NO availability in the presence of hypercholesterolemia and other risk factors appears to be an important link between risk factors and atherosclerosis. This chapter reviews the evidence that hypercholesterolemia and other dyslipidemias are associated with decreased NO availability.

## Hypercholesterolemia and Coronary Heart Disease

Following early identification of the presence of cholesterol in atheroma, Anitschkow[1] observed that atherosclerotic lesions could be induced in susceptible animals by a high-saturated fat and -cholesterol diet, and that lesions regressed when a low-fat and -cholesterol diet was resumed. The landmark Framingham Heart Study, initiated in 1948, followed more than 5000 men and

From Panza JA, Cannon RO III (eds): *Endothelium, Nitric Oxide, and Atherosclerosis* ©Futura Publishing Co, Inc, Armonk, NY, 1999.

women who initially were without cardiovascular disease.[2] This study demonstrated that hypercholesterolemia increases the risk of cardiovascular events and originated the concept of coronary risk factors. The Seven Countries Study and the Multiple Risk Factor Intervention Trial found continuous, graded relationships between serum cholesterol and coronary heart disease risk, although societies appear to lie on different cholesterol-risk curves.[3,4] The strongest evidence that dyslipidemias are related causally to the development of coronary heart disease is derived from clinical lipid-lowering trials.[5–9] The Lipid Research Clinics Coronary Primary Prevention Trial and the Helsinki Heart Trial found 19%–34% reductions in cardiovascular events in hypercholesterolemic men treated with cholestyramine and gemfibrozil, repectively.[5–7] During the past two decades, numerous coronary angiographic trials ulilizing different means of cholesterol lowering have found reductions consistently in disease progression and appearance of new lesions and an increase in disease regression. Major cardiovascular events also have been found to decrease within months of starting treatment, despite the 1–2 years necessary to demonstrate anatomic changes. This association supports the concept of plaque stabilization possibly brought about by improvements in endothelial function.[8] In the past 5 years, three large secondary prevention trials (Scandinavian Simvastatin Survival Study, Cholesterol and Recurrent Events Trial, and Long-Term Intervention with Pravastatin in Ischemic Disease Trial) and two large primary prevention trials (West of Scotland Coronary Prevention Study and Air Force/Texas Coronary Atherosclerosis Study) employing 3-hydroxy-3-methylglutaryl coenzyme A (HMG-CoA) reductase inhibitors found major cardiovascular event reductions ranging from 24% to 40%.[9]

## Endothelium-Dependent Vasoregulation

Key regulatory functions of the endothelium include conduit and resistance vessel tone, platelet activation, monocyte adhesion, thrombogenesis, lipid processing, and vessel growth.[13–18,23–30] In performing these regulatory functions, the endothelium appears to be involved centrally in the development of atherosclerosis, hypertension, and heart failure. The process of vasoregulation provides an important means for assessing NO availability. Vasoregulation is accomplished by a balance among endothelium-derived relaxing factors and contracting factors released in response to local mechanical stimuli (eg, shear stress and stretch), metabolic conditions (eg, oxygen tension), platelet and coagulation-derived products (eg, thrombin), and receptor-mediated agonists [eg acetylcholine (ACh), bradykinin, serotonin, and substance P]. Vasorelaxing factors generally have antithrombogenic and antiproliferative effects and the reverse is true for contracting factors. The predominate relaxing factor is NO or a NO adduct, possibly in the form of a nitrosothiol or nitrosoheme. Prostacyclin and endothelium-derived hyperpolarizing factor are secondary vasodilators. NO is derived from the amino acid L-arginine by the oxidation of the guanidine-nitrogen terminal through the action of NO synthase (NOS), leaving citrulline as a by-product. NOS exists in several isoforms in endothelial cells, platelets, macrophages, vascular smooth muscle cells, nerves, and the brain. Gene expression of endothelial NOS is activated constitutively, calcium dependent, and can be up-regulated by shear stress and estrogen. The activity of NOS is inhibited by the circulating amino acid asymmetrical dimethylarginine (ADMA), the levels of which are increased in hypercholesterolemia, peripheral atherosclerosis, and renal failure. NOS can be inhibited pharmacologically by analogues of L-arginine such as L-$N^G$-monomethyl arginine (L-NMMA) and L-nitroarginine methylester (L-NAME), which compete on the catalytic site of the enzyme with L-arginine. Infusions of NOS inhibitors produce vasoconstriction, decreased blood flow, and sustained hypertension, although the effects are regionally variable. NO is a diffusible free radical with a half-life of only a few seconds. NO vasodilates locally by activating smooth muscle cell guanylate cyclase, leading to increased production of cyclic guanosine monophosphate (cGMP).

Endothelial cells also release prostacyclin and a hyperpolarizing factor in response to the same stimuli that release NO.[13–18,31,32] These factors activate cyclic-adenosine monophosphate (cAMP) and potassium channels, respectively. Prostacyclin contributes predominantly to platelet inactivation although its inhibitory effects are enhanced synergistically by NO. The existence of an endothelium-dependent hyperpolarizing factor has been postulated because vascular smooth muscle cells become hyperpolarized during NO–independent relaxation. Hyperpolarizing factor appears to be a labile arachidonic acid metabolite.

## Endothelium-Derived Contracting Factors

The endothelium also releases several contracting factors, including endothelin-1, the vasoconstrictor prostanoids thromboxane $A_2$ and protaglandin $H_2$, oxygen free radicals such as superoxide anion and angiotensin II (Ang II) through the activity of angiotensin-converting enzyme (ACE).[13–18,33–35] Endothelial cells exclusively produce one of three isoforms of endothelin. At low concentrations, endothelin-1 is a vasodilator, but at higher concentrations, it is a potent vasoconstrictor. In general, vasomotor tone is regulated by the endothelium as a balance between NO and endothelin-1 and Ang II production. The endothelium also produces thromboxane $A_2$ and prostaglandin $H_2$ through the cyclooxygenase pathway. Receptors for these substances are found on both vascular smooth muscle cells and platelets, the stimulation of which tends to counteract the effects of NO. ACE, which both converts Ang I to Ang II and inactivates bradykinin also is expressed on the endothelial cell membrane. Ang II has several proatherosclerotic effects, including the promotion of LDL oxidation, macrophage activation, smooth muscle cell proliferation, matrix formation, and thrombogenesis. Ang II also stimulates the production of endothelin-1 and plasminogen activator inhibitor-1. An important vasocontracting product of both endothelial and smooth muscle cells is the oxygen–free–radical superoxide anion. In the presence of hypercholesterolemia, cigarette smoking, atherosclerosis, and hypertension, superoxide anion production is increased. This appears to lead to a decrease in NO availability through the combination of superoxide anion with NO, which procedes more rapidly than the reaction of superoxide anion with superoxide dismutase. A major source of vascular superoxide anion and hydrogen peroxide, another reactive oxygen species, is a membrane-bound, reduced nicotinamide-adenine dinucleotide (NADH)–dependent oxidase, which is up-regulated by Ang II. This effect may be an important link between hypertension and atherosclerosis.

## Measurement of Nitric Oxide Availability

Although reponsible for numerous regulatory actions, endothelial function is assessed most commonly as the vasodilatory response to pharmacologic or mechanical stimuli.[23,36–43] Numerous endothelium-dependent agonists have been identified, including ACh, serotonin, bradykinin, thrombin, and substance P.[31] Each acts through a membrane receptor with signal transduction operating through G-proteins. Alternatively, increased blood flow (shear stress) has been used as a mechanical means for stimulating the endothelium. In vitro, endothelial function is measured most commonly as vascular ring tension in response to varying concentrations of ACh or other endothelial stimuli.

Clinically, vasoregulation has been measured in both the coronary and the peripheral circulations using changes in vessel diameter as an index of conduit vessel endothelial function and changes in blood flow as an index of resistance vessel endothelial function.[36–43] The three most common clinical techniques are (1) quantitative angiographic measurement of changes in coronary artery diameter and/or blood flow in response to intracoronary infusions of varying concentrations of ACh, serotonin, or substance P; (2) ultrasound measurement of changes in brachial artery diameter following induction of hyperemia with blood pressure cuff occlusion (flow-mediated dilation); and (3) venous plethysmographic measurement of forearm blood flow following intra-arterial infusion of a cholinergic stimulus (eg, methacholine). Acetylcholine-induced coronary vasodilation has been shown to correlate weakly but significantly with flow-mediated brachial artery vasodilation.[44] The normal coronary artery response to ACh is vasodilation. In the presence of endothelial dysfunction, vasoconstriction is observed, probably because of an unopposed direct smooth muscle cell response to ACh. Distal coronary artery infusions of a vasodilator (eg, adenosine) to increase blood flow with measurement of changes in proximal coronary artery diameter also have been used to assess flow-mediated endothelial function.[37,38] Flow-mediated vasoconstriction has been demonstrated in the coronary circulation during exercise and is thought to be an important cause of ischemia in the setting of coronary heart disease and syndrome X.[45,46]

Flow-mediated vasodilation (FMV) also has been assessed noninvasively in peripheral arteries. As a manifestation of shear stress-induced NO release, the brachial artery normally dilates 5%–15% following release of an arterial occlusion (FMV).[42,43] NOS inhibition completely eliminates this vasodilatory response in the peripheral arteries but may have a lesser effect in coronary resistance vessels.[47,48] An abnormal response consists of lesser vasodilatation or occasionally vasoconstriction. Flow-mediated brachial artery vasodilatory responses vary inversely with arterial diameter. The normal response of a 3-mm artery is approximately 15% vasodilation, whereas a 5-mm artery normally may vasodilate only approximately 5%. The use of 5 minutes of upper arm occlusion produces more postocclusion hyperemia and FMV than does 5 minutes of lower arm occlusion. The upper arm occlusion technique appears to better separate patients with and without risk factors, including hypercholesterolemia. Measurements of endothelial function vary depending on technique and location. In conduit vessels including the coronary circulation, distal arteries tend to be more vasoactive than more proximal, larger vessels.[40,49-51] Especially in the setting of atherosclerosis, endothelium-dependent responses tend to vary regionally, even in the same vessel.[52-54] NO appears to contribute significantly to basal tone in conduit and resistance vessels but may have a lesser effect on endothelium-dependent agonist response in resistance vessels.[49] NO also appears to contribute to the sustained hyperemia observed after ischemic stimulus but has little effect during peak hyperemia.[55] Finally, risk factors may affect the endothelial response to one agonist but may not affect the response to another agonist. For example, hypercholesterolemia impairs the vasodilatory response to ACh but not to bradykinin.[50]

## Dyslipidemias and Endothelial Function

All of the the traditional coronary risk factors have been shown to be associated with abnormal endothelial function in patients with and without atherosclerotic disease by angiography and ultrasound.[13-15,56-69] Moreover, endothelial function has been demonstrated to improve rapidly even in patients with coronary artery disease following risk factor modification in the form of cholesterol lowering, smoking cessation, exercise, estrogen replacement, homocysteine lowering, and ACE inhibition in atherosclerotic vessels (Table 1).[70-74] Both coronary and brachial artery endothelial dysfunction have been observed to correlate in multivariate analysis with the presence of traditional risk factors, including advanced age, male gender, hypercholesterolemia, cigarette smoking, hypertension, diabetes mellitus, high-homocysteine levels, high-fat diet, inactivity, and family history of premature coronary heart disease. The magnitude of endothelial dysfunction has been shown to correlate with the number of risk factors present.[58,65] Aging is an independent risk factor for endothelial dysfunction. A decline in flow-mediated endothelial function has been noted in men more than approximately 40 years old and in women more than approximately 55 years old. Endothelial cells survive approximately 30 years and regenerated cells appear to have reduced function.

### Hypercholesterolemia

Considerable experimental and clinical data suggest that elevated total and LDL cholesterol levels are associated with impaired endothelium-dependent vasodilation, independent of the presence of coronary artery dis-

Table 1
**Factors Associated with Endothelial Dysfunction
and Interventions Demonstrated to
Improve Endothelial Function**

| Factors Associated with Endothelial Dysfunction | Interventions Improving Endothelial Function |
|---|---|
| Increased age | L-Arginine |
| Male gender | Estrogen |
| Family history CHD | Antioxidants |
| Smoking | Smoking cessation |
| Increased cholesterol | Cholesterol lowering |
| Low HDL cholesterol | ACE inhibitors |
| Hypertension | Exercise |
| Diabetes mellitus | Homocysteine lowering |
| Obesity | |
| High-fat meal | |
| Increased homocysteine | |

Adapted with permission from Reference 78.

Abbreviations: ACE, angiotensin-converting enzyme; CHD, coronary heart disease; HDL, high density lipoprotein.

ease.[58,74–80] Hypercholesterolemia impairs both conduit and resistance vessel function. Clinical investigations have found inverse relationships between cholesterol and both coronary and peripheral endothelium-dependent vasodilation that extends down to a cholesterol level of approximately 150 mg/dL (Figure 1). Even short periods of hypercholesterolemia have been found to impair vascular function. Feeding rabbits a high-cholesterol diet for 2 weeks

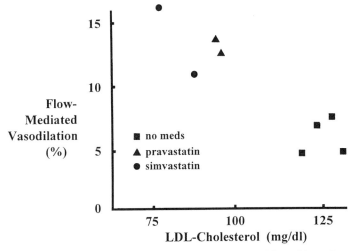

**Figure 1.** Brachial artery flow-mediated vasodilation (FMV) and low-density lipoprotein (LDL) cholesterol measured in seven healthy, normocholesterolemic, middle-aged men before, during, and after simvastatin and pravastatin therapy.

has been found to impair endothelium-dependent vasodilation and increase ischemic myocardial damage.[74] In this study, adverse effects of the diet were reduced substantially by concomitant lovastatin administration. Modified (oxidized) LDL impairs endothelial function more than does native LDL based on in vitro vasodilator responses.[81–86] The offending component of LDL appears to be lysolecithin. Certain types of LDL are more prone to oxidation. Small, dense LDL as occurs in the metabolic syndrome of insulin resistance, dyslipidemia, hypertension, and truncal obesity tends to have a low vitamin E content, oxidizes easily, and is taken up rapidly by macrophages. Oxidized lipoprotein(a) impairs endothelial function more than does oxidized native LDL. Clinical studies assessing both coronary and peripheral endothelium-mediated vasodilation have shown an impaiment of NO availability in the presence of borderline and elevated cholesterol.[48,87,88] The susceptibility of LDL to oxidation correlates better with impairment in endothelial function than does the cholesterol level.[84,86] High-density lipoprotein (HDL) reduces the inhibitory effect of LDL on endothelium-mediated vasodilation and has been shown to vary inversely with clinical measures of endothelial function.[89,90] Hypercholesterolemia increases endothelial adhesion molecule expression and platelet aggregability and adhesion, as well as vasomotion.[91–94]

## Postprandial Triglycerides

A high-fat diet impairs vascular function through at least three mechanisms: elevation of serum LDL and VLDL, direct impairment of endothelial

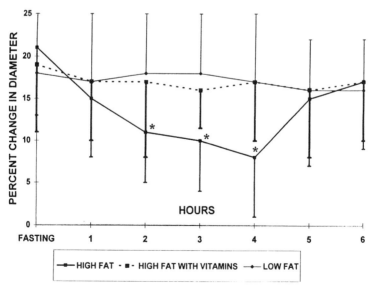

**Figure 2.** Brachial artery FMV measured before and after three isocaloric meals (high fat, high fat with vitamins C and E, and no fat) in 20 healthy, normocholesterolemic, young and middle-aged men and women. Adapted with permission from Reference 96.

function, and increased thrombogenicity. A single high-fat meal recently has been demonstrated to reduce flow-mediated brachial artery vasodilation during the 2–6 hour postprandial period (Figure 2).[95] This adverse effect is reduced substantially by concomitant administration of vitamins C and E along with the high-fat meal.[96] The offending lipid fraction appears to be triglyceride-rich chylomicron remnants, and monounsaturated, polyunsaturated, and saturated fats have been shown to have similar effects. Similar findings have been reported with intravenous triglyceride and free fatty acid administration.[97,98] An exception to this adverse effect of dietary fat on endothelial function is fish oil. Endothelial function has been reported to be improved by chronic fish oil administration in both experimental and clinical studies.[99,100] Fish oil also has been demonstrated to reduce endothelial superoxide production. Increases in coagulation factor VIIa also have been reported following dietary administration of most types of high-fat meals.[101] The impact of fasting as opposed to postprandial hypertriglyceridemia remains controversial. Fasting hypertriglyceridemia has been shown to be associated with reduced dipyridamole-induced coronary hyperemia but not with ACh-induced forearm hyperemia.[102,103] Acute hyperglycemia (locally administered) also appears to impair forearm methacholine-induced vasodilation.[104]

### Very Low-Density Lipoprotein Remnants

VLDL remnant lipoproteins recently have been shown to be associated with impairments of both coronary conduit and resistance vessel vasodilation to ACh.[105,106] By multivariate analysis, remnant lipoproteins concentrations isolated by immunoaffinity mixed gel containing anti–apolipoprotein (anti–apo)-A-I and anti–B-100 monoclonal antibodies correlated better with endothelial function than did LDL cholesterol.

# Interventions

### Cholesterol-Lowering Trials

Following the initial demonstration that lovastatin improves endothelial function in cholesterol-fed rabbits, to date 15 clinical trials have reported the effect of cholesterol lowering on endothelial function using a variety of therapies in patients with a wide range of cholesterol levels (Table 2).[70–73,107–117] Methods of lowering cholesterol have included HMG-CoA reductase inhibitors, bile acid sequestrants, fibric acid derivatives, niacin, and LDL apheresis. Initial mean cholesterol levels in these studies have ranged from 195 to 354 mg/dL. Both angiographically normal and atherosclerotic vessels have been studied, with comparable improvements in both groups. Studies of flow-mediated brachial artery vasodilation following HMG-CoA reductase administration have found similar changes in groups with and without coronary artery disease (Figure 3).[73,109,117] Of the 15 trials, 12 have shown statistically significant improvements in endothelial function as measured by ACh-induced

Table 2
**Studies of the Effect of Cholesterol Lowering on Endothelial Function**

| Reference | CAD | Mean Cholesterol | Technique | Intervention | Months | Result |
|---|---|---|---|---|---|---|
| Egashira[70] | Yes | 272 | CV | Prava | 6 | (+) |
| Anderson[71] | Yes | 209 | CV | Lova/Cho | 12 | (±) |
| Treasure[72] | Yes | 226 | CV | Lova | 6 | (+) |
| Seiler[110] | Yes | 300 | CV | Beza | 7 | (+) |
| Yeung[113] | Yes | 230 | CV | Simva | 6 | (−) |
| Drury[73] | Yes | 209 | BV | Prava | 54 | (+) |
| Tamai[114] | Yes | 195 | FP | Apheresis | 1 h | (+) |
| O'Driscoll[115] | Yes | 254 | FP | Simva | 1 | (+) |
| Andrews[116] | Yes | 202 | BV | Gem/Nia/Cho | 30 | (−) |
| Leung[108] | No | 239 | CV | Cho | 6 | (+) |
| Stroes[112] | No | 354 | FP | Simva/Coles | 3 | (+) |
| Vogel[109] | No | 200 | BV | Simva | 0.5–3 | (+) |
| Goode[111] | No | 373 | AR | Unspec | 10 | (+) |
| Vogel[117] | No | 198 | BV | Prava | 1–7 d | (−) |
| | | | | | 0.5–3 | (+) |
| John[117a] | No | 273 | FP | Fluva | 6 | (+) |

Abbreviations: AR, excised arterial ring; Beza, bezafibrate; BV, brachial vasodilation; CAD, coronary artery disease; Cho, cholestyramine; Chol, cholesterol; Coles, colestipol; CV, coronary vasodilation; Fluva, fluvastatin; FP, forearm plethymography; Gem, gemfibrozil; Nia, niacin; Prava, pravastatin; Prob, probucol; Simva, simvastatin; Unspec, unspecified drugs; (+), significant improvement; (±), borderline improvement (p = 0.08) with lovastatin and cholestyramine, significant improvement with lovastatin and probucol; (−), no improvement.

coronary vasodilation, flow-mediated brachial artery vasodilation, methacholine brachial artery plethysmography, or in vitro vascular ring vasodilation in excised vessels. One trial did not show an improvement with an HMG-CoA reductase inhibitor,[113] one did not show an improvement with combination therapy,[116] and one showed a trend toward improvement ($P = 0.08$) with

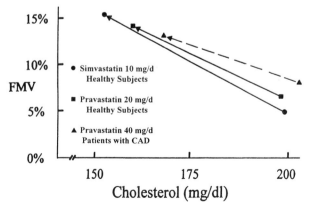

**Figure 3.** Changes in brachial artery FMV and cholesterol measured in middle-aged subjects with and without coronary heart disease before and during simvastatin or pravastatin therapy. Adapted with permission from References 73, 109, and 117.

cholesterol lowering alone (lovastatin + cholestyramine), which reached statistical significance in those subjects receiving both cholesterol lowering (lovastatin) and antioxidant therapy (probucol) (see following text).[71] An improvement in endothelial function was found within 1 hour of cholesterol lowering by LDL apheresis and within 2 weeks of starting an HMG-CoA reductase inhibitor. Improvements in endothelial function have been reported to correlate better with decreased susceptibility of LDL to oxidation than LDL levels.[84,86] Improvements in endothelial function have been observed with reductions of borderline elevated cholesterol levels in the 200 mg/dL range with HMG-CoA reductase inhibitors, suggesting that this level is not ideal[79,80,109,114,117] Whether HMG-CoA reductase inhibitors have direct vascular effects beyond cholesterol lowering remains a controversial issue. In vitro studies have demonstrated a direct effect of lovastatin on LDL susceptibility to oxidation and a reduction in cellular adhesion molecule expression.[118,119] Improvements in endothelial function with cholesterol lowering also have also been shown to improve myocardial perfusion as measured by positron emission tomography, digital radiography, and ST segment monitoring.[120–123] Current opinion also holds that an improvement in endothelial function with cholesterol lowering is an important component of plaque stabilization thought to be a major factor in the decrease in cardiovascular events observed in the recent clinical trials.[8]

## L-Arginine, L-Nitroarginine Methylester and L-$N^G$-Monomethyl Arginine

Administration of the NO precursor L-arginine and the NOS inhibitors L-NAME and L-NMMA have been used as means for evaluating NO availability. In humans, intracoronary L-arginine administration has been shown to improve endothelium-dependent vasodilation in dysfunctional coronary segments in patients with atherosclerosis, coronary risk factors, and microvascular angina.[46,88,124–126] In healthy men, the oral administration of L-arginine was found to improve platelet aggregation, but not endothelium-dependent vasodilation.[127] A lack of improvement in coronary endothelial function after L-arginine infusion also has been reported in patients with advanced atherosclerosis.[128]Intravenously administered L-arginine has been reported to improve brachial artery FMV in hypercholesterolemic and cigarette-smoking young subjects without established coronary heart disease but not in diabetic subjects.[129] The L-arginine administration also reduces monocyte adhesion molecule expression [intercellular adhesion molecule 1(ICAM-1)] in cultured cells and cigarette smokers.[130,131] Inhibition of NOS by L-NMMA has been shown to increase adhesion molecule expression.[130]

The oral administration of L-arginine has been shown to decrease intimal thickening and atherosclerosis progression in LDL receptor knockout mice fed high-cholesterol diets[132] and in hypercholesterolemic rabbits with[133–135] and without[136] balloon vascular injury. Associated improvements in vasodilator endothelial function also have been reported and also have been observed during dietary regression of atherosclerosis in monkeys.[137] Whether L-arginine may have long-term effects remains in question. Six months of oral L-arginine (9 g/day) administration has been shown to improve blood flow responses to ACh in atherosclerotis subjects.[138] However, after 14 weeks of dietary L-arginine administration in a hypercholesterolemic rabbit model, no differences were observed in endothelium-dependent vasodilation and the progression of atherosclerosis was not reduced in female animals nor at certain vascular sites.[139] The chronic administration of NOS by L-NAME administration has been shown to accelerate neointimal formation and atherosclerosis progression in the chosterol-fed rabbit model.[140,141] Associated impairment of endothelial function also was found, which was not reversed by inhibition of thromboxane $A_2$ and prostaglandin $H_2$. These studies demonstrate that NO is a directly antiatherosclerotic molecule independent of changes in cholesterol.[19-21]

## Antioxidants

Several observational studies of dietary and supplemental antioxidant intake have shown inverse correlations with coronary heart disease incidence.[142] This relationship is strongest for vitamin E, which attaches to both LDL and lipid membranes and prevents oxidation. Supporting these observations are the Cambridge Heart Antioxidant Study (CHAOS), which found a significant reduction in cardiovascular events with vitamin E administration in coronary heart disease patients and the Lyon Diet Heart Trial, which also demonstrated the benefit of a Mediterranean diet high in fruits and vegetables.[143,144] The adverse event reduction in both of these trials was unassociated with changes in serum cholesterol levels. In contrast, β-carotene does not inhibit LDL oxidation and has not been found to decrease cardiovascular events in clinical trials.[145] These findings support the concept that coronary risk factors adversely affect the vasculature through an oxidative stress process. Coronary risk factors, including smoking, lack of exercise, increased body mass index, female gender, family history of premature coronary heart disease, and abstinence from alcohol, have been shown to be associated with elevated levels of oxidized LDL.[146] In turn, both endothelium-dependent (ACh) and -independent (dipyridamole) vasodilator responses correlate with the susceptibilty of LDL to oxidation.[81,84,86] Modification of proteins other than LDL also appear to be associated with atherosclerosis.[147]

In experimental models, a reduction in superoxide anion production by dietary cholesterol lowering has been shown in cholesterol-fed rabbits.[148] Decreases in lipid peroxidation and slowing of the progression of atherosclerosis with both cholesterol lowering and antioxidant vitamin E administration have been reported.[118] In clinical studies, the combined administration of vitamins C and E and β-carotene reduces the susceptibility of LDL to oxidation[149] but may not be superior to vitamin E administration alone.[150] Short-term studies of antioxidant vitamin administration have demonstrated improvements in endothelial function, but most long-term studies have reported negative results. Vitamin C infusion has been shown to reverse both brachial and coronary endothelial dysfunction in patients with coronary heart disease and hypertension.[151,152] Decreases in monocyte adhesion molecule expression also have been reported in smokers following 10 days of oral vitamin C supplementation.[153] In contrast, decreases in adhesion molecule expression have been found in smokers following administration of L-arginine but not with vitamin C.[131] Similarly, an investigation employing plethysmographic measurement of forearm vasodilation did not find an improvement in hypercholesterolemic patients treated with vitamins C and E and $\beta$-carotene for 1 month.[154] Conflicting data also exist for the potent antioxidant probucol. Although probucol reduces the development of experimental atherosclerosis and improves endothelial function in combination with cholesterol lowering, it has not been found to decrease the progression of peripheral vascular disease.[71,155]

# Endothelium–Lipid Interactions

The endothelium and lipoproteins are involved in several complex interactions. The endothelium is involved in lipid breakdown and uptake through the expression of LDL receptors and lipoprotein lipase. Through the hydrolysis of triglycerides, the latter releases free fatty acids. Triglyceride-rich chylomicron remnants, free fatty acids, and VLDL remnants recently have been shown to impair endothelial function.[95–98,105,106] A decrease in NO availability appears to be the central defect in hypercholesterolemia based on the finding that NOS inhibition (L-NMMA) reduces endothelium-dependent vasodilation in normocholesterolemic patients more than in hypercholesterolemic patients.[48,87,88] Cholesterol lowering in humans has been shown to increase NO availability.[156] Evidence exists for alterations of both NO production and destruction in hypercholesterolemia. In contrast to experimental atherosclerosis, in which NO production is increased, in human atherosclerotic aortic tissue, endothelial NOS expression and NO release have been shown to be reduced.[157,158] Oxidized LDL has been found to decrease the platelet uptake of L-arginine and reduce NOS expression.[118] L-arginine restores endothelial function induced by oxidized LDL, suggesting an impairment in NOS and/or decreased L-arginine availablility.[118] In most but not all clinical studies, L-arginine infusion has been shown to improve impaired endothelium-dependent vasodilation, including that caused by hypercholesterolemia.[125,126,159,160] The issue of NOS substrate availability in hypercholesterolemia remains controversial because the concentration of L-arginine exceeds the $K_m$ of NOS. Several explanations have been offered for the improvement in endothelial function by L-arginine in hypercholesterolemia, including inhibition of substrate availability by ADMA, decreased microdomain concentration of L-arginine, and insulin release by L-arginine with subsequent vasodilation. Hypercholesterolemia is associated with increases in ADMA, which decreases NOS activity.[16]

Increased superoxide radical production has been demonstrated in cholesterol-fed rabbits.[161] Removal of the endothelium increased superoxide production in the normocholesterolemic animals but substantially reduced it in the hypercholesterolemic animals. Reduction in cholesterol feeding normalizes superoxide anion production.[162] Hypothetically, superoxide and other oxygen free radicals such as hydrogen peroxide and hydroxyl radical can combine with and deactivate NO. A major source of vascular superoxide anion and hydrogen peroxide, another reactive oxygen species, is a membrane-bound, reduced NADH-dependent oxidase, which is up-regulated by Ang II.[22] The reaction between NO and superoxide radical is considerably faster than that between superoxide radical and superoxide dismutase, which may explain why the in vivo administration of superoxide dismutase was not found to improve endo-thelial function in hypercholesterolemic patients.[163] In vitro, superoxide has been shown to restore endothelial function in the presence of oxidized lipopro-tein(a).[83] The concept that hypercholesterolemia and/or atherosclerosis-associated endothelial dysfunction is caused by increased NO destruction is supported by observations that NO production is not reduced in these condi-tions,[157] that changes in coronary endothelial function correlate with changes in susceptibility of LDL to oxidation,[84,86] that endothelial dysfunction and adhesion molecule production are improved by the administration of the an-tioxidant vitamin C,[96,151–154] and that the antioxidant drug probucol improves endothelial function beyond that achieved with cholesterol reduction.[71] Data opposing this concept exist, however. NO production has been found to be reduced in human aortic atherosclerotic tissue.[156] Clinical trials have shown no improvement in endothelial function with administration of antioxidant vitamins[142] or superoxide dismutase[163] and no reduction in the progression of femoral atherosclerosis with probucol.[155] Reduced high-density cholesterol and elevated total to high-density cholesterol ratios also have also been reported to be associated with endothelial dysfunction, possibly because of the antioxidant properties of HDL.[90]

These data underscore the close but complex relationship that exists between dyslipidemias and vascular biology. At the same time, they provide a mechanistic understanding of the impressive benefits that have been observed in the recent clinical trials of cholesterol lowering.

# References

1. Anitschkow N. Experimental atherosclerosis in animals. In: Cowdry EV, ed. *Arteriosclerosis: A Survey of the Problem*. New York: Macmillan; 1933:271–322.
2. Gordon T, Kannel WB. Premature mortality from coronary heart disease. The Framinghan Heart Study. *JAMA* 1971;215:1617–1625.
3. Keys A, Araranis C, Blackburn H, et al. Epidemiologic studies related to coronary heart disease: Characteristics of men aged 40–59 in seven countries. *Acta Med Scand* 1967;180(suppl 460):1–392.
4. The Multiple Risk Factor Intervention Trial research group. Mortality rates after 10.5 years for participants in the Multiple Risk Factor Intervention Trial. Findings related to a priori hypothesis of the trial. *JAMA* 1990;263:1795–1801.
5. Lipid Research Clinics Program. The Lipid Research Clinics coronary primary prevention trial results. I. Reduction in incidence of coronary heart disease. *JAMA* 1984;25:351–364.
6. Lipid Research Clinics Program. The Lipid Research Clinics coronary primary prevention trial results. II. The relationship of reduction in incidence of coronary heart disease to cholesterol lowering. *JAMA* 1984;25:365–374.
7. Frick MH, Elo O, Haapa K, et al. Helsinki Heart Study: Primary-prevention trial with gemfibrozil in middle-aged men with dyslipidemia. Safety of treatment,

changes in risk factors, and incidence of coronary heart disease. *N Engl J Med* 1987;317:1237–1245.

8. Brown BG, Zhao X-Q, Sacco DE, et al. Lipid lowering and plaque regression. New insights into prevention of plaque disruption and clinical events in coronary disease. *Circulation* 1993;87:1781–1789.

9. Gotto AM Jr. Results of recent large cholesterol-lowering trials and their implications for clinical management. *Am J Cardiol* 1997;79:1663–1669.

10. Ross R. The pathogenesis of atherosclerosis. *N Engl J Med* 1986;314:488–500.

11. Steinberg D, Parthasarathy S, Carew TE, et al. Beyond cholesterol. Modifications of low-density lipoprotein that increase its atherogenicity. *N Engl J Med* 1989; 320:915–924.

12. Segrest JP, Anantharamaiah GM. Pathogenesis of atherosclerosis. *Curr Opin Cardiol* 1994;9:404–410.

13. McGorisk GM, Treasure CB. Endothelial dysfunction and coronary heart disease. *Curr Opin Cardio.* 1996;11:341–350.

14. Abrams J. Role of endothelial dysfunction in coronary artery disease. *Am J Cardiol* 1997;79:2–9.

15. Vogel RA. Coronary risk factors, endothelial function, and atherosclerosis: A review. *Clin Cardiol* 1997;20:426–432.

16. Luscher TF, Barton M. Biology of the endothelium. *Clin Cardiol* 1997;20(suppl II):3–10.

17. Celermajer DS. Endothelial dysfunction: Does it matter? Is it reversible? *J Am Coll Cardiol* 1997;30:325–333.

18. Gibbons GH. Endothelial function as a determinant of vascular function and structure: A new theraputic target. *Am J Cardiol* 1997;79:3–8.

19. Cooke JP, Tsao PS. Is NO an endogenous antiatherosclerotic molecule? *Arterioscler Thromb* 1994;14:653–655.

20. Candipan RC, Wang B-Y, Buitrago R, et al. Regression or progression. Dependency on vascular nitric oxide. *Arterioscler Thromb Vasc Biol* 1996;16:44–50.

21. Wever RMF, Luscher TF, Cosentino F, et al. Atherosclerosis and the two faces of endothelial nitric oxide synthase. *Circulation* 1998;97:108–112.

22. Harrison DG. Endothelial function and oxidant stress. *Clin Cardio* 1997;20(suppl II):11–17.

23. Furchgott RF, Zawadzki JV. The obligatory role of endothelial cells in the relaxation of arterial smooth muscle by acetylcholine. *Nature* 1980;288:373–376.

24. Harrison DG. From isolated vessels to the catheterization laboratory. Studies of endothelial function in the coronary circulation of humans. *Circulation* 1989;80: 703–706.

25. Vane JR, Anggard EE, Botting RM. Regulatory functions of the vascular endothelium. *N Engl J Med* 1990;323:27–36.

26. Lerman A, Burnett JC Jr. Intact and altered endothelium in regulation of vasomotion. *Circulation* 1992;86(suppl III):12–19.

27. Flavahan NA. Atherosclerosis or lipoprotein-induced endothelial dysfunction. Potential mechanisms underlying reduction in EDRF/nitric oxide activity. *Circulation* 1992;85:1927–1938.

28. Dzau VJ, Gibbons GH, Cooke JP, et al. Vascular biology and medicine in the 1990's:Scope, concepts, potentials, and perspectives. *Circulation* 1993;87:705–719.

29. Gibbons GH, Dzau VJ. The emerging concept of vascular remodeling. *N Engl J Med* 1994;330:1431–1438.

30. Levine GN, Keaney JF Jr, Vita JA. Cholesterol reduction in cardiovascular disease. Clinical benefits and possible mechanisms. *N Engl J Med* 1995;332:512–521.

31. Flavahan NA, Vanhoutte PM. Endothelium-derived hyperpolarizing factor. *Blood Vessels* 1990;27:238–245.

32. Cohen RA, Vanhouette PM. Endothelium-dependent hyperpolarization. Beyond nitric oxide and cyclic GMP. *Circulation* 1995;92:3337–3349.

33. Lerman A, Hildebrand FL Jr, Margulies KB, et al. Endothelin: A new cardiovascular regulatory peptide. *Mayo Clin Proc* 1990;65:1441–1455.

34. Yanagisawa M. The endothelin system. A new target for theraputic intervention. *Circulation* 1994;89:1320–1322.
35. Gibbons GH. Vasculoprotective and cardioprotective mechanisms of angiotensin-converting enzyme inhibition: The homeostatic balance between angiotensin II and nitric oxide. *Clin Cardiol* 1997;20(suppl II):18–25.
36. Ludmer PL, Selwyn AP, Shook TL, et al. Paradoxical vasoconstriction induced by acetylcholine in atherosclerotic coronary arteries. *N Engl J Med* 1986;315:1046–1051.
37. Cox DA, Vita JA, Treasure CB, et al. Atherosclerosis impairs flow-mediated dilation of human coronary arteries. *Circulation* 1989;80:458–465.
38. Drexler H, Zeiher AM, Wollschlager H, et al. Flow-dependent coronary artery dilatation in humans. *Circulation* 1989;80:466–474.
39. Werns SW, Walton JA, Hsia HH, et al. Evidence of endothelial dysfunction in angiographically normal coronary arteries of patients with coronary artery disease. *Circulation* 1989;79:287–291.
40. Vogel RA. Endothelium-dependent vasoregulation of coronary artery diameter and blood flow. *Circulation* 1993;88:325–327.
41. Celermajer DS, Sorensen KE, Gooch VM, et al. Non-invasive detection of endothelial dysfunction in children and adults at risk of atherosclerosis. *Lancet* 1992;340:1111–1115.
42. Corretti MC, Plotnick GD, Vogel RA. Technical aspects of evaluating brachial artery vasodilation using high-frequency ultrasound. *Am J Physiol* 1995;268:H1397–H1404.
43. Sorensen KE, Celermajer DS, Spiegelhalter DJ, et al. Noninvasive measurement of human endothelium dependent responses: Accuracy and reproducibility. *Br Heart J* 1995;74:247–253.
44. Anderson TJ, Uehata A, Gerhard MD, et al. Close relationship of endothelial function in the human coronary and peripheral circulations. *J Am Coll Cardiol* 1995;26:1235–1241.
45. Zeiher AM, Krause T, Schachinger V, et al. Impaired endothelium-dependent vasodilation of coronary resistance vessels is associated with exercise-induced myocardial ischemia. *Circulation* 1995;91:2345–2352.
46. Egashira K, Hirooka Y, Kuga T, et al. Effects of L-arginine supplementation on endothelium-dependent caronary vasodilation in patients with angina pectoris and normal coronary arteries. *Circulation.* 1996;94:130–134.
47. Joannides R, Haefeli WE, Linder L, et al. Nitric oxide is responsible for flow-dependent dilatation of human peripheral conduit arteries in vivo. *Circulation* 1995;91:1314–1319.
48. Shiode N, Morishima N, Nakayama K, et al. Flow-mediated vasodilation of human epicardial coronary arteries: Effect of inhibition of nitric oxide synthesis. *J Am Coll Cardiol* 1996;27:304–310.
49. Lefroy DC, Crake T, Uren NG, et al. Effect of inhibition of nitric oxide synthesis on epicardial coronary artery caliber and coronary blood flow in humans. *Circulation* 1993;88:43–54.
50. Gilligan DM, Guetta V, Panza JA, et al. Selective loss of microvascular endothelial function in human hypercholesterolemia. *Circulation* 1994;90:35–41.
51. Shiode N, Nakayama K, Morishima N, et al. Nitric oxide production by coronary conductance vessels in hypercholesterolemic patients. *Am Heart J* 1996;131:1051–1057.
52. El-Tamimi H, Mansour M, Wargovich TJ, et al. Constrictor and dilator responses to intracoronary acetylcholine in adjacent segments of the same coronary artery in patients with coronary artery disease. *Circulation* 1994;89:45–51.
53. Penny WF, Rockman H, Long J, et al. Heterogeneity of vasomotor response to acetylcholine along the human coronary artery. *J Am Coll Cardiol* 1995;25:1046–1055.

54. Kuo L, Davis MJ, Chilian WM. Longitudinal gradients for endothelium-dependent and independent vascular responses in the coronary microcirculation. *Circulation* 1995;92:518–525.

55. Tagawa T, Imaizumi T, Endo T, et al. Role of nitric oxide in reactive hyperemia in human forearm vessels. *Circulation* 1994;90:2285–2290.

56. Reddy KG, Nair RN, Sheehan HM, et al. Evidence that selective endothelial dysfunction may occur in the absence of angiographic or ultrasound atherosclerosis in patients with risk factors for atherosclerosis. *J Am Coll Cardiol* 1994;23:833–843.

57. Mano T, Masuyama T, Yamamoto K, et al. Endothelial dysfunction in the early stage precedes appearance of intimal lesions assessable with intravascular ultrasound. *Am Heart J* 1996;131:231–238.

58. Vita JA, Treasure CB, Nabel EG, et al. Coronary vasomotor responses to acetylcholine relates to risk factors for coronary artery disease. *Circulation* 1990;81:491–497.

59. Seiler C, Hess M, Buechi M, et al. Influence of serum cholesterol and other coronary risk factors on vasomotion of angiographically normal coronary arteries. *Circulation* 1993;88(pt 1):2139–2148.

60. Panza JA, Casino PR, Kilcoyne CM, et al. Role of endothelium-derived nitric oxide in the abnormal endothelium-dependent vascular relaxation of patients with essential hypertension. *Circulation* 1993;87:1468–1474.

61. Celermajer DS, Sorensen KE, Georgakopoulos D, et al. Cigarette smoking is associated with dose-related and potentially reversible impairment of endothelium-dependent dilation in healthy young adults. *Circulation* 1993;88:2149–2155.

62. Johnstone MT, Creager SJ, Scales KM, et al. Impaired endothelium-dependent vasodilation in patients with insulin-dependent diabetes mellitus. *Circulation* 1993;88:2510–2516.

63. Egashira K, Inou T, Hirooka Y, et al. Effects of age on endothelium-dependent vasodilation of resistance coronary artery by acetylcholine in humans. *Circulation* 1993;88:77–81.

64. Celermaher DS, Sorensen KE, Spiegelhalter DJ, et al. Aging is associated with endothelial dysfunction in healthy men years before the age-related decline in women. *J Am Coll Cardiol* 1994;24:471–476.

65. Celermajer DS, Sorensen KE, Bull C, et al. Endothelium-dependent dilation in the systemic arteries of asymptomatic subjects relates to coronary risk factors and their interaction. *J Am Coll Cardiol* 1994;24:1468–1474.

66. Taddei S, Virdis A, Mattei P, et al. Aging and endothelial function in normotensive subjects and patients with essential hypertension. *Circulation* 1995;91:1981–1987.

67. Celermajer DS, Adams MR, Clarkson P, et al. Passive smoking and impaired endothelium-dependent arterial dilatation in healthy young adults. *N Engl J Med* 1996;334:150–154.

68. Heitzer T, Yla-Herttuala S, Kurz S, et al. Cigarette smoking potentiates endothelial dysfunction of forearm resistance vessels in patients with hypercholesterolemia. Role of oxidized LDL. *Circulation* 1996;93:1346–1353.

69. Glasser SP, Selwyn AP, Ganz P. Atherosclerosis: rRisk factors and the vascular endothelium. *Am Heart J* 1996;131:379–384.

70. Egashira K, Hirooka Y, Kai H, et al. Reduction in serum cholesterol with pravastatin improves endothelium-dependent coronary vasomotion in patients with hypercholesterolemia. *Circulation* 1994;89:2519–2524.

71. Anderson TJ, Meredith IT, Yeung AC, et al. The effect of cholesterol-lowering and antioxidant therapy on endothelium-dependent coronary vasomotion. *N Engl J Med* 1995;332:488–493.

72. Treasure CB, Klein JL, Weintraub WS, et al. Beneficial effects of cholesterol-lowering therapy on the coronary endothelium in patients with coronary artery disease. *N Engl J Med* 1995;332:481–487.

73. Drury J, Cohen JD, Veenendrababu B, et al. Brachial artery endothelium dependent vasodilation in patients enrolled in the cholesterol and recurrent events (CARE) study. *Circulation* 1996;94(suppl I):402. Abstract.

74. Osborne JA, Siegman MJ, Sedar AW, et al. Lack of endothelium-dependent relaxation in coronary resistance arteries of cholesterol-fed rabbits. *Am J Physiol* 1989;256:C591–C597.

75. Shimokawa AH, Vanhoutte PM. Hypercholesterolemia causes generalized impairment of endothelium-dependent relaxation to aggregating platelets in porcine arteries. *J Am Coll Cardiol* 1989;13:1402–1408.

76. Kugiyama K, Kerns SA, Morisett JD, et al. Impairment of endothelium-dependent relaxation by lysolecithin in modified low-density lipoproteins. *Nature* 1990;334:160–162.

77. Creager MA, Cooke JP, Mendelsohn ME, et al. Impaired vasodilation of forearm resistance vessels in hypercholesterolemic humans. *J Clin Invest* 1990;86:228–234.

78. Vogel RA, Corretti MC. Estrogens, progestins, and heart disease. Can endothelial function divine the benefit? *Circulation* 1998;97:1223–1226.

79. Steinberg HO, Bayazeed B, Hook G, et al. Endothelial dysfunction is associated with cholesterol levels in the high normal range in humans. *Circulation* 1997;96:3287–3293.

80. Creager MA, Selwyn A. When "normal" cholesterol levels injure the endothelium. *Circulation* 1997;96:3255–3257.

81. Simon BC, Cunningham LD, Cohen RA. Oxidized low density lipoproteins cause contraction and inhibit endothelium-dependent relaxation in the pig coronary artery. *J Clin Invest* 1990;86:75–79.

82. Chin JH, Azhan S, Hoffman BB. Inactivation of endothelial derived relaxing factor by oxidized lipoproteins. *J Clin Invest* 1992;89:10–18.

83. Galle J, Bengen J, Schollmeyer P, et al. Impairment of endothelium-dependent dilation in rabbit renal arteries by oxidized lipoprotein(a). Role of oxygen-derived radicals. *Circulation* 1995;92:1582–1589.

84. Anderson TJ, Meredith IT, Charbonneau F, et al. Endothelium-dependent coronary vasomotion relates to the susceptibility of LDL to oxidation in humans. *Circulation* 1996;93:1647–1650.

85. Chen LY, Mehta P, Mehta JL. Oxidized LDL decreases L-arginine uptake and nitric oxide protein expression in human platelets. Relevance of the effect of oxidized LDL on platelet function. *Circulation* 1996;93:1740–1746.

86. Raitakari OT, Pitkanen O-P, Lehtimaki T, et al. In vivo low density lipoprotein oxidation relates to coronary reactivity in young men. *J Am Coll Cardiol* 1997;30:97–102.

87. Casino PR, Kilcoyne CM, Quyyumi AA, et al. The role of nitric oxide in endothelium-dependent vasodilation of hypercholesterolemic patients. *Circulation* 1993;88:2541–2547.

88. Quyyumi AA, Mulcahy D, Andrews NP, et al. Coronary vascular nitric oxide activity in hypertension and hypercholesterolemia. *Circulation* 1997;95:104–110.

89. Matsuda Y, Hirata K, Inoue N, et al. High density lipoprotein reverses inhibitory effect of oxidized low density lipoprotein on endothelium-dependent arterial relaxation. *Circ Res* 1993;72:1103–1109.

90. Kuhn FE, Mohler ER, Reagan K, et al. Effects of high-density lipoprotein on acetylcholine-induced coronary vasoreactivity. *Am J Cardiol* 1991;68:1425–1430.

91. Hackman A, Abe Y, Insull W, et al. Levels of soluble adhesion molecules in patients with dyslipidemia. *Circulation* 1996;93:1334–1338.

92. Sampietro T, Tuomi M, Ferdeghini M, et al. Plasma cholesterol regulates soluble cell adhesion molecule expression in familiar hypercholesterolemia. *Circulation* 1997;96:1381–1385.

93. Lacoste L, Lam JYT, Hung J, et al. Hyperlipidemia and coronary disease. Correction of the increased thrombogenic potential with cholesterol reduction. *Circulation* 1995;92:3172–3177.

94. Nofer J-R, Tepel M, Kehrel B, et al. Low-density lipoproteins inhibit the $Na^+/H^+$ antiport in human platelets. A novel mechanism enhancing platelet activity in hypercholesterolemia. *Circulation* 1997;95:1370–1377.

95. Vogel RA, Corretti MC, Plotnick GD. Effect of a single high-fat meal on endothelial function in healthy subjects. *Am J Cardiol* 1997;79:350–354.

96. Plotnick GD, Corretti MC, Vogel RA. Effect of antioxidant vitamins on the transient impairment of endothelium-dependent vasoactivity following a single high-fat meal. *JAMA* 1997;278:1682–1686.

97. Lundman P, Eriksson M, Schenck-Gustafsson K, et al. Transient triglyceridemia decreases vascular reactivity in young, healthy men without risk factors for coronary heart disease. *Circulation* 1997;96:3266–3268.

98. Steinberg HO, Tarshoby M, Monestel R, et al. Elevated circulating free fatty acids impair endothelium-dependent vasodilation. *J Clin Invest* 1997;100:1230–1239.

99. Malis CD, Leaf A, Varadarajan GS, et al. Effects of dietary ω3 fatty acids on vascular contractility in preanoxic and postanoxic aortic rings. *Circulation* 1991; 84:1393–1401.

100. Goode GK, Garcia S, Heagerty AM. Dietary supplementation with marine fish oil improves in vitro small artery endothelial function in hypercholesterolemic patients. *Circulation* 1997;96:2802–2807.

101. Larsen LF, Bladbjerg E-E, Jespersen J, et al. Effects of dietary fat quality and quantity on postprandial activation of blood coagulation factor VII. *Arterioscler Thromb Vasc Biol* 1997;17:2904–2909.

102. Chowienczyk PJ, Watts GF, Wierzbicki AS, et al. Preserved endothelial function in patients with severe hypertriglyceridemia and low functional lipoprotein lipase activity. *J Am Coll Cardiol* 1997;29:964–968.

103. Yokoyama I, Ohtake T, Momomura S-I, et al. Impaired myocardial vasodilation during hyperemic stress with dipyridamole in hypertriglyceridemia. *J Am Coll Cardiol* 1998;31:1568–1574.

104. Williams SB, Goldfine AB, Timimi FK, et al. Acute hyperglycemia attenuates endothelium-dependent vasodilation in humans in vivo. *Circulation* 1998;97:1695–1701.

105. Kugiyama K, Doi H, Motoyama T, et al. Association of remnant lipoprotein levels with impairment of endothelium-dependent vasomotor function in human coronary arteries. *Circulation* 1998;97:2519–2526.

106. Masuoka H, Ishikura K, Kamei S, et al. Predictive value of remnant-like particles cholesterol/high-density lipoprotein cholesterol as a new indicator of coronary artery disease. *Am Heart J* 1998;136:226–230.

107. Osborne JA, Lento PH, Siegfried MR, et al. Cardiovascular effects of acute hypercholesterolemia. Reversal with lovastatin treatment. *J Clin Invest* 1989;83:465–473.

108. Leung W-H, Lau C-P, Wong C-K. Beneficial effect of cholesterol-lowering therapy on coronary endothelium-dependent relaxation in hypercholesterolaemic patients. *Lancet* 1993;341:1496–1500.

109. Vogel RA, Corretti MC, Plotnick GP. Changes in flow-mediated brachial artery vasoactivity with lowering of desirable cholesterol levels in healthy middle-aged men. *Am J Cardiol* 1996;77:37–40.

110. Seiler C, Suter TM, Hess OM. Exercise-induced vasomotion of angiographically normal and stenotic coronary arteries improves after cholesterol-lowering drug therapy with bezafibrate. *J Am Coll Cardiol* 1995;26:1615–1622.

111. Goode GK, Heagerty AM. In vitro responses of human peripheral small arteries in hypercholesterolemia and effects of therapy. *Circulation* 1995;91:2898–2903.

112. Stroes ESG, Koomans HA, de Bruin TWA, et al. Vascular function in the forearm of hypercholesterolaemic patients off and on lipid-lowering medication. *Lancet* 1995;346:467–471.

113. Yeung A, Hodgson JMcB, Winniford M, et al. Assessment of coronary vascular reactivity after cholesterol lowering. *Circulation* 1996;94(suppl I):402. Abstract.

114. Tamai O, Matsuoka H, Itabe H, et al. Single LDL aphesesis improves endothelium-dependent vasodilatation in hypercholesterolemic humans. *Circulation* 1997;95: 76–82.

115. O'Driscoll G, Green D, Taylor RR. Simvastatin, an HMG-coenzyme. A reductase inhibitor, improves endothelial function within 1 month. *Circulation* 1997;95: 1126–1131.

116. Andrews TC, Whitnet EJ, Green G, et al. Effect of gemfibrozil ± niacin ± cholestyramine on endothelial function in patients with serum low-density lipoprotein cholesterol levels *Am J Cardiol.* 1997;80:831–835.

117. Vogel RA, Corretti MC, Plotnick GD. The mechanism of improvement in endothelial function by pravastatin: Direct effect or through cholesterol lowering. *J Am Coll Cardiol* 1998;31:60A.

117a.John S, Schlaich M, Langenfeld M, et al. Increased bioavailability of nitric oxide after lipid-lowering therapy in hypercholesterolemic patients. *Circulation* 1998; 98:211–216.

118. Chen L, Haught WH, Yang B, et al. Preservation of endogenous antioxidant activity and inhibition of lipid peroxidation as common mechanisms of antiatherosclerotic effects of vitamin E, lovastatin and amlodipine. *J Am Coll Cardiol* 1997;30:569–575.

119. Weber C, Erl W, Weber KSC, et al. HMG-CoA reductase inhibitors decrease CD11b expression and CD11b-dependent adhesion to endothelium and reduce increased adhesiveness of monocytes isolated from patients with hypercholesterolemia. *J Am Coll Cardiol* 1997;30:1212–1217.

120. Gould KL, Ornish D, Scherwitz L, et al. Changes in myocardial perfusion abnormalities by positron emission tomography after long-term, intense risk factor modification. *JAMA* 1995;274:894–901.

121. van Boven AJ, Jukema JW, Zwinderman AH, et al. Reduction of transient myocardial ischemia with pravastatin in addition to the conventional treatment in patients with angina pectoris. *Circulation* 1996;94:1503–1505.

122. Aengevaeren WRM, Uijen GRH, Jukema JW, et al. Functional improvement by pravastatin in the regression growth evaluation statin study (REGRESS). *Circulation* 1997;96:429–435.

123. Andrews TC, Raby K, Barry J, et al. Effect of cholesterol reduction on myocardial ischemia in patients with coronary disease. *Circulation* 1997;95:324–328.

124. Drexler H, Zeiher AM, Meinzer K, et al. Correction of endothelial dysfunction in coronary microcirculation of hypercholesterolaemic patients by L-arginine. *Lancet* 1991;338:1546–1550.

125. Creager MA, Gallagher SJ, Girerd XJ, et al. L-arginine improves endothelium-dependent vasodilation in hypercholesterolemic humans. *J Clin Invest* 1992;90: 1248–1253.

126. Quyyumi AA, Dakak N, Diodati JG, et al. Effect of L-arginine on human coronary endothelium-dependent and physiologic vasodilation. *J Am Coll Cardiol* 1997;30: 1220–1227.

127. Adams MR, Forsyth CJ, Jessup W, et al. Oral L-arginine inhibits platelet aggregation but does not enhance endothelium-dependent vasodilation in healthy young men. *J Am Coll Cardiol* 1995;26:1054–1061.

128. Otsuji S, Nakajima O, Waku S, et al. Attenuation of acetylcholine-induced vasoconstriction by L-arginine is related to the progression of atherosclerosis. *Am Heart J* 1995;129:1094–1100.

129. Thorne S, Mullen MJ, Clarkson P, et al. Early endothelial dysfunction in adults at risk from atherosclerosis: Different responses to L-arginine. *J Am Coll Cardiol* 1998;32:110–116.

130. Adams MR, Jessup W, Hailstones D, et al. L-arginine reduces human monocyte adhesion to vascular endothelium and endothelial expression of cell adhesion molecules. *Circulation* 1997;95:662–668.

131. Adams MR, Jessup W, Celermajer DS. Cigarette smoking is associated with increased human monocyte adhesion to endothelial cells: Reversibility with oral L-arginine but not vitamin C. *J Am Coll Cardiol* 1997;29:491–497.
132. Aji W, Ravalli S, Szabolcs M, et al. L-arginine prevents xanthoma development and inhibits atherosclerosis in LDL recptor knockout mice. *Circulation* 1997;95: 430–437.
133. Cooke JP, Singer AH, Tsao P, et al. Anti-atherogenic effects of L-arginine in the hypercholestyerolemic rabbit. *J Clin Invest* 1992;90:1168–1172.
134. Wang B-W, Candipan RC, Arjomandi M, et al. Arginine restores nitric oxide activity and inhibits monocyte accumulation after vascular injury in hypercholesterolemic rabbits. *J Am Coll Cardiol* 1996;28:1573–1579.
135. Hamon M, Vallet B, Bauters C, et al. Long-term administration of L-arginine reduces intimal thickening and enhances neoendothelium-dependent acetylcholine relaxation after arterial injury. *Circulation* 1994;90:1357–1362.
136. Boger RH, Bode-Boger SM, Brandes RP, et al. Dietary L-arginine reduces the progression of atherosclerosis in cholesterol-fed rabbits. *Circulation* 1997;96: 1282–1290.
137. Benzuly KH, Padgett RC, Kaul S, et al. Functional improvement precedes structural regression of atherosclerosis. *Circulation.* 1994;89:1810–1818.
138. Lerman A, Burnett JC, Higano ST, et al. Long-term L-arginine supplementation improves small-vessel coronary endothelial function in humans. *Circulation* 1998; 97:2123–2128.
139. Jcrcmy RW, McCarron H, Sullivan D. Effects of dietary L-arginine on atherosclerosis and endothelium-dependent vasodilation in the hypercholesterolemic rabbit. Response according to treatment duration, anatomic site, and sex. *Circulation* 1996;94:498–506.
140. Cayette AJ, Palacino JJ, Cohen RA. Chronic inhibition of nitric oxide production accelerates neointimal formation and impairs endothelial function in hypercholesterolemic rabbits. *Arterioscler Thromb* 1994;14:753–759.
141. Naruse K, Shimizu K, Muramatsu M, et al. Long-term inhibition of NO synthesis promotes atherosclerosis in the hypercholesterolemic rabbit thoracic aorta. $PGH_2$ does not contribute to impaired endothelium-dependent relaxation. *Arterioscler Thromb* 1994;14:746–752.
142. Jha P, Flather M, Lonn E, et al. The antoxidant vitamins and cardiovascular disease. A critical review of epidemiologic and clinical trial data. *Ann Intern Med* 1995;123:860–872.
143. Stephens NG, Parsons A, Schofield P, et al. Randomised controlled trial of vitamin E in patients with coronary disease: Cambridge Heart Antioxidant Study (CHAOS). *Lancet* 1996;347:781–786.
144. de Longeril M, Salen P, Martin J-L, et al. Effect of a mediterranean type of diet on the rate of cardiac complications in patients with coronary artery disease. Insights into the cardioprotective effects of certain nutriments. *J Am Coll Cardiol* 1996; 29:1103–1108.
145. Diaz MN, Frei B, Vita JA, et al. Antioxidants and heart disease. *N Engl J Med* 1997;337:408–416.
146. Mosca L, Rubenfire M, Tarshis T, et al. Clinical predictors of oxidized low-density lipoprotein in patients with coronary artery disease. *Am J Cardiol* 1997;80:825–830.
147. O'Brien KD, Alpers CE, Hokanson JE, et al. Oxidation-specific epitopes in human coronary atherosclerosis are not limited to oxidized low-density lipoprotein. *Circulation* 1996;94:1216–1225.
148. Ohara Y, Peterson TE, Sayegh HS, et al. Dietary correction of hypercholesterolemia in the rabbit normalizes endothelial superoxide anion production. *Circulation* 1995;92:898–903.
149. Mosca L, Rubenfire M, Mandel C, et al. Antioxidant nutrient supplementation reduces the susceptibility of low density lipoprotein to oxidation in patients with coronary artery disease. *J Am Coll Cardiol* 1997;30:392–399.

150. Jilal I, Grundy SM. Effect of combined supplementation with α-tocopherol, ascorbate, and beta carotene on low-density lipoprotein oxidation. *Circulation* 1993;88: 2780–2786.
151. Levine GN, Frei B, Koulouris SN, et al. Ascorbic acid reverses endothelial vasomotor dysfunction in patients with coronary artery disease. *Circulation* 1996;93: 1107–1113.
152. Solzbach U, Hornig B, Jeserich M, et al. Vitamin C improves endothelial dysfunction of epicardial coronary arteries in hypertensive patients. *Circulation* 1997;96: 1513–1519.
153. Weber C, Erl W, Weber K, et al. Increased adhesiveness of isolated monocytes to endothelium is prevented by vitamin C intake in smokers. *Circulation.* 1996;93: 1488–1492.
154. Gilligan DM, Sack MN, Guetta V, et al. Effect of antioxidant vitamins on low density lipoprotein oxidation and impaired endothelium-dependent vasodilation in patients with hypercholesterolemia. *J Am Coll Cardiol* 1994;24:1611–1617.
155. Walldius G, Erikson U, Olsson AG, et al. The effect of probucol on femoral atherosclerosis: The Probucol Quantitative Regression Trial (PQRST). *Am J Cardiol* 1994;74:875–883.
156. John S, Schlaich M, Langenfeld M, et al. Increased bioavailability of nitric oxide after lipid-lowering in hypercholesterolemic patients. *Circulation* 1998;98:211–216.
157. Minor R Jr, Myers PR, Guerra R Jr, et al. Diet-induced atherosclerosis increases the release of nitrogen oxides from rabbit aorta. *J Clin Invest* 1990;86:2109–2116.
158. Oemar BS, Tschudi MR, Godoy N, et al. Reduced endothelial nitric oxide synthase expression and production in human atherosclerosis. *Circulation* 1998;97:2494–2498.
159. Casino PR, Kilcoyne CM, Quyyumi AA, et al. Investigation of decreased availability of nitric oxide precursor as the mechanism for impaired endothelium-dependent vasodilation in hypercholesterolemic patients. *J Am Coll Cardiol* 1994; 23:844–850.
160. Chauhan A, More RS, Mullins PA, et al. Aging-associated endothelial dysfunction is reversed by L-arginine. *J Am Coll Cardiol* 1996;28:1796–1804.
161. Ohara Y, Pederson TE, Harrison DG. Hypercholesterolemia increases endothelial superoxide production. *J Clin Invest* 1993;91:2546–2551.
162. Ohara Y, Peterson TE, Sayegh HS, et al. Dietary correction of hypercholesterolemia normalizes endothelial superoxide anion production. *Circulation* 1995;92: 898–903.
163. Garcia CE, Kilcoyne CM, Cardillo C, et al. Evidence that endothelial function in patients with hypercholesterolemia is not due to increased extracellular nitric oxide breakdown by superoxide anions. *Am J Cardiol* 1995;76:1157–1161.

## Chapter 14

# Nitric Oxide Activity in the Human Coronary Circulation

*Arshed A. Quyyumi, MD*

## Introduction

Experimental data in vitro and in animals indicate that the vascular endothelium plays an important role in maintaining blood vessel tone by releasing different dilator and constrictor substances.[1] Endothelium-derived relaxing factors (EDRFs) are produced in response to a variety of receptor-dependent and -independent pharmacologic probes including acetylcholine (ACh), substance P, bradykinin (Bk), adenosine diphosphate (ADP), and calcium ionophore, and also in response to physiological phenomena such as increases in shear stress.[1–4] One important EDRF has been characterized as nitric oxide (NO), or a compound closely related to NO.[5,6] Studies of human coronary endothelial function have relied largely on stimulating production of EDRFs with ACh,[7–10] but whether this is an accurate reflection of the state of the endothelium in general and of NO bioactivity in particular is unknown, because ACh also is capable of producing hyperpolarizing factor and prostaglandins. Furthermore, the results of animal experiments investigating NO activity in the coronary vasculature are conflicting. For example, some studies have suggested the presence of NO activity at rest and with pharmacologic agents in the coronary vasculature, whereas others have not.[11,12] The only human study conducted before ours suggested that NO activity did not contribute to resting coronary microvascular tone, contributed minimally to epicardial tone, and negligibly to ACh-mediated coronary vasodilation.[13] These investigations highlighted the importance of differences in species, in vascular beds, in the agonists and inhibitors employed, and between in vitro and in vivo data and together emphasize the crucial need for in vivo studies to delineate the physiological and pathophysiological role of NO in the human coronary and peripheral circulation.

From Panza JA, Cannon RO III (eds): *Endothelium, Nitric Oxide, and Atherosclerosis* ©Futura Publishing Co, Inc, Armonk, NY, 1999.

# Basal Nitric Oxide Activity in the Human Coronary Vasculature

In normal subjects with angiographically smooth coronary arteries, epicardial coronary arteries progressively constricted and coronary blood flow decreased with increasing doses of L-$N^G$-monomethyl arginine (L-NMMA), a competitive inhibitor of NO synthase (NOS), indicating tonic basal NO activity in the coronary epicardial and microvascular circulation (Figure 1).[14] The constrictor effects of L-NMMA were reduced in patients with either risk factors for atherosclerosis such as hypercholesterolemia, hypertension, diabetes, aging, or smoking, and those with atherosclerosis, indicating that basal NO activity in the coronary vasculature is reduced in

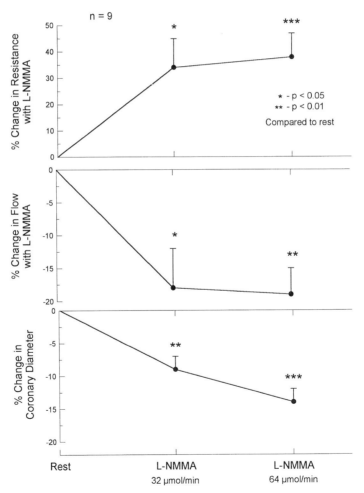

**Figure 1.** Changes in coronary vascular resistance, blood flow, and epicardial diameter with increasing concentrations of L-$N^G$-monomethyl arginine (L-NMMA). Data represent means ± SEM, * = $P < 0.025$, ** = $P < 0.01$ compared with the rest. Adapted with permission from Reference 14.

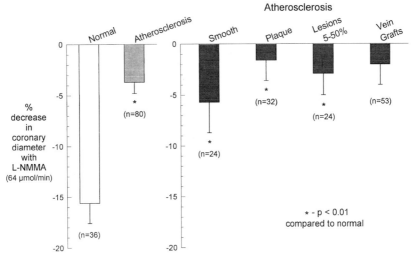

**Figure 2.** The effect of L-NMMA on epicardial coronary vasomotion in patients with normal coronary arteries without risk factors (open column), those with varying severity of coronary atherosclerosis, and in vein grafts (shaded column). Decreased constriction with L-NMMA represents reduced nitric oxide (NO) activity in the latter.

these patients. There was no difference between proximal, mid-, and distal coronary segments of the epicardial coronary arteries in the magnitude of depression in NO activity, and there was no correlation between the angiographic severity of the atherosclerotic stenosis and the effect of L-NMMA (Figure 2).[15] Thus, even angiographically smooth epicardial segments had a depressed response to L-NMMA, suggesting that the NO defect may precede angiographic development of atherosclerosis. Saphenous vein grafts also did not constrict significantly with L-NMMA, indicating low basal NO activity in vein grafts even though they were arterialized for many years.[16] Moreover, the depression in NO activity did not correlate with the age of the vein graft. Internal mammary artery grafts constricted significantly and by a greater magnitude than vein grafts and native arteries indicating greater basal NO activity in internal mammary conduits. This may explain why arterial conduits have longer survival free of atherosclerotic complications than either vein grafts or native coronary arteries.

## Endothelium-Independent Function and Specificity of L-$N^G$-Monomethyl Arginine

To ensure that the coronary vascular abnormalities observed with endothelium-dependent agonists were due to abnormalities of endothelial function and are not a reflection of smooth muscle function in patients with atherosclerosis or risk factors, we have studied coronary epicardial and microvascular function with endothelium-independent agents such as sodium nitroprusside or adenosine. Coronary epicardial and microvascular dilation was similar with sodium nitroprusside and adenosine in normal controls, in patients with atherosclerosis, and in those with only risk factors, except for a mild reduction in atherosclerotic vessel dilation in response to sodium nitroprusside in segments 30% stenosed. The L-NMMA did not inhibit vasodilation in response to sodium nitroprusside or adenosine, and L-arginine infusion (160 μmoL/min) was successful in reversing the constrictor effects of L-NMMA. This indicated that the abnormal reactivity observed with ACh was specific for the endothelium in the presence of preserved smooth muscle function, and that the effects of L-NMMA were specific for competitive inhibition of NO synthesis from L-arginine.[14,15,17]

To exclude the possibility that the lack of constrictor response to L-NMMA in saphenous vein grafts and atherosclerotic coronary arteries is caused by an inability of these vessels to constrict, we examined the effect of phenylephrine in saphenous vein grafts and internal mammary artery conduits. Vein grafts and native coronary arteries constricted with phenylephrine but not with L-NMMA, although the magnitude of constriction was less than internal mammary arterial conduits, indicating that the lack of responsiveness to L-NMMA in vein grafts and native arteries was caused by reduced NO activity and not by reduced sensitivity to constrictor stimuli.[18]

# Pharmacologic Release of Nitric Oxide from Human Coronary Vasculature

ACh, substance P, and Bk, commonly used endothelium-dependent vasodilators, not only release NO but probably stimulate production of other EDRFs and endothelium-derived constricting factors (EDCFs) and also may have direct smooth muscle effects. With the use of L-NMMA we and others have demonstrated that, at least partly, the vasodilation with these agonists is secondary to release of NO from the coronary epicardial and microcirculation.[17,19]

Studies examining the effects of ACh and substance P in the coronary circulation have reported depressed dilator responses in patients with hypertension, hypercholesterolemia, diabetes, smokers, elderly, and those with other risk factors for atherosclerosis.[7,14,15,17,20–22] Indeed, the abnormality in epicardial ACh responses appears to correlate with the magnitude to which low-density lipoprotein (LDL) is oxidizable in the blood, suggesting that patients with greater oxidant stress, presumably in the vessel wall, have greater disturbance of endothelial stimulatory function.[23] In addition, the severity of epicardial and coronary microvascular dysfunction in response to ACh correlates with the number of risk factors patients are exposed to, with function being more depressed in those exposed to several risk factors, implying that combined or repeated injury to the vascular endothelium is able to precipitate greater damage.[21,22]

# Comparison of Acetylcholine, Substance P, and Bradykinin Responses

Although the vascular responses in the human coronary circulation to ACh are abnormal in patients with risk factors or those with atherosclerosis, it is not known whether this abnormality uniformly extends to other, nonmuscarinic stimulators of the endothelium. To investigate this, we compared coronary epicardial and microvascular responses with ACh to those with substance P and Bk. Substance P produced predominant epicardial coronary dilation, whereas the dilating effect of ACh was mainly microvascular.[17] The L-NMMA suppressed epicardial and coronary microvascular dilation in response to both agents but not to sodium nitroprusside, suggesting that both substance P and ACh promote release of NO. The presence of either atherosclerosis or its risk factors without angiographic atherosclerosis significantly inhibited epicardial and microvascular dilation in response to both substance P and ACh. Epicardial dilation with substance P following L-NMMA was similar in patients both with and without risk factors and atherosclerosis, indicating that the depressed response to substance P in those with risk factors or those with established atherosclerosis at baseline is due to impaired NO release. However, there was no significant correlation between the magnitude of epicardial or microvascular responses with ACh and those with either substance P or Bk.[17,19]

Thus, like ACh, substance P- and Bk-induced coronary vascular dilation is at least partly due to stimulation of NO release. Furthermore, atherosclerosis and risk factors in the presence of angiographically normal coronary arteries are both associated with depression of basal and pharmacologically stimulated activity of NO that is not restricted to muscarinic receptors. Finally, the magnitude of depression in endothelial NO release by different activators of the vascular endothelium is variable.

The findings of a poor correlation between the responses to ACh, substance P, and Bk in the human coronary and peripheral circulations could be caused by several of the following factors: (1) risk factors differentially affect endothelial surface receptors; (2) the second messengers mediating the effect of these agents on NOS are affected variably by atherosclerosis and its risk factors; and (3) these pharmacologic agents differentially release other endothelium-dependent vasodilators and constrictors, independent of NO, such as endothelium-derived hyperpolarizing factor (EDHF), and constrictor or dilator prostaglandins.

To investigate the role of prostaglandin release to vasodilation by ACh and substance P, we studied the effects of aspirin, a cyclooxygenase inhibitor that is known to suppress release of prostaglandins in patients with and in patients without atherosclerosis. ACh, but not substance P–induced vasodilation, was lower in patients with atherosclerosis compared with those with only risk factors.[24] Aspirin had no baseline effect in either group, but improved ACh-mediated vasodilation only in patients with atherosclerosis, suggesting that cyclooxygenase-dependent EDCFs impair ACh-induced peripheral vasodilation in patients with atherosclerosis and provides an explanation for the lack of a strong correlation between ACh- and substance P–induced vasodilation. These findings also imply that aspirin, possibly because of inhibition of cyclooxygenase-dependent free radical production,[25] may lead to an increase in vascular NO availability and result in improved vasodilation during stress, fewer thrombotic episodes, and inhibition of progression of atherosclerosis. These observations provide a pathophysiological basis for the beneficial effects of aspirin in atherosclerosis.

The mechanisms underlying the observed depression of NO activity in humans have not been studied in detail. However, experimental animal models of atherosclerosis, hypercholesterolemia, hypertension, and diabetes have demonstrated that, among the many biological changes that appear in the vessel wall in these conditions, reduced bioavailability of NO in a setting of increased superoxide anion levels seems to be a uniform underlying abnormality. Increased free radicals in the vascular wall, generated from oxidized LDL (eg, oxidize NO to nitrite, to nitrate, and also to peroxynitrite that is known to be toxic to tissues) lead to the generation of more free radicals as well as to activation of cytokines. Thus, the reduction in basal and stimulated NO activity observed in these conditions is accompanied paradoxically by excess generation of NO, which then is catabolized to nonbiologically active nitrogen oxides. This was demonstrated in vessels from hypercholesterolemic rabbits in whom total nitrogen oxide production was increased, whereas biological NO activity was reduced.[26–28]

Several other mechanisms have been proposed for the observed abnormalities of NO in patients with risk factors for atherosclerosis. Among these are an effect of these risk factors on signaling pathways involving G-proteins. This was highlighted by studies in which ACh responses were depressed in the forearm vasculature of patients with hypercholesterolemia, but Bk responses were unaffected.[29] A direct effect of oxygen free radicals in down-regulating endothelial constitutive NOS (ecNOS) also has been demonstrated, and the presence of naturally occurring inhibitors of L-arginine, for example L-glutamine and asymmetric dimethyl L-arginine (ADMA), may also be important in competing for L-arginine binding sites with ecNOS.[30,31] Reduced cofactors such as tetrahydrobiopterin have been proposed as another important condition in the down-regulating production of NO.[32,33] Clinical studies designed to investigate specific strategies to counteract these potential triggers in humans have begun to shed light on the importance of each of these mechanisms.

## Does Nitric Oxide Contribute to Physiological Abnormalities of Vascular Vasodilator Function?

To assess whether NO is contributing to physiological coronary epicardial, microvascular vasodilation, and peripheral vasodilation during metabolic stress, the effect of L-NMMA was studied on vasomotor function during cardiac pacing, forearm exercise, and reactive hyperemia.[34–36]

In a study of patients with chest pain and normal coronary angiograms, we demonstrated impaired atrial pacing–induced coronary vasodilation in some patients. Moreover, the response to pacing correlated with the response to ACh. Thus, patients with depressed metabolic vasodilation (in response to pacing-induced increase in MVO2) also had depressed endothelium-dependent vasodilation, and vice versa. This result suggested that release of EDRF may contribute to metabolic coronary vasodilation, and that endothelial dysfunction leads to impaired vasodilator responses to physiological stimuli.[37]

To investigate the contribution of NO to human coronary epicardial and microvascular dilation during conditions of increasing myocardial oxygen requirements, we studied the effect of inhibiting NO synthesis with L-NMMA on coronary vasodilation during cardiac pacing in patients with angiographically normal coronary arteries without risk factors and also in those with normal coronary angiograms and risk factors for atherosclerosis.[34] Significant inhibition of epicardial and microvascular vasodilation was observed, such that epicardial coronary arteries constricted with pacing after L-NMMA in normal subjects. In patients with risk factors for atherosclerosis, there was no significant vasodilation of epicardial coronary arteries during pacing and microvascular vasodilation was depressed compared with controls; these changes were unaffected by L-NMMA, indicating that this depressed vasodilation was secondary to reduced contribution of NO to physiological vasodilation (Figure 3). Thus, coronary microvascular dilation in response to increasing myocardial oxygen requirements, believed to be due to release of a variety of humoral factors and to the accumulation of local metabolites, also is partly dependent on the stimulation of NO in the coronary microvascular endothelium. Coronary epicardial vasodilation during stress appears largely to be caused by release of NO in the epicardial coronary arteries. Patients with endothelial dysfunction caused by exposure to risk factors for atherosclerosis have reduced contribution of NO to coronary vasodilation during stress, and this may contribute to myocardial ischemia in these patients by limiting epicardial and microvascular coronary vasodilation.

During intermittent handgrip exercise, L-NMMA significantly inhibited forearm vasodilation, such that forearm vascular resistance was 26% higher after L-NMMA. The degree of reduction in ACh-mediated vasodilation with L-NMMA correlated with the degree of reduction in exercise vasodilation.[35]

Myogenic, neurogenic, and local factors are believed to contribute to vasodilation during exercise and reactive hyperemia. Previous investigators have studied the role of NO in conductance vessel dilation, but the contribution of NO to reactive hyperemia of the microvessels has been a subject of controversy in experimental animals and human studies. Based on the understanding that NO release is stimulated by increasing shear stress, we hypothesized that NO contributes to the reactive hyperemic response and that endothelial dysfunction in atherosclerosis will reduce this contribution (Figure 4).[36] The entire hyperemic response including peak hyperemia was reduced by L-NMMA in normal subjects. In contrast, atherosclerotic patients had no inhibition of peak hyperemia with L-NMMA, suggesting that the contribution of NO to hyperemia was reduced in patients with atherosclerosis or its risk factors.

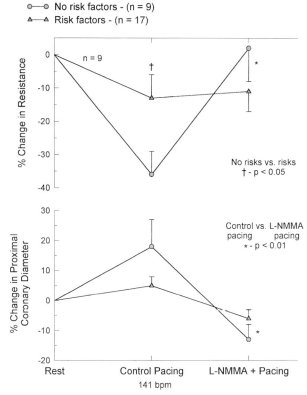

**Figure 3.**  Effect of L-NMMA on the pacing-induced changes in coronary vascular resistance and epicardial coronary artery diameter. Patients without risk factors are depicted in circles and those with risk factors in triangles. Adapted with permission from Reference 34.

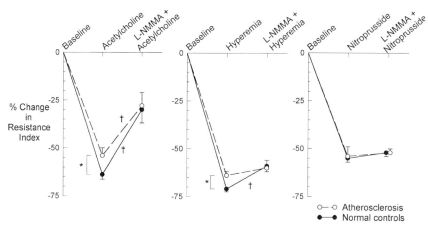

**Figure 4.**  The percent change in femoral vascular resistance index in patients with atherosclerosis or its risk factors (– – –) compared with normal controls (——) during acetylcholine (ACh), sodium nitroprusside, and peak reactive hyperemia are compared before and after L-NMMA. * = $P < 0.05$ normal controls vs. atherosclerosis. † = $P < 0.002$ pre- vs. post-L-NMMA Adapted with permission from Reference 36.

Thus, NO contributes to exercise-induced dilation and to all phases of the reactive hyperemic response in the normal human peripheral vasculature. In addition, patients with atherosclerosis or its risks have abnormal NO bioactivity in response to pharmacologic and physiological (reactive hyperemia) stimulation. This reduced vasodilation during physiological stress in atherosclerosis may contribute to or exacerbate hypertension and ischemia.

# Interaction Between Platelets and Nitric Oxide In Vivo

Endothelial NO not only diffuses into the vascular smooth muscle layer causing cyclic guanosine monophosphate (cGMP)–mediated dilation, but also is released luminally, where it potently inhibits platelet adhesion and, to a lesser extent, platelet aggregation by increasing cytosolic levels of cGMP.[38–40] In whole blood, where the half-life of NO is attenuated by hemoglobin and other oxidants, the platelet inhibitory effects are demonstrated less easily and have not been confirmed in humans.[41]

We studied the effects of ACh on agonist-stimulated ex vivo whole blood platelet aggregation in the human peripheral circulation. Whole blood platelet aggregation in response to collagen and ADP was measured by ex vivo impedance aggregometry in blood drawn from the femoral vein in patients without atherosclerosis during infusions of ACh into the femoral artery to stimulate release of NO. This response was compared with that of patients with atherosclerosis.[42] To investigate whether endothelial NO under resting conditions contributes to platelet cGMP levels and to test whether the observed antiplatelet effect of ACh is due to NO-mediated increase in platelet cGMP levels, we performed a study in which platelet cGMP content was measured in blood drawn from the coronary sinus before and after intracoronary L-NMMA, ACh, and nitroprusside.[43]

There was no baseline arterio–venous difference in platelet aggregation.[42] However, significant inhibition of agonist-stimulated whole blood platelet aggregation was observed in femoral venous blood during arterial infusion of ACh; compared with baseline, platelet aggregation was lower with collagen and ADP (Figure 5). Platelet aggregation returned toward baseline 10 minutes after discontinuation of ACh infusion. Although there was significant attenuation of collagen-induced platelet aggregation in both groups, the magnitude of inhibition was lower in patients with atherosclerosis, compared with those without atherosclerosis. A significant correlation was present between the percentage change in flow velocity with ACh and the percentage decrease in collagen-induced platelet aggregation with ACh, suggesting that patients with greater vasodilation with ACh also had greater inhibition of platelet aggregation, and vice versa.

L-NMMA had no effect on platelet cGMP content during in vitro incubation but in vivo produced the expected increase in coronary vascular resistance and reduced platelet cGMP content by 8% ± 5%, indicating that luminal release of NO under resting conditions contributes to inhibition of platelet

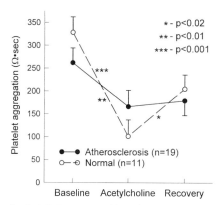

**Figure 5.** Whole blood platelet aggregation in response to collagen or adenosine diphosphate in femoral venous blood in patients with (●----●) and without (○----○) atherosclerosis at baseline, during intraarterial ACh (30 mg/min), and 10 minutes after recovery. (* = $P < 0.02$, ** = $P < 0.01$, *** = $P < 0.001$). Adapted with permission from Reference 42.

adhesion and aggregation to the vessel wall. There was a $21\% \pm 8\%$, increase in platelet cGMP content with ACh. Patients without risk factors for atherosclerosis had greater vasodilation of the coronary circulation with ACh and a greater increase in platelet cGMP content when compared with patients with atherosclerosis and its risk factors. Sodium nitroprusside, an exogenous donor of NO, produced a larger increase in platelet cGMP level, but the magnitude of increase was not significantly different between patients with and without atherosclerosis.

These studies demonstrate that tonic release of NO from the vascular endothelium contributes to platelet cGMP content, and the stimulation of luminal release of NO contributes to inhibition of platelet aggregation by a cGMP-dependent mechanism. This capacity of the normal endothelium is impaired in patients with atherosclerosis and its risk factors and may contribute to the increased incidence of thrombotic coronary and peripheral vascular events in this population.

# Conclusions

Several other local and systemic vasoactive mediators also are likely to regulate endothelial NO activity. For example, norepinepherine, angiotensin II, and endothelin may directly or indirectly (by causing vasoconstriction) affect NO bioavailability. Thus, individuals with a higher rate of activity in these vasoconstrictors may be at increased risk of vascular dysfunction when they are subjected to conventional risk factors such as hypercholesterolemia, hypertension, or diabetes that also depress NO activity. The influence of local dilators such as insulin and Bk and their effect on NO activity needs to be better defined. Finally, in the near future, the influence on vascular NO activity of genetic factors and new environmental risk factors such as hyperhomocysteinemia and infections, which are considered to be instrumental in predisposing to atherosclerosis, will become better defined.

# References

1. Furchgott RF, Zawadzki JV. The obligatory role of the endothelial cells in the relaxation of arterial smooth muscle by acetylcholine. *Nature* 1980;288:373–376.
2. De Mey JG, Claeys M, Vanhoutte PM. Endothelium-dependent inhibitory effects of acetycholine, adenosine triphosphate, thrombin and arachidonic acid in the canine femoral artery. *J Pharmacol Exp Ther* 1982;222:166–173.
3. Holtz J, Forstermann U, Pohl U, et al. Flow-dependent, endothelium-mediated dilation of epicardial coronary arteries in conscious dogs: Effects of cyclooxygenase inhibition. *J Cardiovasc Pharmacol* 1984;6:1161–1169.
4. Cox DA, Vita JA, Treasure CB, et al. Atherosclerosis impairs flow-mediated dilatation of coronary arteries in humans. *Circulation* 1989;80:458–465.
5. Palmer RM, Ferrige AG, Moncada S. Nitric oxide release accounts for the biological activity of endothelium-derived relaxing factor. *Nature* 1987;327:524–526.
6. Ignarro LJ, Byrns RE, Buga GM, et al. Endothelium-derived relaxing factor from pulmonary artery and vein possesses pharmacologic and chemical properties identical to those of nitric oxide radical. *Circ Res* 1987;61:866–879.
7. Ludmer PL, Selwyn AP, Shook TL, et al. Paradoxical vasoconstriction induced by acetylcholine in atherosclerotic coronary arteries. *N Engl J Med* 1986;315:1046–1051.
8. Zeiher AM, Drexler H, Wollschläger H, et al. Modulation of coronary vasomotor tone in humans. Progressive endothelial dysfunction with different early stages of coronary atherosclerosis. *Circulation* 1991;83:391–401.
9. Hodgson JM, Marshall JJ. Direct vasoconstriction and endothelium-dependent vasodilation. Mechanism of acetylcholine effects on coronary flow and arterial diameter in patients with non-stenotic coronary arteries. *Circulation* 1989;79:1043–1051.
10. Newman CM, Maseri A, Hackett DR, et al. Responses of angiographically normal and atherosclerotic left anterior descending coronary arteries to acetylcholine. *Am J Cardiol* 1990;66:1070–1076.
11. Parent R, Pare R, Lavallee M. Contribution of nitric oxide to dilation of resistance coronary vessels in conscious dogs. *Am J Physiol* 1992;262:H10–H16.
12. Ishizaka H, Okumura K, Yamabe H, et al. Endothelium-derived nitric oxide as a mediator of acetylcholine-induced coronary vasodilation in dogs. *J Cardiovasc Pharmacol* 1991;18:665–669.
13. Lefroy DC, T Crake T, Uren NG, et al. Effect of inhibition of nitric oxide synthesis on epicardial coronary caliber and coronary blood flow in humans. *Circulation* 1993;88:43–54.
14. Quyyumi AA, Dakak N, Andrews NP, et al. Nitric oxide activity in the human coronary circulation: Impact of risk factors for coronary atherosclerosis. *J Clin Invest* 1995;95:1747–1755.
15. Quyyumi AA, Dakak N, Mulcahy D, et al. Impaired release of nitric oxide from atherosclerotic human coronary vasculature. *J Am Coll Cardiol* 1997;29:308–317.
16. Mulcahy D, Husain S, Andrews NP, et al. In vivo nitric oxide activity in human saphenous vein grafts. *Circulation* 1995;92:I642.
17. Quyyumi AA, Mulcahy D, Andrews NP, et al. Coronary vascular nitric oxide activity in hypertension and hypercholesterolemia: Comparison of acetylcholine and substance P. *Circulation* 1997;95:104–110.
18. Prasad A, Zalos G, Mincemoyer R, et al. Nitric oxide activity in arterial and venous bypass grafts. *J Am Coll Cardiol* 1998;31(suppl 1):460A.
19. Prasad A, Husain S, Mincemoyer R, et al. Coronary endothelial dysfunction in humans improves with angiotensin converting enzyme inhibition. *Circulation* 1996;94(suppl 1):I61.
20. Quyyumi AA, Cannon RO, Panza JA, et al. Endothelial dysfunction in patients with chest pain and normal coronary arteries. *Circulation* 1992;86:1864–1871.

21. Egashira K, Inou T, Hirooka Y, et al. Impaired coronary blood flow response to acetylcholine in patients with coronary risk factors and proximal atherosclerotic lesions. *J Clin Invest* 1993;91:29–37.
22. Vita JA, Treasure CB, Nabel EG, et al. Coronary vasomotor response to acetylcholine relates to risk factors or coronary artery disease. *Circulation* 1990;8l:49l-497.
23. Anderson TJ, Meredith T, Charbonneau F, et al. Endothelium-dependent coronary vasomotion relates to the susceptibility of LDL to oxidation in humans. Circulation 1996;93:1647–1650.
24. Husain S, Andrews NP, Mulcahy D, et al. Aspirin improves endothelial dysfunction in atherosclerosis. *Circulation* 1988;97:716–720.
25. Tesfamariam B, Cohen RA. Free radicals mediate endothelium cell dysfunction caused by elevated glucose. *Am J Physiol* 1992;263:H321–H326.
26. Minor RL, Myers PR, Guerra R Jr, et al. Diet-induced atherosclerosis increases the release of nitrogen oxides from rabbit aorta. *J Clin Invest* 1990;86:2109–2116.
27. Cosentino F, Hishikawa K, Katusic ZS, et al. High glucose increases nitric oxide synthase expression of superoxide anion generation in human aortic endothelial cells. *Circulation* 1997;96:25–28.
28. Wiztum JL. The oxidation hypothesis of atherosclerosis. *Lancet* 1994;344:793–795.
29. Gilligan DM, Guetta V, Panza JA, et al. Selective loss of endothelial function in human hypercholesterolemia. *Circulation* 1994;90:35–41.
30. Arnal J-F, Münzel T, Venema RC, et al. Interactions between L-arginine and L-glutamine change endothelial nitric oxide production. An effect independent of nitric oxide synthase substrate availability. *J Clin Invest* 1995;95:2565–2572.
31. Bode-Boger SM, Boger RH, Kienke S, et al. Elevated L-arginine/dimethylarginine ratio contributes to enhanced systemic NO production by dietary L-arginine in hypercholesterolemic rabbits. *Biochem Biophys Res Commun* 1996;219:598–603.
32. Schini-Kerth VB, Vanhoutte PM. Nitric oxide synthases in vascular cells. *Exp Physiol* 1995;80:885–905.
33. Werner-Felmayer G, Werner ER, Fuchs D, et al. Tetrahydrobiopterin-dependent formation of nitrite and nitrate in murine fibroblasts. *J Exp Med* 1990;172:1599–1607.
34. Quyyumi AA, Dakak N, Andrews NP, et al. Contribution of nitric oxide to metabolic coronary vasodilation in the human heart. *Circulation* 1995;92:320–326.
35. Gilligan DM, Panza JA, Kilcoyne CM, et al. The contribution of endothelium-derived nitric oxide to exercise induced vasodilation in man. *Circulation* 1994;90:2853–2858.
36. Dakak N, Husain S, Mulcahy DM, et al. Contribution of nitric oxide to reactive hyperemia: Impact of endothelial dysfunction and effect of L-arginine. *Hypertension* 1998;32:3–8.
37. Quyyumi AA, Cannon RO III, Panza JA, et al. Endothelial dysfunction in patients with chest pain and normal coronary arteries. *Circulation* 1992;86:1864–1871.
38. Radomski MW, Palmer RMJ, Moncada S. Endogenous nitric oxide inhibits human platelet adhesion to vascular endothelium. *Lancet* 1987;2:1057–1058.
39. Pohl U, Busse R. EDRF increases cyclic GMP in platelets during passage through the coronary vascular bed. *Circ Res* 1989;65:1798–1803.
40. Hogan JC, Lewis MJ, Henderson AH. In vivo EDRF activity influences platelet function. *Br J Pharmacol* 1988;94:1020–1022.
41. Vallance P, Benjamin N, Collier J. The effect of endothelium-derived nitric oxide on ex vivo whole blood platelet aggregation in man. *Eur J Clin Pharmacol* 1992;42:37–41.
42. Diodati JG, Andrews NP, Dakak N, et al. Effect of atherosclerosis on endothelium-dependent inhibition of platelet activation in humans. *Circulation* 1998;98:17–24.
43. Andrews NP, Dakak N, Schenke W, et al. Platelet-endothelium interaction in humans: Changes in platelet cyclic guanosine monophosphate content in patients with endothelial dysfunction. *Circulation* 1994;90:I397.

## Chapter 15

# Endothelial Vasodilator Dysfunction in Chronic Heart Failure

*Helmut Drexler, MD, and Burkhard Hornig, MD*

## Introduction

The endothelium plays an important role in the control of vascular tone by releasing both vasodilating and vasoconstricting substances.[1] These mechanisms are important both for the regulation of the microvasculature[2–5] and for the larger conduit arteries.[6,7] Patients with chronic heart failure are characterized by increased vasoconstriction and a reduced vasodilator response during exercise. These abnormalities appear to be caused by the triggering of compensatory mechanisms and neurohumoral factors, which have been studied extensively in the past. There is now growing evidence to suggest that the endothelium contributes to the abnormal vasodilator response in chronic heart failure. In particular, the role of endothelium-derived nitric oxide (NO) has received considerable attention. The present chapter summarizes the evidence for a reduced vasodilator capacity of the endothelium in chronic heart failure and focuses on the potential mechanisms underlying this abnormality.

## Impaired Endothelium-Dependent Vasodilation in Heart Failure

The endothelium releases NO in response to a variety of stimuli including increased shear stress during increased blood flow[6,7] or receptor stimulation[1,2] such as muscarinic or bradykinin (Bk) B2 receptors. Following its release and uptake into vascular smooth muscle (VSM) cells, NO stimulates guanylyl cyclase to form cyclic guanosine monophosphate (cGMP) resulting in smooth muscle relaxation and vascular dilatation. Because of the ease with which endothelium-dependent NO-mediated vasodilator function can be assessed by acetylcholine (ACh) or other muscarinic receptor agonists, a number of studies

From Panza JA, Cannon RO III (eds): *Endothelium, Nitric Oxide, and Atherosclerosis* ©Futura Publishing Co, Inc, Armonk, NY, 1999.

have used regional (ie, intra-arterial) infusions of ACh and measured the resulting vasodilation. With the assumption that a diminished vasodilator response to ACh reflects endothelial dysfunction,[2,3] evidence for an impaired endothelium-dependent vasodilator response was found in the microcirculation of the myocardium,[8] leg,[9] and forearm.[10–13] These data are compatible with the view that the impairment of endothelium-dependent NO-mediated vasodilator function is a generalized phenomenon in patients with chronic heart failure. Although the diminished peripheral vasodilator capacity may be important for the reduced tissue perfusion during physical exercise and, therefore, is likely to contribute to impaired exercise capacity, the disturbance of microvascular dilatation in the coronary circulation might result in ischemia and further myocardial damage and dysfunction in chronic heart failure.

The studies cited so far tested endothelium-dependent vasodilator capacity but did not evaluate the importance of endothelium-derived NO in the maintenance of basal vascular tone. The regional infusion of $N$-monomethyl-L-arginine (L-NMMA), a selective inhibitor of NO synthase (NOS), can be used to assess the importance of endothelium-derived NO for the maintenance of basal vascular tone.[14] With the use of brachial artery infusions of L-NMMA, it was shown that resistance vessels from patients with chronic heart failure showed greater vasoconstriction in response to removal of NO-mediated vasodilation by L-NMMA as compared with control subjects.[12] Therefore, in contrast to stimulated NO-dependent vasodilation, the contribution of NO to basal tone appears to be preserved or even enhanced in forearm resistance vessels of patients with severe chronic heart failure.[12] Interestingly, peripheral venous nitrate, the product of NO metabolism in blood, also has been found to increase in heart failure,[15,16] a finding compatible with enhanced basal NO production in severe chronic heart failure. However, these results were obtained in a small group of patients and further studies are needed to better define the importance of endothelium-derived NO for the regulation of basal vascular tone in heart failure patients.

Although numerous studies have focused on endothelial function of resistance vessels, the measurement of diameter of large conduit arteries now can be obtained accurately by ultrasound techniques,[6,7] that is, at baseline and in response to increases in flow (eg, during reactive hyperemia). This approach confirmed that flow-dependent dilation in humans is, to a large extent, caused by the endothelial release of NO. By using this approach, it was shown that flow-dependent vasodilation of the radial artery was attenuated significantly in patients with chronic heart failure.[7] Interestingly, this impairment was similar in patients with dilated and ischemic cardiomyopathies and was significantly greater in the nondominant arm. Importantly, after blockade of NOS by L-NMMA, flow-dependent forearm vasodilation was similar in control subjects and patients, suggesting that the impairment in patients was mostly due to reduced NO/bioavailability.[7] Taken together, endothelial dysfunction is not only present in the microcirculation of patients with heart failure but also in large conduit vessels. Because large arteries are more than just passive conduits,[17] it is tempting to speculate that such an impairment of flow-mediated vasodilation during exercise might lead to increased impedance to left ventricular ejection and, thereby, contribute to the hemodynamic derangements characteristic of chronic heart failure.

# Mechanisms of Endothelial Vasodilator Dysfunction in Heart Failure

Animal experiments suggest that endothelial dysfunction is a progressive, time-dependent process that probably plays a minor role early in heart failure. Rats in whom heart failure was induced by coronary ligation and subsequent myocardial infarction demonstrated no evidence of endothelial dysfunction at week 1, but a reduced ACh response of thoracic aortic rings was evident after 4 and 16 weeks as compared with sham-operated control rats.[18] Moreover, endothelial dysfunction in the rat infarct model appears to emerge only in rats with large infarcts, markedly impaired left ventricular systolic function, and evidence of heart failure.[19]

A number of factors might be responsible for the impaired NO-dependent vasodilation in chronic heart failure and many of these aspects have been studied in humans.

# Nitric Oxide Synthase in Heart Failure

The reduced endothelium-dependent NO–mediated vasodilator response to ACh may be caused by a reduced activity of the NO-forming enzyme NOS. Because pulsatile flow[20] and the associated shear stress[21,22] are important regulators of NO production, it is possible that the reduced cardiac output and stroke volume act as the link to impaired endothelial vasodilator function in chronic heart failure. Recent experimental evidence supports this possibility. In dogs with heart failure, NOS gene expression was reduced markedly in endothelial cells from the thoracic aorta as compared with control animals. In addition, there was a marked reduction in endothelial cell NOS protein and nitrate production. Interestingly, this down-regulation of NOS was accompanied by a similar down-regulation of endothelial cyclooxygenase-1 in heart failure dogs.[23] Moreover, NO production from cardiac microvessels isolated from patients with end-stage heart failure undergoing transplantation appeared to be reduced as compared with nitrite production from the microvascular of normal hearts,[24] and the gene expression of endothelial NOS (eNOS) is reduced in the failing human heart.[25] Taken together, these studies indicate that endothelial NO (eNO) production is reduced in patients with chronic heart failure, possibly through reduced gene expression of vascular eNOS. Consistent with the concept, a reduced release of NO in response to receptor or flow-stimulated conditions has been noted in patients with chronic heart failure.[7,10–12] By using a high-resolution ultrasound wall–tracking system for measurement of radial artery diameter and blood flow, we have demonstrated in patients with chronic heart failure that flow-dependent, endothelium-mediated dilation is reduced because of a severely reduced availability of NO compared with normals.[7] Recent experimental data have demonstrated that eNOS gene expression is regulated by shear stress,[22] raising the possibility that chronically reduced blood flow in chronic heart failure possibly leads to reduced NOS gene expression.

## Impact of Cytokines

Increased levels of cytokines, particularly tumor necrosis factor-$\alpha$ (TNF-$\alpha$) are increased in severe heart failure[26] and may represent one mechanism leading to impaired endothelium-mediated vasodilation caused by diminished availability of NO.[27] Experimental evidence suggests that TNF-$\alpha$ can inhibit the stimulated release of NO[28] and can also impair the stability of the eNOS mRNA[29] by shortening its half-life. TNF-$\alpha$ also increases VSM production of superoxide anion which decreases the half-life of NO.[30] Thus, TNF-$\alpha$ may inhibit endothelium-dependent NO-mediated vasodilation by decreasing the NO bioavailability through either enhanced destruction or reduced synthesis by NOS, although little data are available in human studies. Interestingly, TNF-$\alpha$ concentrations were closely correlated with forearm blood flow responses to brachial artery infusions of ACh.[27] However, more data are needed to better define the role of cytokines in the pathogenesis of endothelial dysfunction in humans.

## Inactivation of Nitric Oxide

Another mechanism that appears to play a role in the development of endothelial dysfunction in chronic heart failure is an enhanced inactivation of NO. It has recently been shown that the production of oxygen free radicals is enhanced with chronic heart failure,[31] raising the possibility that increased degradation of NO by radicals leads to endothelial dysfunction in these patients. Observations from our laboratory suggest that this mechanism is relevant in vivo, since the antioxidant ascorbic acid improved and nearly normalized endothelium-mediated vasodilation in patients with chronic heart failure by increasing the availability of NO.[32] Using the forearm model established in our laboratory, we demonstrated that ascorbic acid improved flow-dependent dilation of the radial artery, especially the portion mediated by endothelial release of NO. This effect of the antioxidant ascorbic acid was demonstrated after acute as well as chronic treatment.[33] So far the underlying mechanism(s) leading to increased production of oxygen free radicals in chronic heart failure is not elucidated completely. However, there is experimental evidence that the redox state of the vascular wall is influenced by angiotensin II, which increases the production of superoxide anions in VSM cells caused by activation of nicotinamide-adenine dinucleotide/nicotinamide-adenine-dinucleotide phosphate (NADH/NADPH)-driven oxidases.[33] In addition, there is experimental evidence that TNF-$\alpha$ activates angiotensinogen gene expression (the only known precursor of angiotensin II)[34] raising the possibility that elevated cytokine plasma levels have the potential to induce the angiotensin II–driven synthesis of oxygen free radicals in chronic heart failure. Further sources for increased radical formation in chronic heart failure may include the failing cardiac myocyte[35,36] and leukocytes.[37]

# Renin–Angiotensin System in Chronic Heart Failure

Another mechanism involved in endothelial dysfunction in chronic heart failure might be an activation of the angiotensin-conversion enzyme (ACE) [38] caused by activation of the renin–angiotensin system. The ACE is identical to the kininase II that is responsible for the degradation of endogenous Bk. Therefore, an activated ACE would not only increase angiotensin II but also enhance the inactivation of Bk. Bk is a very potent vasodilating peptide that exerts its vasodilating properties through endothelial release of NO,[39] prostacyclin,[40] and endothelium-derived hyperpolarizing factor (EDHF).[39] Indeed, there is experimental evidence that long-term treatment with ACE inhibitors improves aortic endothelial dysfunction.[41]

It is well established that the circulating and tissue renin–angiotensin system is activated in heart failure. Therefore, activation of ACE in heart failure might be associated with a reduced Bk-mediated endothelial release of NO, prostacyclin, and EDHF leading to impaired endothelium-mediated vasodilation, which might be reversed by ACE inhibitors. In fact, numerous experimental studies have indicated strongly that Bk tissue levels are altered in heart failure and that ACE inhibitors can improve Bk availability. Moreover, there appears to exist a specific interaction of ACE inhibitors with the Bk receptor. Interestingly, the Bk B2 receptor can act as an inverse receptor,[42] which also may play a role in interventions with ACE inhibitors. By using a specific Bk receptor antagonist, we have shown recently, for the first time in humans, that Bk is involved in the regulation of vascular tone in vivo,[43] consistent with previous experimental observations. Moreover, the beneficial effects of ACE inhibitors are related to Bk and/or a Bk receptor–mediated mechanism.[44] Recently,we have shown that ACE inhibitors improve but do not totally restore impaired endothelium-dependent relaxation in patients with chronic heart failure.[45] This improvement was attributed exclusively to increased availability of NO. However, it should be noted that the Bk-related effects of ACE inhibitors on endothelial function were examined only after acute administrations in these series of studies. More recently, we have confirmed that ACE inhibitors improve endothelial vasodilator dysfunction in patients with chronic heart failure after long-term treatment. Before initiation of ACE inhibition, the impaired endothelium-mediated flow-dependent dilation was restored by vitamin C; after 4 weeks of treatment with an ACE inhibitor; flow-dependent dilation was improved without additional beneficial effect of vitamin C. This observation suggests that the beneficial effect of chronic ACE inhibition on endothelium-dependent vasodilator function also may include reduced formation of superoxide anions by NADPH oxidase (Fig-

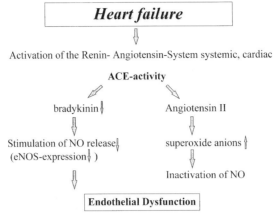

**Figure 1.** Potential mechanisms by which an activated renin angiotensin system can alter endothelial functions.

ure 1). Thus, considering the specific pathophysiology of endothelial dysfunction in heart failure (ie, activation of ACE; angiotensin II–induced radical formation), ACE inhibition represents a promising concept to improve the impaired endothelium-mediated vasodilation in chronic heart failure.

The impact of ACE inhibitors on endothelial function in patients with chronic heart failure also has been examined in peripheral resistance vessels by determining ACh-induced responses. Data obtained in patients with chronic heart failure suggest that the increase in forearm blood flow elicited by acute administration of enalapril is mediated by prostaglandins, because the effect of enalapril was attenuated after pretreatment with indomethacin and aspirin,[46] whereas the contribution of Bk and NO remained uncertain. More recent data from Nakamura and coworkers[47] have shown that the ACh-induced increase in forearm blood flow was enhanced by enalaprilat in normal individuals and patients with mild heart failure, whereas such an effect was not observed in patients with severe heart failure. Because coadministration of aspirin blunted the beneficial effect of enalaprilat in patients with mild heart failure (whereas L-NMMA had no effect), Nakamura et al[47] proposed that the beneficial effect of enalaprilat in ACh-induced increase in blood flow is modulated by factors derived from prostaglandin metabolism.

# Alterations of Signal Transduction in Chronic Heart Failure

Abnormalities in vasodilator responsiveness studies with the use of ACh also might be explained by a defect at the muscarinic receptor level or its signal transduction pathway. The majority of patients with heart failure have underlying ischemic heart disease and risk factors that are known to affect adversely the vascular response to ACh.[2,3,48] However, a reduced response to ACh also was found in chronic heart failure patients with nonischemic cardiomyopathy and without risk factors.[49] Because ACh has direct smooth muscle–contracting properties,[1] the response to this agonist represents the net effects of the release of vasodilating substances from the endothelium and direct smooth muscle vasoconstriction. Accordingly, the use of a pure endothelium-dependent vasodilator without effects on VSM might provide a more clear picture of endothelial vasodilator capacity. Substance P is a peptide that stimulates NOS through a different endothelial receptor, for example, the tachykinin receptor,[50] and has no direct effects on smooth muscle cells. Substance P has been shown to dilate epicardial coronary arteries and coronary microvessels in humans[51] and forearm resistance and conductance vessels.[52] This vasodilator effect can be attenuated significantly by the NOS inhibitor L-NMMA in normal subjects.[53] Interestingly, ACh-induced dilation of forearm resistance vessels was reduced significantly in patients with chronic heart failure, whereas the increase in forearm blood flow in response to substance P was not impaired. Similarly, intracoronary infusions of ACh caused significantly less of an increase in coronary blood flow in heart failure patients as compared with control subjects, whereas substance P resulted in similar increases in coronary blood flow in both groups.[54] Furthermore, the epicardial vasodilator response to substance P also was similar in both groups.[54] Therefore, these studies are compatible with the concept that chronic heart failure may be associated with a specific abnormality of the muscarinic receptor and/or postreceptor coupling mechanisms, which could contribute to the observed reduction of the response to ACh. These data also suggest that substance P may be a better pharmacologic probe than ACh to investigate eNO dependent vasodilation. Nevertheless, results obtained with stimulation of NO release through another nonmuscarinic receptor suggest that the abnormality in chronic heart failure patients is not likely to be explained solely by a defect at the muscarinic receptor level. Vasodilation in response to stimulation of vasopressin type II (V2) receptors[55] is dependent on eNO release and can be blocked by L-NMMA but not by indomethacin.[56,57] When the V2 receptor agonist desmopressin was infused into the brachial artery of heart failure patients and control subjects, the ensuing vasodilation was attenuated significantly in patients.[58] Moreover, inhibition of NO synthesis by L-NMMA reduced desmopressin responses to a significantly greater extent in control subjects as compared with patients.[58] Accordingly, these data are compatible with the view that impaired endothelium-dependent vasodilation in patients with chronic heart failure is not limited to a specific defect of the muscarinic receptor or its signal transduction pathway.

## L-Arginine Utilization in Chronic Heart Failure

Brachial artery infusions of L-arginine have been shown to augment the forearm vasodilator response to ACh in normal subjects.[3,59] The effects of intra-arterial L-arginine on the response to ACh also have been studied in patients with heart failure.[59] L-arginine augmented the vasodilator response to

ACh in normal subjects, except at the highest dose. In contrast, in patients with chronic heart failure, L-arginine also augmented the vasodilator response to the highest dose of ACh. Moreover, L-arginine did not affect the postischemic increase in forearm blood flow after upper arm occlusion in normal subjects; however, it significantly increased postischemic blood flow in patients with chronic heart failure.[59]

Supplementation with L-arginine in patients with chronic heart failure has yielded conflicting results. Doses between 5.6 and 20 g/d for 4–6 weeks failed to augment the response to muscarinic receptor stimulation.[13,60] Also, it did not enhance reactive hyperemia.[61] However, oral L-arginine improved functional status, as indicated by increased distances during a 6-minute walk test and lower scores on the Living With Heart Failure questionnaire in one study[60] but not in the other.[13] Although the mechanism(s) by which L-arginine may work is still unsettled, a recent experimental study suggests that increased aysmmmetrical dimethyl L-arginine (ADMA) is increased in heart failure and can be overcome by additional L-arginine supplementation.[61] Our own observations suggest that ADMA levels are elevated only in a subset of patients and appear to be associated with impaired functional capacity (H. Drexler and B. Hornig, unpublished observations, 1998)

## Abnormalities of Smooth Muscle Responsiveness in Chronic Heart Failure

Beyond impaired endothelium-dependent responses, it is possible that the response of the underlying smooth muscle to NO is altered in severe chronic heart failure. NO stimulates guanylyl cyclase in VSM cells and the resultant increase in cGMP leads to vasodilatation. It is conceivable that a reduced responsiveness of this system to NO stimulation also could contribute to endothelial vasodilator dysfunction. This possibility has been tested in most studies by assessing the vasodilator response to arterial infusion of a direct NO donor (eg, nitroglycerin or sodium nitroprusside). In this regard, a reduced response to nitroglycerin was observed by Zelis et al[62] in their landmark study of the peripheral circulation in 1968. Although many more recent studies did not find significant differences in the vascular responses to direct-acting NO donors, the opposite observation also has been reported. Thus, nitroglycerin resulted in a significantly smaller increase in mean blood flow velocity of the superficial femoral artery after intra-arterial infusion in patients with chronic heart failure as compared with control subjects.[9] In addition, brachial artery infusions of nitroglycerin caused significantly less forearm resistance vessel dilatation in chronic heart failure patients as compared with control subjects.[11] Therefore, a reduced VSM responsiveness to NO-dependent cGMP-mediated vasodilation also may contribute to this apparent endothelial vasodilator dysfunction, at least in some patients.

Finally, ACh also stimulates production of endothelium-derived vasoactive substances originating from the cyclooxygenase metabolic pathway.[63–65] This possibility was tested in a study of the forearm circulation in which patients with chronic heart failure showed a blunted response to ACh as compared with control subjects.[11] When these experiments were repeated after cyclooxygenase inhibition with indomethacin, the vasodilator response to ACh was unchanged in normal subjects but significantly increased in patients. Despite this improvement, the response still was significantly attenuated compared with normal subjects.[11] In addition, intra-arterial infusion of sodium nitroprusside in chronic heart failure patients treated with aspirin resulted in significantly greater vasodilatation as compared with patients not pretreated with aspirin.[66] Both findings are compatible with the view that an abnormal production of cyclooxygenase-dependent vasoconstricting factor(s) seems to be present in the peripheral circulation of patients with chronic heart failure. Such an effect may blunt the vasodilatory effects of both endogenous NO liberated by endothelial agonists such as ACh as well as of exogenous NO derived from NO donors.

Thus, there is abundant evidence that chronic heart failure is associated with impaired endothelium-dependent microvascular and larger conduit vessel vasodilator dysfunction. Although much of this impairment can be attributed to reduced NO bioavailability, the precise mechanism(s) underlying this defect remains to be established. Nevertheless, it appears that the impaired endothelial function in chronic heart failure is multifactorial, including reduced expression of eNOS (ie, secondary to reduced flow and shear stress), L-arginine substrate limitations, activated renin-angiotensin system (increased ACE activity reducing local Bk levels), and probably, enhanced degradation of NO caused by inactivation by free radical molecules (Figure 2).

## Potential Functional Implications for Patients with Chronic Heart Failure

Because endothelial vasodilator function is involved in the control of tissue perfusion, the question arises whether impaired exercise-induced re-

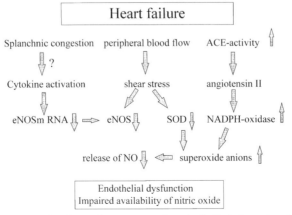

**Figure 2.** Factors involved in the impaired endothelial function in chronic heart failure.

lease of NO contributes to reduced aerobic exercise capacity in patients with chronic heart failure. Moreover, it would be important to know whether improved endothelial function increases exercise capacity in chronic heart failure. If so, the endothelium would represent an important therapeutic target in these patients.

The beneficial effects of physical training in patients with chronic heart failure are established and are associated with improved endothelial vasodilator function. Several mechanisms have been proposed to account for the clinical benefit of training, including improvement in left ventricular diastolic function, autonomic balance, and ventilatory and/or skeletal muscle function. In particular, skeletal muscle atrophy, impaired metabolism, and reduced oxidative capacity appear to contribute to the reduced exercise capacity in chronic heart failure. Exercise training improves force of contraction, metabolism of skeletal muscle, and oxidative capacity of skeletal muscle. Force of contraction in skeletal muscle is modulated by NO through reduced $Ca^{2+}$ activation of actin filaments resulting in decreased myofibrillar calcium sensitivity.[67] Skeletal muscle fibers express two isoforms of NOS; neuronal and endothelial. In chronic heart failure, expression of the inducible NOS has been shown to emerge in skeletal muscle of patients.[68] Therefore, increased NO availability within skeletal muscle may reduce contractile force in these patients. Moreover, endogenous NO released from microvascular endothelium plays an important role in the modulation of cellular respiration in skeletal muscle.[69] The suppression of tissue $O_2$ consumption in response to Bk (presumably stimulating endothelial release of NO) is blunted in skeletal muscle from dogs with heart failure,[70] indicating a defective endogenous NO-mediated modulation of tissue $O_2$ consumption in skeletal muscle after the development of heart failure. It is conceivable that defective NO biosynthesis in skeletal muscle blood vessels can be improved by physical training. Interestingly, preservation of endothelial vasodilator function by physical training is associated with preserved resting hemodynamics and alleviation of clinical manifestations of heart failure,[71] suggesting that the beneficial effects of physical training in heart failure are mediated in part by endothelial mechanisms.

The significant relationship between improvement of endothelial function and exercise capacity supports the notion that improved endothelial function contributes to increased exercise capacity. However, improved endothelial function can account only for a small incremental increase in exercise capacity. Therefore, it is not clear how an improvement in peripheral endothelium-mediated vasodilation may contribute to exercise capacity. A complex physiology exists for hyperemia, exercise, and NO. The role of NO in exercise-induced increases in blood flow and/or reactive hyperemia remains controversial and the effects of inhibition of NO synthesis in this respect are modest at best. Increases in flow during exercise or following arterial occlusion are mediated by several mechanisms and blockade of several systems are necessary to attenuate reactive hyperemia. In normal individuals, peak vasodilatory capacity can be increased by physical training without influencing basal or stimulated activity of the NO dilator system,[72] although exercise training undoubtedly augments eNO synthesis and flow-dependent dilation of skeletal muscle arterioles through NO and prostaglandins.[73] Following physical training, an increase in flow reserve or reactive hyperemia has been observed both in animals and in humans. In fact, physical training in patients has been associated with increases in skeletal muscle blood flow during exercise, reactive hyperemia, and peak oxygen consumption possibly by enhancing vascular conduction and growth.[74] However, increased metabolic vasodilation in response to arterial occlusion may not be associated necessarily with increased training-induced endothelium-dependent vasodilation during exercise in chronic heart failure. Indeed, a recent study observed that the increased vasodilatory responses following arterial occlusion and endothelium-dependent stimuli following physical training in patients with chronic heart failure do not correlate, suggesting that the determinants of peak reactive hyperemia and endothelium-dependent vasodilation are not linked.[75] However, increased NO availability during exercise provided by physical training may contribute to exercise capacity without affecting total increases in skeletal muscle blood flow, by affecting the distribution of blood flow within skeletal muscle.

In chronic heart failure, skeletal muscle underperfusion emerges predominantly in oxidative working muscle.[76] Inhibition of NO synthesis and release by L-nitroarginine methylester (L-NAME) is most effective in limiting blood flow to oxidative working muscle, but the inhibitory effect of L-NAME on blood flow in these muscle fibers appears to be attenuated in chronic heart failure.[77] Thus, redistribution of blood flow within skeletal muscle appears to emerge in heart failure caused by endothelial dysfunction possibly secondary to chronic deconditioning. It may be speculated that improved oxygen delivery with physical training is related partially to the reversal of impaired endothelium-dependent relaxation within oxidative muscle fibers. In this respect, it is noteworthy that neuronal NOS activity can be up-regulated by endurance training.[78]

NO also is involved in the central regulation of sympathetic outflow, raising the possibility that both neuronal and endothelial NO synthesis may contribute to the regulation of vasomotor tone.[79] It is possible that the sympathoinhibitory effects of NO may be reduced in chronic heart failure and thus contribute to sustained sympathetic activation.

Other interventions targeting the endothelium have been studied in chronic heart failure. L-arginine, the substrate of NO, is associated with improvement in endothelial function and a moderate increase in exercise capacity.[61] ACE inhibition has been shown to improve endothelium-dependent vasodilation.[45,66] Accordingly, it is conceivable that the related beneficial effect of ACE inhibitors on exercise-induced blood flow and exercise capacity in heart failure[80] is, in part, caused by improved endothelium-dependent vasodilation. Antioxidants, such as vitamin C, are effective in restoring endothelium-dependent vasodilation;[32] however, their potential to improve exercise capacity has not been determined.

Thus, endothelial dysfunction may play a role in redistribution of blood flow during exercise and adversely affect exercise capacity. Conditions, such as chronic heart failure, that reduce endothelium-derived NO availability also impair the normal exercise-induced blood flow response. This, in turn, may lead to diminished exercise capacity.

# References

1. Vane JR, Änggard EE, Botting RM. Regulatory functions of the endothelium. *N Engl J Med* 1990;323:27–36.
2. Linder L, Kiowski W, Buhler FR, et al. Indirect evidence for release of endothelium-derived relaxing factor in human forearm circulation in vivo. Blunted response in essential hypertension. *Circulation* 1990;81:1762–1767.
3. Panza JA, Casino PR, Kilcoyne CM, et al. Role of endothelium-derived nitric oxide in the abnormal endothelium-dependent vascular relaxation of patients with essential hypertension. *Circulation* 1993;87:1468–1474.
4. Kiowski W, Lüscher TF, Linder L, et al. Endothelin-1-induced vasoconstriction in humans. Reversal by calcium channel blockade but not by nitrovasodilators or endothelium-derived relaxing factor. *Circulation* 1991;83:469–475.
5. Haynes WG, Webb DJ. Contribution of endogenous generation of endothelin-1 to basal vascular tone. *Lancet* 1994;344:852–854.
6. Joannides R, Haefeli WE, Linder L, et al. Nitric oxide is responsible for flow-dependent dilatation of human peripheral conduit arteries in vivo. *Circulation* 1995;91:1314–1319.
7. Hornig B, Maier V, Drexler H. Physical training improves endothelial function in patients with chronic heart failure. *Circulation* 1996;93:210–214.
8. Treasure CB, Vita JA, Cox DA, et al. Endothelium-dependent dilation of the coronary microvasculature is impaired in dilated cardiomyopathy. *Circulation* 1990;81:772–779.
9. Katz SD, Biasucci L, Sabba C, et al. Impaired endothelium-mediated vasodilation in the peripheral vasculature of patients with congestive heart failure. *J Am Coll Cardiol* 1992;19:918–925.
10. Kubo SH, Rector TS, Bank AJ, et al. Endothelium-dependent vasodilation is attenuated in patients with heart failure. *Circulation* 1991;84:1589–1596.
11. Katz SD, Schwarz M, Yuen J, et al. Impaired acetylcholine-mediated vasodilation in patients with congestive heart failure. Role of endothelium-derived vasodilating and vasoconstricting factors. *Circulation* 1993;88:55–61.
12. Drexler H, Hayoz D, Munzel T, et al. Endothelial function in chronic congestive heart failure. *Am J Cardiol* 1992;69:1596–1601.
13. Chin DJ, Kaye DM, Lefkovits J, et al. Dietary supplementation with L-arginine fails to restore endothelial function in forearm resistance arteries of patients with severe heart failure. *J Am Coll Cardiol* 1996;27:1207–1213.
14. Vallance P, Collier J, Moncada S. Effects of endothelium-derived nitric oxide on peripheral arteriolar tone in man. *Lancet* 1989;2:997–1000.
15. Winlaw DS, Smythe GA, Keogh AM, et al. Increased nitric oxide production in heart failure. *Lancet* 1994;344:373–374.
16. Habib F, Dutka D, Crossman D, et al. Enhanced basal nitric oxide production in heart failure: another failed counter-regulatory vasodilator mechanism? *Lancet* 1994;344:371–373.
17. Ramsey MW, Jones CJH. Large arteries are more than passive conduits. *Br Heart J* 1994;72:3–4.
18. Teerlink JR, Clozel M, Fischli W, et al. Temporal evolution of endothelial dysfunction in a rat model of chronic heart failure. *J Am Coll Cardiol* 1993;22:615–620.
19. Drexler H, Lu W. Endothelial dysfunction of hindquarter resistance vessels in experimental heart failure. *Am J Physiol* 1992;262:H1640–H1645.
20. Rubanyi G, Romero CJ, Vanhoutte PM. Flow-induced release of endothelium-derived relaxing factor. *Am J Physiol* 1986;250:H1145–H1149.
21. Buga GM, Gold ME, Fukuto JM, et al. Shear-stress induced nitric oxide release from endothelial cells grown on beads. *Hypertension* 1991;17:187–192.
22. Uematsu M, Ohara Y, Navas JP, et al. Regulation of endothelial cell nitric oxide synthase mRNA expression by shear stress. *Am J Physiol* 1995;269:C1371–C1378.
23. Smith CJ, Sun D, Hoegler C, et al. Reduced gene expression of vascular endothelial NO synthase and cyclooxygenase-1 in heart failure. *Circ Res* 1996;78:58–64.

24. Kichuk MR, Seyedi N, Zhang X, et al. Regulation of nitric oxide production in human coronary microvessels and the contribution of local kinin formation. *Circulation* 1996;94:44–51.
25. Drexler H, Kästner A, Strobel A, et al. Expression, activity, and functional significance of inducible nitric oxide synthase in the failing human heart. *J Am Coll Cardiol* 1998;32:955–963.
26. Katz SD, Ramanath R, Berman JW, et al. Pathophysiological correlation of increased serum tumor necrosis factor in patients with chronic heart failure. Relation to nitric oxide dependent vasodilation in the forearm circulation. *Circulation* 1994; 90:12–16.
27. Aoki N, Siegfried M, Lefer AM. Anti-EDRF effect of tumor necrosis factor in isolated, perfused cat carotid arteries. *Am J Physiol* 1989;256(suppl):H1509–H1512.
28. Yoshimuzi M, Perella MA, Burnett JC, et al. Tumor necrosis factor down regulates an endothelial nitric oxide synthase mRNA by shortening its half-life. *Circ Res* 1993;73:205–209.
29. Levine B, Kalman J, Mayer L, et al. Elevated circulating levels of tumor necrosis factor in severe chronic heart failure. *N Engl J Med* 1990;323:236–241.
30. Matsubara T, Ziff M. Increased superoxide anion release from human endothelial cells in response to cytokines. *J Immunol* 1986;137:3295–3298.
31. Belch JJF, Bridges AB, Scott N, et al. Oxygen free radicals and congestive heart failure. *Br Heart J* 1991;65:245–248.
32. Hornig B, Arakawa N, Kohler C, et al. Vitamin C improves endothelial function of conduit arteries in patients with chronic heart failure. *Circulation* 1998;97:363–368.
33. Griendling KK, Minieri CA, Ollerenshaw JD, et al. Angiotensin II stimulates NADH and NADPH oxidase activity in cultured vascular smooth muscle cells. *Circ Res* 1994;74:1141–1148.
34. Brasier AR, Li J, Wimbish KA. Tumor necrosis factor activates angiotensinogen gene expression by the RelA transactivator. *Hypertension* 1996;27:1009–1017.
35. Mohazzab HKM, Zhang X, Kichuk MR, et al. Potential sites and changes of superoxide anion production in failing and nonfailing explanted human cardiac myocytes. *Circulation* 1995;92(suppl I):32. Abstract.
36. Sole M, Schimmer J, Goldstein D, et ak. Oxidative stress contributes to decompensation of the failing heart. *Circulation* 1995;92(supp I):31. Abstract.
37. Prasad K, Kalra J, Bharadwaj B. Phagocytic activity in blood of dogs with chronic heart failure. *Clin Invest Med* 1987;10:1354–1357.
38. Studer R, Reinecke H, Müller B, et al. Increased angiotensin-I converting enzyme gene expression in the failing human heart. *J Clin Invest* 1994;94:301–310.
39. O'Kane KPJ, Webb DJ, Collier JG, et al. Local L-N-mono-methyl-arginine attenuates the vasodilator action of bradykinin in the human forearm. *Br J Clin Pharmacol* 1994;38:311–315.
40. Barrow SE, Dollerey CT, Heavey DJ, et al. Effect of vasoactive peptides on prostacyclin synthesis in man. *Br J Pharmacol* 1986;87:243–247.
41. Ramsey MW, Goodfellow J, Jones CJ, et al. Endothelial control of arterial distensibility is impaired in chronic heart failure. *Circulation* 1995;92:3212–3219.
42. Leeb-Lundberg LM, Mathis SA, Herzig MCS. Antagonists of bradykinin that stabilze a G-protein uncoupled sate of the B2 receptor act as inverse agonists in rat myometrial cells. *J Biol Chem* 1994;269:25970–25973.
43. Groves P, Kurz S, Just H, et al. Role of endogenous bradykinin in human coronary vasomotor control. *Circulation* 1995;92:3424–3430.
44. Hornig B, Kohler C, Drexler H. Role of bradykinin in mediating vascular effects of ACE-inhibitors in in humans. *Circulation* 1997;95:1115–1118.
45. Hornig B, Arakawa N, Haussmann D, et al. Differential effects of quinaprilat, and enalprilat on endothelial function of conduit arteries in patients with chronic heart failure circulation. *Circulation* 1998;98:2842–2848.

46. Hirsch H, Bijou R, Yuen J, et al. Enalapril-induced vasodilation is attenuated by indomethacin in congestive heart failure and completely abolished in normal subjects. *Circulation* 1993;88:I293.
47. Nakamura M, Funokoshi T, Arakawa N, et al. Effect of angiotensin-converting enzyme inhibitors on endothelium-dependent peripheral vasodilation in patients with chronic heart failure. *J Am Coll Cardiol* 1994;24:1321–1327.
48. Creager MA, Cooke JP, Mendelsohn ME, et al. Impaired vasodilation of forearm resistance vessels in hypercholesterolemic humans. *J Clin Invest* 1990;86:228–234.
49. Nakamura M, Yoshida H, Arakawa N, et al. Endothelium-dependent vasodilatation is not selectively impaired in patients with chronic heart failure secondary to valvular heart disease and congenital heart disease. *Eur Heart J* 1996;17:1875–1881.
50. Saito R, Nonaka S, Konishi H, et al. Pharmacological properties of the tachykinin receptor subtype in the endothelial cell and vasodilation. *Ann N Y Acad Sci* 1991;632:457–459.
51. Crossman DC, Larkin SW, Fuller RW, et al. Substance P dilates epicardial coronary arteries and increases coronary blood flow in humans. *Circulation* 1989;80:475–484.
52. McEwan JR, Benjamin N, Larkin S, et al. Vasodilatation by calcitonin gene-related peptide and by substance P: A comparison of their effects on resistance and capacitance vessels of human forearms. *Circulation* 1988;77:1072–1080.
53. Panza JA, Casino PR, Kilcoyne CM, et al. Impaired endothelium-dependent vasodilation in patients with essential hypertension: Evidence that the abnormality is not at the muscarinic receptor level. *J Am Coll Cardiol* 1994;23:1610–1616.
54. Holdright DR, Clarke D, Fox K, et al. The effects of intracoronary substance P and acetylcholine on coronary blood flow in patients with idiopathic dilated cardiomyopathy. *Eur Heart J* 1994;15:1537–1544.
55. Hirsch AT, Dzau VJ, Majzoub JA, et al. Vasopressin-mediated forearm vasodilation in normal humans. Evidence for a vascular vasopressin V2 receptor. *J Clin Invest* 1989;84:418–426.
56. Liard JF. L-NAME antagonizes vasopressin V2-induced vasodilatation in dogs. *Am J Physiol* 1994;266:H99–H106.
57. Tagawa T, Imaizumi T, Shiramoto M, et al. V2 receptor-mediated vasodilation in healthy humans. *J Cardiovasc Pharmacol* 1995;25:387–392.
58. Rector TS, Bank AJ, Tschumperlin LK, et al. Abnormal desmopressin-induced forearm vasodilatation in patients with heart failure: Dependence on nitric oxide synthase activity. *Clin Pharmacol Ther* 1996;60:667–674.
59. Hirooka Y, Imaizumi T, Tagawa T, et al. Effects of L-arginine on impaired acetylcholine-induced and ischemic vasodilation of the forearm in patients with heart failure. *Circulation* 1994;90:658–668.
60. Rector TS, Bank AJ, Mullen KA, et al. Randomized, double-blind, placebo-controlled study of supplemental oral L-arginine in patients with heart failure [see Comments]. *Circulation* 1996;93:2135–2141.
61. Feng Q, Lu X, Fortin AJ, et al. Elevation of an endogenous inhibitor of nitric oxide in experimental congestive heart failure. *Cardiovasc Res* 1998;37:667–675.
62. Zelis R, Mason DT, Braunwald E. A comparison of the effects of vasodilator stimuli on peripheral resistance vessels in normal subjects and in patients with congestive heart failure. *J Clin Invest* 1968;47:960–970.
63. Mombouli JV, Illiano S, Nagao T, et al. Potentiation of endothelium-dependent relaxations to bradykinin by angiotensin-I converting enzyme inhibitors in canine coronary arteries involve both endothelium-derived relaxing and hyperpolarizing factors. *Circ Res* 1992;71:137–144.
64. Katusic ZS, Shepherd JT, Vanhoutte PM. Endothelium-dependent contractions to calcium ionophore A23187, arachidonic acid, and acetylcholine in canine basilar arteries. *Stroke* 1988;19:476–479.
65. Kaiser L, Spickard RC, Olivier NB. Heart failure depresses endothelium-dependent responses in canine femoral artery. *Am J Physiol* 1989;256:H962–H967.

66. Jeserich M, Pape L, Just H, et al. Effect of long-term angiotensin-converting enzyme inhibition on vascular function in patients with chronic congestive heart failure. *Am J Cardiol* 1995;76:1079–1082.
67. Andrade FH, Reid MB, Allen DG, et al. Effect of nitric oxide on single skeletal muscle fibres from the mouse. *J Physiol* 1998;509:577–586.
68. Riede UN, Förstermann U, Drexler H, et al. Inducible nitric oxide synthase in skeletal muscle of patients with chronic heart failure. *J Am Coll Cardiol* 1998;32:964–969.
69. Shen W, Hintze TH Wolin MS. Nitric oxide: An important signaling mechanism between vascular endothelium and parenchymal cells in the regulation of oxygen consumption. *Circulation* 1995;92:1086–1095.
70. Shen W, Wolin MS, Hintze TH. Defective endogenous nitric oxide-mediated modulation of cellular respiration in canine skeletal muscle after the development of heart failure. *J Heart Lung Transplant* 1997;16:1026–1034.
71. Wang J, Yi GH, Knecht M, et al. Physical Training alters the pathogenesis of pacing-induced heart failure through endothelium-mediated mechanisms in awake dogs. *Circulation* 1997;96:2683–2692.
72. Green DJ, Fowler DT, O'Driscoll JG, et al. Endothelium-derived nitric oxide activity in forearm vessels of tennis players. *J Appl Physiol* 1996;81:943–948.
73. Koller A, Huang A, Sun D, et al. Exercise training augments flow-dependent dilation in rat skeletal muscle arterioles. Role of endothelial nitric oxide and prostaglandins. *Circ Res* 1995;76:544–550.
74. Demopoulos L, Testa M, Zulio M, et al. Low level physical training improves peak oxygen consumption in patients with congestive heart failure despite long-term beta adrenergic blockade by enhancing vascular conductance and growth. *J Am Coll Cardiol* 1996;27(suppl A):754-1. Abstract.
75. Katz SD, Yuen J, Bijou R, et al. Training improves endothelium-dependent vasodilation in resistance vessels of patients with heart failure. *J Appl Physiol* 1997;82:1488–1492.
76. Drexler H, Faude F, Hönig S, et al. Blood flow distribution within skeletal muscle during exercise in the presence of heart failure: Effect of milrinone. *Circulation* 1987;76:1344–1352.
77. Hirai T, Zelis R, Musch TI. Effects of nitric oxide synthase inhibition on the muscle blood flow response to exercise in rats with heart failure. *Cardiovasc Res* 1995;30:469–476.
78. Owlya R, Vollenweider L, Trueb L, et al. Cardiovascular and sympathetic effects of nitric oxide inhibition at rest and during static exercise in humans. *Circulation* 1997;96:3897–3903.
79. Balon TW, Nadler JL. Nitric oxide release is present from incubated skeletal muscle preparations. *J Appl Physiol* 1994;77:2519–2521.
80. Drexler H, Banhardt U, Meinertz T, et al. Contrasting peripheral short-term and long-term effects of converting enzyme inhibition in patients with congestive heart failure. A double-blind, placebo-controlled trial. *Circulation* 1989;79:491–502.

*Chapter 16*

# In Vitro Studies of the Human Microcirculation in Cardiovascular Disorders

*Anthony M. Heagerty, MD*

## Introduction

Ever-increasing sophistication in the techniques used to examine any scientific question is a tribute to the ingenuity of man. Clinical science is no exception in this respect, but here our knowledge is enhanced by the integration of information obtained from a variety of disciplines. In consequence, the appreciation that the heart and circulation formed a vital system influenced by nerves and hormones was the first major step in our understanding of how blood perfused our tissues. Next came the desire to know how the circulation becomes disordered in a variety of diseases. George Pickering noted that the observations that first excite wonder usually are made with the eye, either unaided or with its range enlarged by optical instruments. Later comes measurement and with that accuracy and the establishment of quantitative relationships. In this context, much has been learned about the hemodynamics of the human circulation in health and disease using studies of blood flow through the vascular beds of the arm and leg. Newer techniques have complemented this approach and include in vitro investigations of human small arteries taken from a number of sources. This permits both morphological and functional measurements to take place under standardized conditions of test and improve our knowledge of the circulation at the level of the resistance vessel, which is responsible for controlling local blood flow. This chapter summarizes what has been reported in this area using human small blood vessels harvested against a background of cardiovascular disorders including hypertension, hypercholesterolemia, and heart failure. Again, the data have to be interpreted in conjunction with the information obtained from a variety of sources and mindful of the short-falls that all techniques intrinsically possess. Nevertheless, it is clear that the human microcirculation is beginning to

From Panza JA, Cannon RO III (eds): *Endothelium, Nitric Oxide, and Atherosclerosis* ©Futura Publishing Co, Inc, Armonk, NY, 1999.

surrender some of its many properties and to reveal an inherent ability to adapt in the face of adverse conditions often imposed on it as a result of systemic injury either hemodynamically or metabolically imposed.

# Small Arteries and Hypertension

## Structural Changes

An early cross-sectional study of mild hypertension reported that the predominant hemodynamic feature was a high-cardiac output and at this stage the peripheral resistance is low. However, a longitudinal study of the hemodynamics of essential hypertension followed a cohort of patients for 20 years and demonstrated that the high-cardiac index–normal total peripheral resistance pattern changed to a low-cardiac index–high-resistance situation. Blood flow measurements at maximal dilatation have confirmed that indeed there is an increase in minimum vascular resistance in established hypertension. Folkow has performed elegant studies using this methodology and put forward the theory that this increase in resistance is brought about by structural alterations in the arterial wall, which encroach on the lumen, thereby narrowing the small blood vessels that control vascular resistance. Alternative research approaches have sought to confirm these findings by either direct histological examination of arterial segments or in vitro investigations of such small blood vessels, either mounted on wires as isometric ring preparations or on cannulas at fixed pressures followed by morphological measurements.[1,2] Histological studies under standardized conditions have indicated that the media thickness:lumen diameter ratio of small arteries is increased in hypertension. Studies performed on isolated small blood vessels from a number of vascular beds that have been either mounted on wires or in pressure myograph systems also confirm these findings. Indeed, irrespective of the technique used, which could range from plethysmography, wire or pressure myography, or histology, there is remarkable concordance: the percentage increase in the media:lumen ratio either measured or predicted almost exactly matches the blood pressure increase when compared with normotensive control subjects and this appears to be accompanied by a reduction of between 7% and 8% in the vascular lumen diameter.[1]

Confirmation that these techniques are indeed complementary has been provided recently by a study that has demonstrated that minimal vascular resistance when measured in vivo in the forearm in hypertensive patients, correlates closely with the media:lumen ratio of gluteal subcutaneous small arteries examined in vitro.[3]

In this respect, many of the studies that have used isolated segments of human blood vessels have obtained these from biopsies of skin and subcutaneous fat. There are a number of points to examine. The first is whether vessels harvested in such a fashion are representative of the resistance vasculature. The lumen diameter of these arteries usually is approximately 300 $\mu$m. Recent data in conscious unrestrained animals where catheters have been introduced into the mesenteric arcade and pressure measured in vessels of this size would indicate that it is approximately 60% of systemic arterial pressure. In other words, the available data suggest that, indeed, vessels of this size contribute to vascular resistance. The next question is whether such arteries are representative of vascular beds elsewhere in the body. Clearly, the dermal circulation is highly specialized, being important for thermoregulatory control; however, data from the human intestinal vasculature and, more recently, small arteries harvested from explanted hearts all appear to demonstrate that the changes in vascular wall architecture demonstrated in subcutaneous arteries are representative of morphological findings elsewhere.[2]

## The Nature of the Structural Alteration in Small Arteries in Hypertension

For many years the increased media:lumen ratio of small arteries has been interpreted as being synonymous with some form of growth response predominantly as a result of the rising pressure. However, when Short[4] perfused and fixed the mesenteric arcades from hypertensive and normotensive patients at post mortem and divided the vessels into deciles on the basis of size, he was unable to detect an increase in medial cross-sectional area. In consequence, he ascribed the changes that clearly were observed in the media:lumen ratio as caused by a "contracture" brought about by raised blood pressure and not by a hypertrophy or hyperplasia of any tissue elements found within the vascular wall. More recently, Korsgaard and coworkers[5] have carried out studies of segments of small arteries and confirmed that there is no evidence for hyperplasia in hypertension although there is a small contribution from hypertrophy. Nevertheless, the predominating feature of the vasculature at this level of the circulation in hypertension appears to be a rearrangement of the existing tissue around a small lumen, the so-called remodeling phenomenon. There are experimental models of hypertension, such as the Ren-2 transgenic rat, which demonstrate almost complete remodeling with no contribution from hypertrophy, whereas in others, such as in aortic coarctation hypertension, there is evidence of hypertrophy as the major contributor to structural alterations with a small contribution from remodeling.[2]

## The Importance of Remodeling in the Maintenance of Hypertension

The circulation is an integrated system comprising a number of highly specialized vascular beds exposed to a number of pressor and dilator stimuli that influence blood pressure from second to second. However, if small arteries serve as resistance vessels then a structural narrowing of the vascular lumen should lead to enhanced vascular reactivity and the maintenance of a higher pressure. Studies of forearm blood flow performed at maximum dilatation would appear to confirm this contention, but it is important to realize that the conditions under which these vascular beds are being examined are entirely different from those normally observed; all vasoconstrictor tone has been abolished from the forearm and in consequence the vasculature is pharmacologically stimulated in a situation that must permit any structural alterations to exert profound influence over any other, thereby producing an increase in vascular reactivity.[2,6]

Recently, Izzard and coworkers[7] investigated the morphological and contractile characteristics of distal mesenteric arteries from spontaneously hypertensive rats (SHR) and Wistar-Kyoto (WKY) control animals at a distending pressure of 63% of the mean aortic pressure of each rat using a pressure arteriograph. The wall:lumen ratios obtained were compared with those observed when the pressures were set at 100 mm Hg. Experiments were carried out at 5 weeks of age when the blood pressure was rising and 20 weeks when it was established. The mean aortic pressure of SHR was increased significantly at 5 weeks compared with that of WKY and was further increased at 20 weeks. It was of interest that when set at 63% of mean aortic pressure, no difference in the wall:lumen ratio of these vessels was observed between strains at 5 weeks. At 20 weeks of age, the wall:lumen ratio of SHR arteries was increased significantly compared with that observed in WKY vessels. When activated with norepinephrine there was no evidence of an increase in vascular reactivity. In other words, these studies provide no evidence for an increased contractility to vasoconstrictor stimuli when arteries are examined at physiological pressures. Nevertheless, the criticism could be leveled that this is an examination of one vascular bed under specific conditions of testing. But Marks et al[8] were unable to demonstrate an increase in pressor responsiveness either to norepinephrine or to angiotensin II when chronically hypertensive rats were infused with these hormones despite well-established structural changes. Such findings have been confirmed by others and to avoid the criticism that many of these whole animal studies have been performed on anesthetized rats, the most recent reports have been carried out on conscious animals.[9]

In summary, all investigations of the human vasculature in hypertensive patients have demonstrated changes in arterial wall architecture and the major component of this appears to be remodeling. Careful review of published data would suggest that this is brought about almost completely by an increased pressure load rather than pressor-independent mechanisms, and that the changes are secondary to the blood pressure rather than a pathogenetic mechanism. There is little evidence to support the theory that these changes maintain blood pressure once it has been established. However, they are widespread and found in vital organs such as the heart and are associated with a reduction in coronary vascular reserve, implying if they are not reversed even when blood pressure is controlled, they may explain some of the mortality and morbidity associated with blood pressure in terms of coronary events, despite rigorous treatment programs.

# Endothelial Function and Hypertension

Studies of arteries of the arterial function of genetically hypertension-prone rats have demonstrated an impairment of endothelium-dependent dilation. Panza and coworkers[10] investigated whether patients with essential hypertension have similar abnormalities of endothelium-dependent vascular relaxation. They studied the response of the forearm vasculature to acetylcholine (ACh) and sodium nitroprusside and measured the responses by strain gauge plethysmography. They demonstrated that there was a highly significant reduction in the responses of blood flow and vascular resistance to ACh in hypertensive patients but no difference between groups in the response of blood flow and vascular resistance to sodium nitroprusside. Using pressure arteriography Falloon and Heagerty[11] confirmed that endothelium-dependent relaxation to ACh was reduced significantly in small arteries obtained by gluteal biopsy from hypertensive patients but that the endothelium-independent relaxation response to sodium nitroprusside was similar. However, Cockcroft and colleagues,[12] using forearm blood flow assessments and admittedly a much larger cohort than the previous studies, were unable to confirm these findings. At first glance it appears difficult to reconcile these discrepant reports. However, the cohorts examined by Cockcroft et al[12] had identical cholesterol levels, whereas those of the hypertensive patients in the study by Panza et al[10] were raised slightly and cholesterol was not measured by Falloon and Heagerty.[11] In other words, it is possible that hyperlipidemia, which often is associated with hypertension, might be confounding the findings. It is of interest that SHRs fed a high-cholesterol diet develop impaired endothelium-dependent relaxation compared with WKY animals.[13] Almost certainly there are contributions from the aging process as well as blood pressure in these animals as time goes by, but a high cholesterol certainly appears to accelerate the deterioration in endothelium-dependent relaxation (see following text). The contribution of the aging process to impairment of vascular endothelium-dependent relaxation also has been the subject of human studies; using forearm blood flow measurements, an impairment with increasing age was evident by the fourth decade, although endothelium-independent vasodilatation was not influenced. Age, total cholesterol, and low-density lipoprotein (LDL) cholesterol were univariate predictors of endothelium-dependent vasodilatation, although mean blood pressure was not.[14]

In summary, studies of endothelium-dependent vasodilatation in hypertension would suggest that this parameter is normal if careful provision is made for possible confounding factors such as dyslipidemia and age. It is also important to point out that there is an overwhelming body of evidence to suggest that vasoconstrictor function in the circulation of hypertensive patients is normal.

## Cholesterol and the Endothelium in Small Arteries

In small arteries that form the proximal resistance vasculature, atheromatous plaques are not observed. Nevertheless, evidence has accumulated from both experimental animals and studies of selected human vascular beds that hypercholesterolemia can have a profound effect on the dilator function of such vessels. For example, in the human heart, recent indirect evidence has been reported that hypercholesterolemia causes impairment of endothelium-dependent dilatation in intramyocardial small blood vessels.[15] Also a study of forearm blood flow has demonstrated blunted responses to both methacholine and nitroprusside in hypercholesterolemia suggesting that hyperlipidemia can both compromise endothelium-dependent dilatation and have a direct action on smooth muscle function. There is the intriguing possibility that such phenomena may precede atheroma formation in upstream medium-size and large arteries, while representing a widespread abnormality in the peripheral vasculature that persists and interferes with vascular tone and pressure homeostasis. Certainly there is evidence for changes in aortic compliance and endothelial function in young adults and children with hyperlipidemia and some evidence that blood pressure is higher in such individuals. In addition, when taken in conjunction with evidence that endothelium-dependent relaxation declines with age, one begins to see a picture emerging of how multiple cardiovascular risk factors may affect adversely the circulation and cause premature atherosclerosis.

Recently, further reports have been published that indicate that endothelial dysfunction in hyperlipidemia can be reversed with treatment: Two studies in humans have reported that reduction of serum cholesterol can improve epicardial coronary artery dilatation and coronary blood flow.[15]

Using subcutaneous small arteries obtained from gluteal biopsies, we have demonstrated that untreated patients with a total serum cholesterol of 7.5 mmol/L despite 3 months of a standard step-one diet have impaired significantly relaxation to ACh, again confirming the abnormality of embarrassed endothelium-dependent dilatation. In addition, we also demonstrated a direct effect of hyperlipidemia on smooth muscle relaxation because dose-response curves to sodium nitroprusside also showed a reduction in relaxation. Although this study was small it was of interest that the hypercholesterolemic patients had a higher blood pressure than matched controls. [15]

More than half of the cohort of patients underwent successful treatment of their hyperlipidemia according to European Atherosclerosis Society guidelines with significant reduction in both total and LDL cholesterol. These individuals agreed to undergo a second biopsy. The average time for treatment to normalize the lipid profile was 10 months. It was of interest that the previously impaired endothelium-dependent relaxation was restored completely to normal as was the response to sodium nitroprusside; furthermore, blood pressure fell significantly.[15]

We have extended these studies to intramyocardial small arteries harvested from explanted hearts removed at transplantation. The same pattern was observed and, as with peripheral small arteries, there was a very strong correlation between the degree of endothelial dilator impairment and total cholesterol.[16]

The mechanism by which an abnormal lipid profile impairs arterial function has been the subject of considerable attention. It is important to consider that although endothelium-dependent dilatation is most affected, endothelium-independent relaxation also is influenced, albeit to a lesser extent. With respect to endothelium-dependent relaxation, it would appear that there must be a reduced bioavailability of nitric oxide (NO), which is synthesized from the substrate L-arginine. It has been demonstrated that an infusion of L-arginine can restore endothelium-dependent relaxation to normal levels in hypercholesterolemic rabbits. Similar findings have been reported in the human coronary circulation and the forearm vasculature. However, in our studies, preincubation in vitro with L-arginine only slightly improved endothelium integrity.[15]

Also, it has been reported that hypercholesterolemia produces an increase in the release of nitrosylated compounds from the rabbit aorta. In consequence, it would appear that there is evidence that NO synthesis is enhanced in hypercholesterolemia but that its degradation is more rapid or it is released in a less bioactive form. Ultimately, the vasodilatation induced by such factors occurs by the same mechanism activated by endothelium-independent agonists such as sodium nitroprusside, that is, stimulation of guanylate cyclase within vascular myocytes and the formation of a nitrosylporphyrin complex. Therefore, the activity of guanylate cyclase may be affected directly by hypercholesterolemia as a result of a change in the redox state of the vascular smooth muscle. Evidence also is emerging implicating hypercholesterolemia in the genesis of free radicals, which again may influence NO metabolism and as a result, dilator status.

The precise lipid fraction responsible for these phenomena is thought to be oxidized LDL. Recently, it has been reported that oxidized LDL can attenuate endothelium-dependent relaxation in vitro and that this can be overcome by high-density lipoprotein (HDL). Furthermore, HDL cholesterol improves abnormal vasoconstriction in human coronary arteries and high levels of oxidized LDL can generate free-radical species from endothelial cells. Finally, as indicated above, superoxide anions are released from vessels from hypercholesterolemic animals and can inactive NO.

In terms of dietary improvement in lipid profiles, these have been relatively disappointing when compared with the effects that can be achieved using drug therapy. Nevertheless, regimens that include marine fish oil supplements have been demonstrated to be potentially useful in the prevention and treatment of coronary heart disease. Several mechanisms have been proposed for these effects, including favorable changes in serum lipid profile, lowering blood pressure, inhibiting platelet aggregation, and prolonging bleeding time. Also, there is evidence that such supplements may well produce vasodilator prostaglandins, which in themselves, may influence vascular function.

In a recent study of hypercholesterolemic patients randomized to receive fish oil capsules containing 18% eicosapentanoic and 12% docosahexanoic acid or placebo there was partial improvement in the endothelial dysfunction already described; however, an influence of this dietary change on sodium nitroprusside responses was not observed.[17] An effect of antioxidants used as preservatives in the capsules was discounted. The mechanism by which this was brought about is not clear, but probably did not involve an increase in the production of vasodilator prostaglandins, because an improvement in vascular reactivity was not altered by the in vitro application of indomethacin. However, the results were consistent with an influence on endothelium-dependent dilatation and by inference, NO production. Nevertheless, the precise mechanism remains uncertain.

# Cholesterol, Endothelial Dysfunction, and Hypertension

These findings take on a more prominent role when it is recognized that there is evidence of a relation between serum lipids and blood pressure independent of confounding variables such as age and body mass index. Data pooled from 41 000 subjects show a clear-cut relationship between total cholesterol and blood pressure in seven major studies[18] and although information is sparse concerning the effects on blood pressure in lipid-lowering trials designed to examine the effects of lowering lipids on coronary heart disease, what data are available point to small but consistent effects on pressure. The World Health Organization (WHO) study of more than 5000 men with hypercholesterolemia, for example, who were randomized to receive either clofibrate or placebo, demonstrated a 25% reduction in the incidence of hypertension in men treated with clofibrate. Furthermore, the reduction in nonfatal myocardial infarction was greater in those with the largest reductions in cholesterol and higher initial blood pressures. Data from more than 17 000 patients in this respect are available and although small falls in serum cholesterol were achieved, falls in blood pressure were observed, which if extrapolated to the community at large, would reduce the incidence of coronary heart disease.[18]

If one were seeking a unifying hypothesis to explain such findings, then the direct effect of serum lipids on endothelial function appears attractive. Hypercholesterolemia is associated with abnormalities of coronary vascular reserve, which as noted above, can be corrected within minutes with L-arginine by infusion. In addition, there is a loss of normal flow-dependent dilatation in arteries from patients who have hypercholesterolemia and virtually no evidence of atheroma on angiography. This abnormality impairs exercise-induced vascular conductance in coronary vessels.

Our recent in vitro investigations of segments of small intramyocardial blood vessels, harvested from explanted hearts and preconstricted with a thromboxanemimetic, have demonstrated impairment of endothelium-dependent relaxation to ACh and bradykinin in patients with ischemic cardiomyopathy compared with nonischemic cardiomyopathy.[16] With the use of stepwise multivariate analysis, hypercholesterolemia but no other risk factor for atherosclerosis was independently associated with this finding. The magnitude of impairment was proportional directly to the level of serum total cholesterol. There seems to be little doubt that there is a widespread abnormality of circulatory dilator function in the presence of hyperlipidemia.

# Small Arteries and Mild Heart Failure

Two studies have been published that have examined directly small arteries using the gluteal biopsy technique to provide samples for in vitro investigations from patients with heart failure. There is no doubt that the prevalence of heart failure in the population is rising and it carries with it a particularly bad prognosis. Although the primary abnormality is a loss of functioning myocardium, the consequent fall in cardiac output leads to an activation of a number of compensatory neuroendocrine mechanisms such as the sympathetic nervous and renin-angiotensin systems. To maintain blood pressure, these mechanisms produce ionotropic stimulation of the residual myocardium, peripheral vasoconstriction, and fluid retention. Although cardiac output improves in the short term, over a longer period, direct cardiotoxic effects of angiotensin II and norepinephrine with an increase in peripheral vascular resistance contribute to the inevitable progressive decline in cardiac function. The role of the peripheral vasculature in this process is not clarified. High concentrations of catecholamines and renin could influence the function of small blood vessels and there are reports that heart failure is associated with impairment of endothelium-dependent relaxation. Also, there is the intriguing possibility that sympathomimetic amines and angiotensin II could cause structural changes in the vasculature similar to those seen in hypertensive patients. Angus et al[19] examined blood vessels from subcutaneous biopsy taken from patients with severe heart failure and demonstrated impaired endothelium-dependent vasodilatation. Recently, in collaboration with the Department of Cardiovascular Research at Leeds, we have been able to examine a subset of the patients recruited to the Acute Infarction Ramipril Efficacy (AIRE) study.[20] All patients displayed clinical evidence of heart failure, which was defined as at least one of the following: evidence of left ventricular failure, evidence of pulmonary edema, or auscultatory evidence of a third heart sound with persistent tachycardia. It should be pointed out that in accordance with the AIRE study criteria, patients with severe heart failure were excluded. Subjects were assigned randomly to therapy with placebo or ramipril starting 3–10 days after myocardial infarction with a mean duration of treatment of 27 months. Standard therapy was maintained for all patients throughout the trial.

The two groups of patients with mild heart failure were compared with a cohort of control subjects, similarly aged but without any evidence of myocardial infarction or left ventricular dysfunction. Predictably, systolic pressure was significantly higher in these subjects compared with the patients, and patients treated with placebo had higher pressures than those treated with ramipril. It was of interest that the blood vessels from patients treated with ramipril had slightly reduced vascular morphology in the media:lumen ratio than patients on placebo, although this did not achieve statistical significance. However, functionally, the blood vessels performed normally and we could provide no evidence for endothelial dysfunction or changes in vascular contractility. There was a significantly enhanced responsiveness to angiotensin II in patients treated with ramipril, which might reflect the exposure of these vessels in vivo to reduced concentrations of this hormone at the level of the receptor. Beyond this, it would appear that small blood vessels in mild heart failure function relatively normally.

## In Vitro Studies of Small Arteries in Other Cardiovascular Disorders

Although data are emerging with respect to diabetes, there are only small reports of in vitro investigations of small blood vessel function in this disease.

Again, it would appear that endothelium-dependent relaxation is reduced. This probably reflects the dyslipidemia that often is associated with this condition rather than an intrinsic pathogenetic mechanism. Larger cohorts are being examined at present. Given the most recent publications of major population interventions directed at not only controlling the metabolic consequences of diabetes but also reducing complications of this disorder, it would appear that improving circulatory function may well be prognostically important. In consequence, the use of agents to lower blood pressure and control dyslipidemias may well be crucial to improving long-term survival in diabetic patients, as a result of correcting the endothelial dysfunction and morphological changes induced as a result of hypercholesterolaemia and hypertension.

In summary, in vitro investigations over the last 10 years have yielded insights into the way that small blood vessels respond to hypertension, heart failure, and hypercholesterolemia. Endothelial dysfunction appears to be observed consistently in many of these conditions in blood vessels, which do not develop atherosclerotic plaques. The functional change that must be induced in consequence, may well be extremely important in terms of tissue perfusion, especially in organs such as the heart, where coronary vascular reserve undoubtedly is embarrassed. The fact that medication can restore integrity to normal relatively quickly lends further support for the need to be increasingly vigilant in the detection and management of such conditions.

*Acknowledgments:* I am grateful to Mrs. J. Heydon for her assistance in preparing this manuscript.

# References

1. Heagerty AM, Aalkjaer C, Bund SJ, et al. Small artery structure in hypertension: Dual processes of remodeling and growth. *Hypertens* 1993;21:391–397.
2. Heagerty AM, Izzard AS. Small artery changes in hypertension. *J Hypertens* 1995;13:1560–1565.
3. Agabiti Rosei E, Rizzoni D, Castellano M, et al. Media:lumen ratio in human resistance arteries is related to forearm minimal vascular resistance. *J Hypertens* 1995;13:349–355.
4. Short D. Morphology of the intestinal arterioles in chronic hypertension. *Br Heart J* 1966;28:184–192.
5. Korsgaard N, Aalkjaer C, Heagerty AM, et al. Histology of subcutaneous small arteries from patients with essential hypertension. *Hypertens* 1993;22:523–526.
6. Izzard AS, Heagerty AM. Hypertension and the vasculature: Arterioles and the myogenic response. *J Hypertens* 1995;13:1–4.
7. Izzard AS, Bund SJ, Heagerty AM. Increased wall-lumen ratio of mesenteric vessels from the spontaneously hypertensive rat is not associated with increased contractility under isobaric conditions. *Hypertens* 1996;28:604–608.
8. Marks ES, Bing RF, Thurston H, et al. Responsiveness to pressor agents in experimental and renovascular and steroid hypertension. *Hypertens* 1982;4:238–244.
9. Leenen FHH, Yuan B, Tsoporis J, et al. Arterial hypertrophy and pressor responsiveness during development of hypertension in spontaneously hypertensive rats. *J Hypertens* 1994;12:23–32.
10. Panza JA, Quyyumi AA, Brush JE, et al. Abnormal endothelium-dependent vascular relaxation in patients with essential hypertension. *N Engl J Med* 1990;323:22–27.

11. Falloon BJ, Heagerty AM. In vitro perfusion studies of human resistance artery function in essential hypertension. *Hypertens* 1994;24:16–23.
12. Cockcroft JR, Chowienczyk PJ, Benjamin N, et al. Preserved endothelium-dependent vasodilatation in patients with essential hypertension. *N Engl J Med* 1994;330:1036–1040.
13. Capelli-Bigazzi M, Rubattu S, Battaglia C, et al. Effects of high-cholesterol and atherogenic diets on vascular relaxation in spontaneously hypertensive rats. *Am J Physiol* 1997;2273:H647–H654.
14. Gerhard M, Roddy M-A, Creager SJ, et al. Aging progressively impairs endothelium-dependent vasodilatation in forearm resistance vessels of humans. *Hypertens* 1996; 27:849–853.
15. Goode GK, Heagerty AM. In vitro responses of human peripheral small arteries in hypercholesterolaemia and effects of therapy. *Circulation* 1995;91:2898–2903.
16. Cooper A, Heagerty AM. Endothelial dysfunction in human intramyocardial small arteries in atherosclerosis and hypercholesterolaemia. *Am J Physiol* 1998. In press.
17. Goode GK, Garcia S, Heagerty AM. Dietary supplementation with marine fish oil improves in vitro small artery endothelial function in hypercholesterolaemic patients. *Circulation* 1997;96:2802–2807.
18. Goode GK, Miller JP, Heagerty AM. Hyperlipidaemia, hypertension and coronary heart disease. *Lancet* 1995;345:362–364.
19. Angus JA, Ferrier CP, Sudhir D, et al. Impaired contraction and relaxation in skin resistance arteries from patients with congestive heart failure. *Cardiovasc Res* 1993;27:204–210.
20. Stephens N, Drinkhill MJ, Hall AS, et al. Structure and in vitro function of human subcutaneous small arteries in mild heart failure. *Am J Physiol* 1998;274:C1298–C1305.

# Part IV

## Therapeutic Strategies to Improve Endothelial Dysfunction

## Chapter 17

# Endothelium as a Target of the Risk Factors in Cardiovascular Disease

*Scott Kinlay, MBBS, PhD, Andrew P. Selwyn, MD, and Peter Ganz, MD*

## Introduction

Epidemiological studies have shown consistently that several factors measured at one point in time determine the risk of vascular disease over the subsequent years.[1–5] Clinical trials have shown that the reversal of some of these risk factors, most successfully demonstrated with hyperlipidemia, can reduce the complications of atherosclerotic disease.[6–10]

However, it takes many years to establish the links between risk factors and the clinical events. Furthermore, a lack of understanding for the biological mechanisms that explain how the risk factors are related to clinical events delays the widespread acceptance of their causal role. It has been established that many of the conventional and recently proposed risk factors for cardiovascular disease adversely affect the function of the vascular endothelium. In particular, the potential for risk factors to impair the bioavailability of endothelium-derived nitric oxide (EDNO) is shared by all risk factors examined to date.

This review will focus on the role of endothelial dysfunction in the development of clinical events and the effects of risk factors on disturbing endothelial function. An increased understanding of the mechanisms for the effects of risk factors on the endothelium may help to improve current strategies and develop new strategies for the prevention of cardiovascular disease.

## Endothelial Dysfunction and Clinical Events

In healthy arteries, shear stress, acetylcholine (ACh), and other stimuli activate nitric oxide synthase (NOS) within the endothelium and increase the production of NO from L-arginine[11] (Figure 1). NO performs multiple functions

From Panza JA, Cannon RO III (eds): *Endothelium, Nitric Oxide, and Atherosclerosis* ©Futura Publishing Co, Inc, Armonk, NY, 1999.

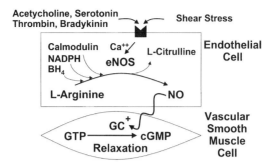

**Figure 1.** The nitric oxide (NO) pathway. Abbreviations: $BH_4$, tetrahydrobiopterin; NADPH, nicotinamide-adenine dinucleotide phosphate; $Ca^{2+}$, calcium ion; eNOS, endothelial NO synthase; GC, guanylate cyclase; GTP, guanosine triphosphate phosphate; cGMP, cyclic guanosine monophosphate.

in the homeostasis of the arterial wall including the regulation of vascular tone, inflammation, and hemostasis.

NO generated by the endothelium induces vasodilation by diffusing to the adjacent vascular smooth muscle where it activates guanylate cyclase.[12,13] Experimental studies have shown that NO regulates inflammation in part by inhibiting the activity of the transcriptional factor nuclear factor–kappa $\beta$ (NF-$\kappa\beta$) and the subsequent expression of cellular adhesion molecules on the surface of the endothelium,[14–16] and inhibiting the expression of the proinflammatory mediators monocyte chemoattractant protein-1, interleukin-6, interleukin-8, and macrophage-colony–stimulating factor.[14,17–19] These cellular adhesion molecules, cytokines, and chemoattractants allow the endothelial cells to capture leukocytes and assist in their migration into the arterial wall. Endothelium-derived NO also reduces platelet aggregation and adhesion and proliferation of vascular smooth muscle.[20–23]

In atherosclerotic arteries, NO bioavailability is reduced,[24] by a combination of decreased production and enhanced degradation.[24–28] As a result, inflammatory cells are recruited into the plaque. T lymphocytes in plaques produce $\gamma$-interferon, which inhibits the production of matrix collagen by intimal smooth muscles cells.[29] Activated macrophages and smooth muscle cells secrete matrix metalloproteinases that can degrade components of the fibrous cap of plaques.[29] The diminished synthesis and enhanced degradation of the matrix components act to weaken the fibrous cap and increase the likelihood of plaque rupture. In the event that plaque rupture occurs, the decreased NO permits platelet activation and extension of thrombus that promotes the development of the acute ischemic syndromes.[11]

Our understanding of the relationship of NO and plaque inflammation stems mostly from experimental studies because accurate methods of assessing and localizing vascular inflammation in humans are lacking. However, valuable insights into the role of endothelium-derived NO in the regulation of vasomotor tone in humans have been provided by the use of modern techniques including quantitative angiography, intravascular ultrasound, and Doppler ultrasound in the cardiac catheterization laboratory and two-dimensional ultrasound and plethysmography of systemic arteries.

In healthy arteries, endothelial NO (eNO) production can be stimulated pharmacologically by infusions of agents such as ACh or serotonin.[30] Increasing blood flow by reactive hyperemia or exercise is a physiological stimulus to the endothelium to produce more NO.[30-35] The released NO diffuses to the medial smooth muscle causing vasodilation. Dilation of conduit arteries can be assessed by angiography and two dimensional ultrasound, whereas dilatation of the microvascular bed is identified by measuring changes in blood flow with Doppler ultrasound or plethysmography. In epicardial (conduit) arteries with reduced NO bioavailability, the direct vasoconstrictor action of ACh is unopposed leading to vasoconstriction of the conduit artery.[24] Similarly, during exercise, reactive hyperemia results in reduced vasodilation of epicardial arteries with reductions of NO permitting adrenergic vasoconstriction to dominate.[31-36]

Studies during cardiac catheterization have shown that epicardial coronary arteries with angiographic evidence of atherosclerosis constrict to ACh or with exercise.[24,31,33,37-39] In contrast, patients free of angiographic disease dilate in response to these stimuli. When superimposed on coronary stenoses, vasoconstriction increases the hemodynamic significance of atherosclerotic lesions and likely contributes to the development of angina.

Studies of coronary and systemic artery endothelium-dependent vasomotion are used to assess the bioavailability of NO in vivo and may provide surrogate measures for the other cellular functions of NO. The evidence that links the coronary risk factors to reductions in NO and endothelial vasomotor dysfunction is discussed below.

## Dyslipidemia

Native low density lipoprotein (LDL) has limited effect on the function of the endothelium. Once modified by oxidation, the apolipoprotein B-100, phospholipid, and other components of this particle are altered.[40-44] The modified LDL particle is bound avidly by scavenger receptors on macrophages in an unregulated fashion.[40-44] The progressive accumulation of oxidized LDL leads to foam cell formation and trapping of LDL within the intima. Experimental studies have shown that oxidized LDL can impair endothelial vasodilator function more effectively than native LDL.

Clinical studies have shown that patients with dyslipidemias may have impaired coronary endothelium-dependent vasomotion even in the absence of angiographically detectable disease. In patients with smooth coronary arteries, the response to ACh infusions is related directly to serum cholesterol levels, with greater vasodilation with lower cholesterol levels[38,45-47] (Figure 2). Small, dense LDL particles are particularly atherogenic and prone to impairing endothelium-dependent dilation.[48] The response of the epicardial arteries also is related to the susceptibility of the LDL particle to oxidation.[49] In contrast, high-density lipoprotein (HDL) cholesterol is a protective factor for both coronary artery disease and endothelium-dependent vasomotion.[50,51]

A potent support for the role of LDL cholesterol in reducing the bioavailability of NO comes from interventional studies that have lowered cholesterol

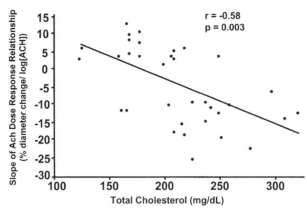

**Figure 2.** Relationship between serum cholesterol levels and endothelium-dependent vasomotion. Reproduced with permission from Reference 45.

levels. These studies have shown that lipid-lowering drugs improve endothelial dysfunction in patients with dyslipidemia. Over a period of 6–12 months, endothelial function was improved in epicardial arteries[52–54] and resistance vessels.[55]

In one study, the addition of the potent antioxidant probucol to lovastatin led to an additional improvement in vasomotor function compared with the placebo group.[53] The degree of improvement was related directly to the extent of antioxidant protection of LDL cholesterol conferred by this drug.[49] Although the beneficial role of other antioxidants has yet to be confirmed, the potential for antioxidants to increase the effectiveness of cholesterol lowering on endothelial function suggests that some synergy may occur between LDL cholesterol and oxidation that could be exploited in preventive therapies.

# Menopause

Prior to menopause, women in western societies have lower rates of heart disease than men. After menopause, the risk of heart disease converges with the risk in men. One explanation for this rise in risk is the loss of estrogen in women after the menopause.[56,57] Several large cohort studies have found that postmenopausal women using estrogen or estrogen and progesterone replacement therapy develop less coronary heart disease than those who do not use hormone replacement therapy.[58–60] However, a recent randomized clinical trial [Heart and Estrogen/Progestin Replacement Study (HERS)][61] showed no advantage of conjugated equine estrogens when combined with medroxyprogesterone acetate over placebo in reducing clinical events in postmenopausal women with coronary artery disease.

Nevertheless, the beneficial effect of acute and chronic estrogens on endothelium-dependent vasomotion was demonstrated initially in oophorectomized primates.[62,63] These results led to studies of the effects of estrogen supplementation on endothelial function in postmenopausal women.

Several studies have examined the effect of the acute administration of intracoronary or intravenous estrogens on coronary vasomotion in postmenopausal women. Intracoronary infusion of estradiol-17β at physiological concentrations improves the epicardial response to ACh, consistent with improvement in endothelial function.[64] This acute effect of estrogens may be restricted to women because another study found that similar improvements in endothelial function were not observed in men receiving infusions of estradiol-17β.[65] The effect of estrogen on blood vessels also may be dependent on the type and dose of estrogen. In one study that used an infusion of supraphysiological concentrations of a synthetic estrogen, ethinyl estradiol, direct vasodilation of the coronary arteries was observed.[66] However, this direct effect was not seen in studies using physiological concentrations of estradiol-17β or of intravenous infusion of Premarin, the estrogen used most often in observational studies of cardiovascular risk. In this study, intravenous Premarin improved endothelium-dependent vasodilation to ACh but had no direct effect on vascular tone.[67]

These investigations have demonstrated beneficial effects of estrogen replacement on endothelial vasomotion within several minutes of administration and therefore cannot be explained by the action of estrogen on the classic intracellular estrogen receptor pathway or by changes in the lipid profile that occur over a much longer time frame. Recently, estradiol-17β has been shown to act rapidly by interaction with a cytoplasmic estrogen receptor but without the need for translocation to the nucleus and gene transcription.[68] A second estrogen receptor (the β-receptor) has been identified[69] and may be the dominant estrogen receptor in endothelial cells. Estrogen also may be acting as an antioxidant. Estradiol-17β shares the hydroxyphenol ring of other antioxidants such as vitamin E and probucol and is capable of behaving as an antioxidant.[70,71] Thus, it is possible that novel receptor pathways and other nonspecific properties could explain the rapid estrogen effect.

The effect of the long-term administration of estrogen on vasomotor function has been investigated conveniently using brachial artery ultrasound to examine the vasodilator response to reactive hyperemia. This brachial artery flow-mediated dilation is mediated by eNO and is correlated closely to the coronary artery responses to ACh in individuals who have had both tests.[72] The brachial artery flow-mediated dilation is modulated by physiological variations in estrogen levels. The brachial artery dilation increases with the rise in estrogen during the midcycle follicular stage of the ovarian cycle and decreases only modestly in the late cycle luteal stage when progesterone and estrogen are both elevated.[73] Furthermore, the decline in brachial flow-mediated dilation corresponds to the time of the menopause[74] and occurs 10 years later than in men.

It remains speculative why the HERS study failed to show a benefit. Possible explanations that need to be investigated include the use of medroxyprogesterone acetate, a synthetic progestin. Interestingly, although natural progesterone does not reduce the benefits of estrogen on endothelial function,[75] the synthetic progestin norethisterone may abolish estrogen's favorable effects.[76] Further studies should clarify this issue.

# Diabetes Mellitus

Diabetes is a risk factor for coronary artery disease, and patients with diabetes have impaired endothelial function. Endothelial function in the coronary arteries of patients with diabetes has been compared with controls.[77] Both groups of patients were free of angiographic evidence of coronary atherosclerosis; however, the patients with diabetes exhibited abnormal coronary vasoconstriction to ACh consistent with endothelial dysfunction. Most other studies of diabetes have examined endothelial function in the microcirculation of the forearm by measuring changes in forearm blood flow to endothelium-dependent and -independent vasodilation stimuli. Endothelial vasomotor responses measured by this approach are impaired in patients with non–insulin-dependent (type II) and insulin-dependent (type I) diabetes mellitus.[78–82] Brachial artery flow-mediated dilation assessed in the conduit artery by ultrasound also is impaired in diabetes mellitus compared with controls.[83] Endothelial dysfunction occurs in patients with diabetes even in the absence of hypercholesterolemia or hypertension[78,79] and can be reproduced in a healthy subject by raising the concentration of glucose in the forearm for several hours.[84,85]

There may be some difference in the pathophysiological processes responsible for the abnormal vasomotion in patients with insulin- and non–insulin-dependent diabetes mellitus.[78,79] Patients with non–insulin-dependent diabetes mellitus have a blunted vasodilation to exogenous NO donors that is not observed in patients with insulin-dependent diabetes mellitus. However, the dilation to a direct smooth muscle dilator (verapamil) is preserved in either group, suggesting inactivation of NO as a more important mechanism for the vasomotor dysfunction in non–insulin-dependent than in insulin-dependent diabetes mellitus.[78]

Recently, the acute administration of vitamin C has been shown to reverse the impaired response to methacholine infusions in patients with non–insulin- and insulin-dependent diabetes mellitus.[81,82] This suggests that the reduced bioavailability of NO in the forearm circulation in diabetes is caused by increased inactivation of NO by oxygen-derived free radicals. If this finding is reproduced in other vascular beds, antioxidants may find a therapeutic role in diabetes.

# Smoking

Cigarette smoking is associated strongly with the development of coronary artery disease and peripheral atherosclerosis and also impairs coronary and peripheral artery endothelial function. Coronary flow-mediated dilation is impaired in smokers compared with nonsmokers, especially in those with evidence of angiographic disease.[86]

In the brachial artery, cigarette smoking is associated strongly with reduced flow-mediated dilation.[87,88] Furthermore, the impairment in brachial artery flow-mediated dilation is greater among heavier smokers than lighter smokers and greater in current than former smokers.[88] Even passive smoking is associated with endothelial vasodilator dysfunction.[89]

Endothelial function in the microcirculation also is impaired in smokers and further impaired smokers who have hypercholesterolemia.[90] Acute infusions of the antioxidant vitamin C are able to reverse the decreased endothelium-dependent vasodilation in smokers[91] suggesting that smoking may impair NO mechanisms by increasing oxidative stress.

## Hypertension

Coronary and peripheral artery endothelial vasomotion is impaired in patients with hypertension compared with controls. Epicardial artery vasodilation to ACh is impaired in patients with hypertension,[92,93] and coronary microvascular dilation to ACh is reduced in those with hypertension or left ventricular hypertrophy caused by hypertension compared with controls.[92,93] Endothelium-dependent vasodilation also is impaired in the systemic arteries of hypertensive patients both in conduit arteries and in the microvasculature.[34,94–96] Hypertension may be a primary result of endothelial vasomotor function or a secondary effect of hypertension. Several observations suggest that a defect in the NO pathway occurs as the principle event in some patients. These include the presence of endothelial vasomotor dysfunction in the prehypertensive offspring of hypertensive patients and its absence in the offspring of normotensive subjects.[97] Furthermore, endothelial dysfunction in hypertensive patients is not reversed universally by all of the antihypertensive agents.

## Other Proposed Risk Factors

The effect of several newer risk factors on endothelial function has been investigated to understand how they may cause vascular disease. These risk factors include hyperhomocyst(e)inemia and lipoprotein(a).

Hyperhomocyst(e)inemia is associated with impaired brachial artery flow-mediated dilation compared with age and sex-matched controls,[98,99] and homocysteine concentrations are related directly to the brachial artery response.[98] Furthermore, methionine loading in normal volunteers, an experimental approach to raising serum homocysteine, rapidly induces endothelial dysfunction in brachial arteries.[100]

Lipoprotein(a) concentrations have been found to be related inversely to coronary endothelium-dependent vasodilation in 30 patients with angiographically normal coronary arteries.[101] If the results of these studies are confirmed, treatments that reverse these factors could be employed to assess their effect on endothelial vasomotion and increase support for their role in the pathogenesis of coronary artery disease.

## Combinations of Multiple Risk Factors

Multiple risk factors impair endothelium-dependent vasomotion to a greater extent than any one risk factor alone. The number of risk factors

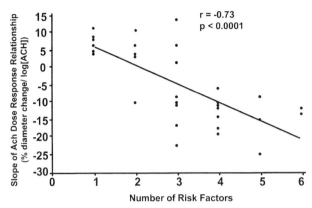

**Figure 3.** Relationship between the number of coronary risk factors and endothelium-dependent vasomotion. Reproduced with permission from Reference 45.

counted in a simple scoring system is associated more strongly with impaired coronary[45] (Figure 3) and brachial artery[34] endothelium-dependent vasodilation than the individual risk factors alone. Thus the analogy between the effect of multiple risk factors on endothelial function and on cardiovascular risk supports the hypothesis that an impairment of eNO availability is one of the principal mechanisms that accounts for the relationship between the risk factors and coronary artery disease.

## Effect of Reversing Coronary Risk Factors on Endothelial Function

Support for the relationship between endothelial function and the clinical coronary artery disease syndromes has arisen from several studies that have reversed coronary risk factors. In recent years several studies have demonstrated that lowering total and LDL cholesterol has a potent effect on improving endothelial function over a period of weeks to months. These included several studies in patients with atherosclerosis where lipid-lowering drugs improve coronary endothelial vasomotion to ACh.[52–55] This intervention improves the conduit artery vasodilation and augments coronary blood flow responses toward normal.

Lipid-lowering medications also reduce ambulatory myocardial ischemia over a similar time frame.[102,103] These changes occur much sooner than that required for the modest changes in lumen diameter noticed in the atherosclerosis regression trials.[104] Therefore it is more likely that the reduction in ischemia is caused by improvement in coronary vasomotion and thereby perfusion rather than by significant changes in coronary stenoses severity.

Several studies in patients with atherosclerosis, diabetes, and smokers suggest that antioxidants can partly reverse the impaired endothelium-dependent vasomotor responses.[53,81,82,105,106] Oxidation of LDL cholesterol and "oxidative stress" within the arterial wall reduces NO bioavailability in experimental studies. However, the evidence that antioxidants may reduce the risk of coronary artery disease remains inconclusive.[107,108]

Support for the therapeutic role of antioxidants will depend on the development of more potent agents, confirmation of their effectiveness in large randomized studies, and investigations addressing the effect of antioxidant supplements on vascular function.

Angiotensin-converting enzyme inhibitors also improve coronary endothelial dysfunction. Angiotensin II has several actions on vascular tissue including increasing the generation of superoxide free radicals by the up-regulation of membrane-bound nicotinamide-adenine dinucleotide (NADH) and nicotinamide-adenine-dinucleotide phosphate (NADPH) oxidases[109,110] and increasing the expression of the potent vasoconstrictor endothelin-1.[111] Superoxide free radicals react with NO to form the vasoinactive product peroxynitrite. In experimental studies, angiotensin-converting enzyme inhibitors reduce superoxide production and restore endothelium-dependent vasorelaxation.[109] In human studies, treatment with an angiotensin-converting enzyme inhibitor for 6 months has been shown to improve coronary endothelial function[112] and to improve endothelium-dependent vasomotion in the forearm.[113]

# Conclusions

Experimental and clinical studies have shown that endothelial dysfunction is associated closely with the development of coronary artery disease and clinical coronary events. The conventional risk factors for coronary artery disease are thought to cause coronary events in part by impairing endothelial function, thereby promoting vasoconstriction, inflammation, thrombosis, and vascular proliferation.

In clinical studies, coronary and systemic endothelium-dependent vasodilation are impaired by these risk factors demonstrating that NO bioavailability is reduced. The assessment of endothelial dysfunction may provide insights into the different effects of risk factors in and among individuals and help develop new strategies to prevent coronary artery disease and its complications.

# References

1. Pekkanen J, Linn S, Heiss G, et al. Ten-year mortality from cardiovascular disease in relation to cholesterol level among men with and without pre-existing cardiovascular disease. *N Engl J Med* 1990;322:1700–1707.
2. Stamler J, Wentworth D, Neaton JD. Is the relationship between serum cholesterol and risk of premature death from CHD continuous and graded? Findings in 356 222 primary screenees of the Multiple Risk Factor Intervention Trial (MRFIT). *JAMA* 1986;256:2823–2828.
3. Stampfer MJ, Sacks FM, Salvini S, et al. A prospective study of cholesterol, apolipoproteins, and the risk of myocardial infarction. *N Engl J Med* 1991;325: 373–381.

4. Manson JE, Colditz GA, Stampfer MJ, et al. A prospective study of obesity and risk of coronary heart disease in women. *N Engl J Med* 1990;322:882–889.

5. Shaper AG, Pocock SJ, Walker M, et al. Risk factors for ischaemic heart disease: The prospective phase of the British Regional Heart Study. *J Epidemiol Community Health* 1985;39:197–209.

6. Lipid Research Clinics Program. The Lipid Research Clinics Coronary Primary Prevention Trial results: I. Reduction in incidence of CHD. *JAMA* 1984;251:351–364.

7. Frick MH, Elo O, Haapa K, et al. Helsinki Heart Study: Primary prevention trial with gemfibrozil in middle-aged men with dyslipidemia. *N Engl J Med* 1987;717:1237–1245.

8. Scandinavian Simvastatin Survival Study Group. Randomized trial of cholesterol lowering therapy in 4444 patients with coronary heart disease: The Scandinavian Simvastatin Survival Study (4S). *Lancet* 1994;344:1383–1389.

9. Sacks FM, Pfeffer MA, Moye LA, et al. The effect of Pravastatin on recurrent coronary events after myocardial infarction in patients with average cholesterol levels. *N Engl J Med* 1996;335:1001–1009.

10. Shepherd J, Cobbe SM, Ford I, et al. Prevention of coronary heart disease with pravastatin in men with hypercholesterolemia. West of Scotland Coronary Prevention Study Group. *N Engl J Med* 1995;333:1303–1307.

11. Selwyn AP, Kinlay S, Creager MA, et al. Cell dysfunction in atherosclerosis and the ischemic manifestations of coronary artery disease. *Am J Cardiol* 1997;79(suppl 5A):17–23.

12. Palmer RM, Ferrige AG, Moncada S. Nitric oxide release accounts for the biological activity of endothelium-derived relaxing factor. *Nature* 1987;327:524–526.

13. Palmer RM, Ashton DS, Moncada S. Vascular endothelial cells synthesize nitric oxide from L-arginine. *Nature* 1988;333:664–666.

14. DeCaterina R, Libby P, Peng H-B, et al. Nitric oxide decreases cytokine-induced endothelial activation. *J Clin Invest* 1995;96:60–68.

15. Tsao P, Buitrago R, Chan JR, et al. Fluid flow inhibits endothelial adhesiveness: Nitric oxide and transcriptional regulation of VCAM-1. *Circulation* 1996;94:1682–1689.

16. Kubes P, Suzuki M, Granger DN. Nitric oxide: An endogenous modulator of leukocyte adhesion. *Proc Natl Acad Sci U S A* 1991;88:4651–4655.

17. Zeiher AM, Fisslthaler B, Schray-Utz B, et al. Nitric oxide modulates the expression of monocyte chemoattractant protein 1 in cultured human endothelial cells. *Circ Res* 1995;76:980–986.

18. Tsao PS, Wang B, Buitrago R, et al. Nitric oxide regulates monocyte chemotactic protein-1. *Circulation* 1997;96:934–940.

19. Peng HB, Rajavashisth TB, Libby P, et al. Nitric oxide inhibits macrophage-colony stimulating factor gene transcription in vascular endothelial cells. *J Biol Chem* 1995;270:17050–17055.

20. Azuma H, Ishikawa M, Sekizaki S. Endothelium-dependent inhibition of platelet aggregation. *Br J Pharmacol* 1986;88:411–415.

21. Hogan JC, Lewis MJ, Henderson AH. In vivo EDRF activity influences platelet function. *Br J Pharmacol* 1988;94:1020–1022.

22. Yao S-K, Ober JC, Krishnaswami A, et al. Endogenous nitric oxide protects against platelet aggregation and cyclic flow variations in stenosed and endothelium-injured arteries. *Circulation* 1992;86:1302–1309.

23. Bassenge E. Antiplatelet effects of endothelium-derived relaxing factor and nitric oxide donors. *Eur Heart J* 1991;12(suppl E):12–15.

24. Ludmer PL, Selwyn AP, Shook TL, et al. Paradoxical vasoconstriction induced by acetylcholine in atherosclerotic coronary arteries. *N Engl J Med* 1986;315:1046–1051.

25. Cox DA, Cohen ML. Effects of oxidized low-density lipoprotein on vascular contraction and relaxation: Clinical and pharmacological implications in atherosclerosis. *Pharmacol Rev* 1996;48:3–19.

26. Liao JK, Shin WS, Lee WY, et al. Oxidized low-density lipoprotein decreases the expression of endothelial nitric oxide synthase. *J Biol Chem* 1995;270:319–324.
27. Liao JK, Clark SL. Regulation of G-protein and $\alpha_{i2}$ submit expression by oxidized low-density lipoprotein. *J Clin Invest* 1995;95:1457–1463.
28. Keaney JF, Vita JA. Atherosclerosis, oxidative stress, and antioxidant protection in endothelium-derived relaxing factor action. *Prog Cardiovasc Dis* 1995;38:129–154.
29. Libby P. Molecular bases of the acute coronary syndromes. *Circulation* 1995: 2844–2850.
30. Meredith IT, Yeung AC, Weidinger FF, et al. Role of impaired endothelium-dependent vasodilation in ischemic manifestations of coronary artery disease. *Circulation* 1993;87(suppl V):V56–V66.
31. Gordon JB, Ganz P, Nabel EG, et al. Atherosclerosis and endothelial function influence the coronary vasomotor response to exercise. *J Clin Invest* 1989;83: 1946–1952.
32. Nabel EG, Selwyn AP, Ganz P. Large coronary arteries in humans are responsive to changes in blood flow: An endothelium-dependent mechanism that fails in patients with atherosclerosis. *J Am Coll Cardiol* 1990;16:349–356.
33. Cox DA, Vita JA, Treasure CB, et al. Atherosclerosis impairs flow-mediated dilation of coronary arteries in humans. *Circulation* 1989;80:458–465.
34. Celermajer DS, Sorensen KE, Bull C, et al. Endothelium-dependent dilation in the systemic arteries of asymptomatic subjects relates to coronary risk factors and their interaction. *J Am Coll Cardiol* 1994;24:1468–1474.
35. Creager MA, Cooke JP, Mendelsohn ME, et al. Impaired vasodilation of forearm resistance vessels in hypercholesterolemic humans. *J Clin Invest* 1990;86:228–234.
36. Lefroy DC, Crake T, Uren NG, et al. Effect of inhibition of nitric oxide synthesis on epicardial coronary artery caliber and coronary blood flow in humans. *Circulation* 1993;88:43–54.
37. Quyyumi AA, Dakad N, Mulcahy D, et al. Nitric oxide activity in the atherosclerotic human coronary circulation. *J Am Coll Cardiol* 1997;29:308–317.
38. Zeiher AM, Drexler H, Wollschläger H, et al. Modulation of coronary vasomotor tone in humans: Progressive endothelial dysfunction with different early stages of coronary atherosclerosis. *Circulation* 1991;83:391–401.
39. Gage JE, Hess OM, Murakami T, et al. Vasoconstriction of stenotic coronary arteries during dynamic exercise in patients with classic angina pectoris: Reversibility by nitroglycerin. *Circulation* 1986;73:865–876.
40. Steinbrecher UP, Parthasarathy S, Leake DS, et al. Modification of low density lipoprotein by endothelial cells involves lipid peroxidation and degradation of low density lipoprotein phospholipids. *Proc Natl Acad Sci U S A* 1984;81:3883–3887.
41. Morel DW, DiCorleto PE, Chisolm CM. Endothelial and smooth muscle cells alter low density lipoprotein in vitro by free radical oxidation. *Arteriosclerosis* 1984;4: 357–364.
42. Zang HF, Basra HJ, Steinbrecher UP. Effects of oxidatively modified LDL on cholesterol esterifcation in cultured macrophages. *J Lipid Res* 1990;31:1361–1369.
43. Steinbrecher UP. Oxidation of human low density lipoprotein results in esterification of lysine residues of apolipoprotein B by lipid peroxide decomposition products. *J Biol Chem* 1987;262:3605–3608.
44. Fruebis J, Parthasarathy S, Steinberg D. Evidence for concerted reaction between lipid hydroperoxides and polypeptides. *Proc Natl Acad Sci U S A* 1992;89:10588–10592.
45. Vita JA, Treasure CB, Nabel EG, et al. The coronary vasomotor response to acetylcholine relates to risk factors for coronary artery disease. *Circulation* 1990; 81:491–497.
46. Egashira K, Inou T, Hirooka Y, et al. Impaired coronary blood flow response to acetylcholine in patients with coronary risk factors and proximal atherosclerotic lesions. *J Clin Invest* 1993;91:29–37.

47. Quyyumi AA, Dakak N, Andrews NP, et al. Contribution of nitric oxide to metabolic coronary vasodilation in the human heart. *Circulation* 1995;92:320–326.

48. Dyce MC, Anderson TJ, Yeung AC, et al. Indices of LDL particle size closely relate to endothelial function. *Circulation* 1993;88:466.

49. Anderson TJ, Meredith IT, Charbonneau F, et al. Endothelium-dependent coronary vasomotion relates to the susceptibility of LDL to oxidation in humans. *Circulation* 1996;93:1647–1650.

50. Kuhn FE, Mohler ER, Satler LF, et al. Effects of high-density lipoprotein on acetylcholine-induced coronary vasoreactivity. *Am J Cardiol* 1991;68:1425–1430.

51. Zeiher AM, Schachlinger V, Hohnloser SH, et al. Coronary atherosclerotic wall thickening and vascular reactivity in humans. Elevated high-density lipoprotein levels ameliorate abnormal vasoconstriction in early atherosclerosis. *Circulation* 1994;89:2525–2532.

52. Leung WH, Lau CP, Wong CK. Beneficial effect of cholesterol-lowering therapy on coronary endothelium-dependent relaxation in hypercholesterolemia patients. *Lancet* 1993;341:1496–1500.

53. Anderson TJ, Meredith IT, Yeung AC, et al. The effect of cholesterol-lowering and antioxidant therapy on endothelium-dependent coronary vasomotion. *N Engl J Med* 1995;332:488–493.

54. Treasure CB, Klein JL, Weintraub WS, et al. Beneficial effects of cholesterol-lowering therapy on the coronary endothelium in patients with coronary artery disease. *N Engl J Med* 1995;332:481–487.

55. Egashira K, Hirooka Y, Kai H, et al. Reduction in serum cholesterol with pravastatin improves endothelium-dependent coronary vasomotion in patients with hypercholesterolemia. *Circulation* 1994;89:2519–2524.

56. Grodstein F, Stampfer M. The epidemiology of coronary heart disease and estrogen replacement in postmenopausal women. *Prog Cardiovasc Dis* 1995;38:199–210.

57. Stampfer MJ, Colditz GA. Estrogen replacement therapy and coronary heart disease: A quantitative assessment of the epidemiologic evidence. *Prev Med* 1991; 20:47–63.

58. Stampfer MJ, Colditz GA, Willett WC, et al. Postmenopausal estrogen therapy and cardiovascular disease: Ten-year follow-up from the Nurses' Health Study. *N Engl J Med* 1991;325:756–762.

59. Bush TL, Barrett-Connor E, Cowan LD, et al. Cardiovascular mortality and non-contraceptive estrogen use in women: Results from the Lipid Research Clinics Program Follow-up Study. *Circulation* 1987;75:1002–1009.

60. Grodstein F, Stampfer MJ, Manson JE, et al. Postmenopausal estrogen and progestin use and the risk of cardiovascular disease. *N Engl J Med* 1996;335:453–461.

61. Hulley S, Grady D, Bush T, et al. Randomized trial of estrogen plus progestin for secondary prevention of coronary heart disease in postmenopausal women. Heart and Estrogen/progestin Replacement Study (HERS) Research Group *JAMA* 1998; 280:605–613.

62. Williams JK, Adams MR, Herrington DM, et al. Short-term administration of estrogen and vascular responses of atherosclerotic coronary arteries. *J Am Coll Cardiol* 1992;20:452–457.

63. Williams JK, Adams MR, Klopfenstein S. Estrogen modulates responses of atherosclerotic coronary arteries. *Circulation* 1990;81:1680–1687.

64. Gilligan DM, Quyyumi AA, Cannon RO. Effects of physiological levels of estrogen on coronary vasomotor function in postmenopausal women. *Circulation* 1994;89:2545–2551.

65. Collins P, Rosano GMC, Sarrel PM, et al. 17β-estradiol attenuates acetylcholine-induced coronary arterial constriction in women but not men with coronary heart disease. *Circulation* 1995;92:24–30.

66. Reis SE, Gloth ST, Blumenthal RS, et al. Ethinyl estradiol acutely attenuates abnormal coronary vasomotor responses to acetylcholine in postmenopausal women. *Circulation* 1994;89:52–60.

67. Lieberman EH, Gerhard M, Yeung AC, et al. Estrogen improves coronary vasomotor responses to acetylcholine in post-menopausal women. *Circulation* 1993; 88(suppl):I79.

68. Caulin-Glaser T, Garcia-Cardena G, Sarrel P, et al. 17 beta-estradiol regulation of human endothelial cell basal nitric oxide release, independent of cytosolic Ca2+ mobilization. *Circ Res* 1997;81:885–892.

69. Kuiper GG, Enmark E, Pelto-Huikko M, et al. Cloning of a novel receptor expressed in rat prostate and ovary. *Proc Natl Acad Sci U S A* 1996;93:5925–5930.

70. Keaney JF, Shwaery GT, Xu A, et al. 17β-estradiol preserves endothelial vasodilator function and limits low-density lipoprotein oxidation in hypercholesterolemic swine. *Circulation* 1994;89:2251–2259.

71. Sugioka JM, Shimosegawa Y, Nakano MM. Estrogens as natural antioxidants of membrane lipid peroxidation. *FEBS Lett* 1987;210:37–39.

72. Anderson TJ, Gerhard MD, Meredith IT, et al. Systemic nature of endothelial dysfunction in atherosclerosis. *Am J Cardiol* 1995;75:71B–74B.

73. Hashimoto M, Akishita M, Eto M, et al. Modulation of endothelium-dependent flow-mediated dilation of the brachial artery by gender and menstrual cycle. *Circulation* 1995;92:3431–3435.

74. Celermajer DS, Sorensen KE, Spiegelhalter DJ, et al. Aging is associated with endothelial dysfunction in healthy men years before the age-related decline in women. *J Am Coll Cardiol* 1994;24:471–476.

75. Gerhard M, Tawakol A, Haley E, et al. Long-term estradiol therapy with or without progesterone improves endothelium-dependent vasodilation in post-menopausal women. *Circulation* 1996;94(suppl):I279.

76. Sorensen KE, Dorup I, Hermann AP, et al. Combined hormone replacement therapy does not protect women against the age-related decline in endothelium-dependent vasomotor function. *Circulation* 1998;97:1234–1238.

77. Nitenberg H, Valensi P, Sacho R, et al. Impairment of coronary vascular reserve and Ach-induced coronary vasodilation in diabetic patients with angiographically normal coronary arteries and normal left ventricular function. *Diabetes* 1993;43: 1017–1025.

78. Williams SB, Cusco JA, Roddy M-A, et al. Impaired nitric oxide-mediated vasodilation in patients with non-insulin-dependent diabetes mellitus. *J Am Coll Cardiol* 1996;27:567–574.

79. Johnstone MT, Creager SJ, Scales KM, et al. Impaired endothelium-dependent vasodilation in patients with insulin-dependent diabetes mellitus. *Circulation* 1993;88:2510–2516.

80. McVeigh GE, Brennan GM, Johnston GD, et al. Impaired endothelium-dependent and independent vasodilation in patients with type 2 (non-insulin dependent). *Diabetologia* 1992;35:771–776.

81. Ting HH, Timimi FK, Boles KS, et al. Vitamin C improves endothelium-dependent vasodilation in patients with non-insulin dependent diabetes mellitus. *J Clin Invest* 1996;97:22–28.

82. Timimi F, Ting HH, Haley EA, et al. Vitamin C improves endothelium-dependent vasodilation in patients with insulin-dependent diabetes mellitus. *J Am Coll Cardiol* 1998;31:552–557.

83. Clarkson P, Celermajer DS, Donald AE, et al. Impaired vascular reactivity in insulin-dependent diabetes mellitus is related to disease duration and low density lipoprotein cholesterol levels. *J Am Coll Cardiol* 1996;28:573–579.

84. Williams SB, Goldfine AB, Timimi FK, et al. Acute hyperglycemia attenuates endothelium-dependent vasodilation in humans in vivo. *Circulation* 1998. In press.

85. Giugliano D, Marfella R, Coppola L, et al. Vascular effects of acute hyperglycemia in humans are reversed by L-arginine: Evidence for reduced availability of nitric oxide during hyperglycemia. *Circulation* 1997;95:1783–1790.

86. Zeiher AM, Schächinger V, Minners J. Long-term cigarette smoking impairs endothelium-dependent coronary arterial vasodilator function. *Circulation* 1995; 92:1094–1110.

87. Anderson TJ, Uehata A, Gerhard MD, et al. Close relation of endothelial function in the human coronary and peripheral circulations. *J Am Coll Cardiol* 1995;26: 1235–1241.

88. Celermajer DS, Sorensen KE, Georgakopoulos D, et ak. Cigarette smoking is associated with dose-related and potentially reversible impairment of endothelium-dependent dilation in healthy adults. *Circulation* 1993;88:2149–2155.

89. Celermajer DS, Adams MR, Clarkson P, et al. Passive smoking and impaired endothelium-dependent arterial dilation in healthy young adults. *N Engl J Med* 1996;334:150–154.

90. Heitzer T, Ylä-Herttuala S, Luoma J, et al. Cigarette smoking potentiates endothelial dysfunction of forearm resistance vessels in patient with hypercholesterolemia: Role of oxidized LDL. *Circulation* 1996;93:1346–1353.

91. Heitzer T, Just H, Münzel T. Antioxidant vitamin C improves endothelial dysfunction in chronic smokers. *Circulation* 1996;94:6–9.

92. Treasure CB, Manoukian SV, Klein JL, et al. Epicardial coronary artery responses to acetylcholine are impaired in hypertensive patients. *Circ Res* 1992;71:776–781.

93. Brush JE, Faxon DP, Salmon S, et al. Abnormal endothelium-dependent coronary vasomotion in hypertensive patients. *J Am Coll Cardiol* 1992;19:809–815.

94. Panza JA, Quyyumi AA, Brush JE, et al. Abnormal endothelium-dependent vascular relaxation in patients with essential hypertension. *N Engl J Med* 1990;323; 22–27.

95. Gerhard M, Roddy M-A, Creager SJ, et al. Aging progressively impairs endothelium-dependent vasodilation in forearm resistance vessels of humans. *Hypertension* 1996;27:849–853.

96. Taddei S, Virdis A, Mattei P, et al. Hypertension causes premature aging of endothelial function in humans. *Hypertension* 1997;29:736–743.

97. Taddei S, Virdis A, Mattei P, et al. Defective L-arginine-nitric oxide pathway in offspring of essential hypertensive patients. *Circulation* 1996;94:1298–1303.

98. Tawakol A, Omland T, Gerhard M, et al. Hyperhomocyst(e)inemia is associated with impaired endothelium-dependent vasodialation in humans. *Circulation* 1997;95:1119–1121.

99. Woo KS, Chook P, Lolin YI, et al. Hyperhomocyst(e)inemia is a risk factor for arterial endothelial dysfunction in humans. *Circulation* 1997;96:2542–2544.

100. Bellamy MF, McDowell IFW, Ramsey MW, et al. Hyperhomocysteinemia after an oral methionine load acutely impairs endothelial function in healthy adults. *Circulation* 1998;98:1848–1852.

101. Tsurumi Y, Nagashima H, Ichikawa K, et al. Influence of plasma lipoprotein(a) levels on coronary vasomotor response to acetylcholine. *J Am Coll Cardiol* 1995; 26:1242–1250.

102. Andrews TC, Raby K, Barry J, et al. Effect of cholesterol reduction on myocardial ischemia in patients with coronary disease. *Circulation* 1997;95:324–328.

103. van Boven AJ, Jukema JW, Zwinderman AH, et al. Reduction of transient myocardial ischemia with pravastatin in addition to the conventional treatment in patients with angina pectoris. REGRESS Study Group. *Circulation* 1996;94:1503–1505.

104. Kinlay S, Selwyn AP, Delagrange D, et al. Biological mechanisms for the clinical success of lipid-lowering in coronary artery disease and the use of surrogate end-points. *Curr Opin Lipidol* 1996;7:389–397.

105. Ting HH, Timimi FK, Haley EA, et al. Vitamin C improves endothelium-dependent vasodilation in forearm resistance vessels of humans with hypercholesterolemia. *Circulation* 1997;95:2617–2622.

106. Levine GN, Frei B, Koulouris SN, et al. Ascorbic acid reverses endothelial vaso-motor dysfunction in patients with coronary artery disease. *Circulation* 1996;93: 1107–1113.
107. Stephens NG, Parsons A, Schofield PM, et al. Randomised controlled trial of vitamin E in patients with coronary disease: Cambridge Heart Antioxidant Study (CHAOS). *Lancet* 1996;347:781–786.
108. The alpha-tocopherol beta carotene cancer prevention group. The effect of vitamin E and beta carotene on the incidence of lung cancer and other cancers in male smokers. *N Engl J Med* 1994;330:1029–1035.
109. Rajagopalan S, Kurz S, Münzel T, et al. Angiotensin II mediated hypertension in the rat increases vascular superoxide production via membrane NADH/NADPH oxidase activation: Contribution to alterations of vasomotor tone. *J Clin Invest* 1996;97:1916–1923.
110. Griendling K, Ollerenshaw JD, Minieri CA, et al. Angiotensin II stimulates NADH and NADPH activity in cultured vascular smooth muscle cells. *Circ Res* 1994;74:1141–1148.
111. Ruschitzka FT, Lüscher TF. Is there a rationale for combining angiotensin-converting enzyme inhibitors and calcium antagonists in cardiovascular disease? *Am Heart J* 1997;134:S31–S47.
112. Mancini GBJ, Henry GC, Macaya C, et al. Angiotensin-converting enzyme inhibition with Quinapril improves endothelial vasomotor dysfunction in patients with coronary artery disease: The TREND study (Trial on Reversing Endothelial Dysfunction). *Circulation* 1996;94:258–265.
113. Nakamura M, Funakoshi T, Arakawa N, et al. Effect of angiotensin-converting enzyme inhibitors on endothelium-dependent peripheral vasodilation in patients with chronic heart failure. *J Am Coll Cardiol* 1994;24:1321–1327.

## Chapter 18

# Oxidant Stress and Endothelial Function in Patients with Risk Factors for Atherosclerosis

*Mark A. Creager, MD*

## Introduction

Endothelium-derived nitric oxide (NO) contributes to the normal regulation of vascular tone in healthy humans,[1,2] whereas endothelium-dependent vasodilation, and by implication the bioavailability of endothelium-derived NO, is reduced in patients with atherosclerosis.[3–5] In addition to regulating vasomotor activity, endothelium-derived NO inhibits leukocyte adhesion to the endothelium, platelet aggregation, and vascular smooth muscle growth.[6–11] Atherosclerosis is accelerated following vascular injury in endothelial NO synthase (eNOS) knockout mice and inhibition of NOS increases atherosclerosis in experimental models of hypercholesterolemia.[12–14] Taken together, studies such as these underscore an important role for NO as a vascular sentry that limits the blood vessel's response to injurious agents. Therefore, diseases and other factors that reduce the availability or activity of NO are more likely to promote atherogenesis. Such is the case with the traditional risk factors for atherosclerosis. Studies in experimental models and in humans have found that endothelium-dependent relaxation is impaired in experimental models and in patients affected by hypercholesterolemia, diabetes mellitus, hypertension, tobacco use, hyperhomocyst(e)inemia, and aging.

Multiple mechanisms have been proposed to explain the abnormalities of endothelium-dependent vasodilation among the various risk factors associated with atherosclerosis including reduced access of L-arginine to eNOS, dysfunction of G-protein receptor coupling, deficiency of eNOS cofactors, decreased production or activity of eNOS, and inactivation of NO by superoxide anion. This chapter will focus specifically on oxidant stress and abnormalities of endothelium-dependent vasodilation in humans with atherosclerosis and its risk factors.

From Panza JA, Cannon RO III (eds): *Endothelium, Nitric Oxide, and Atherosclerosis* ©Futura Publishing Co, Inc, Armonk, NY, 1999.

## Oxidant Stress and Nitric Oxide

NO is inactivated by oxygen-derived free radicals, particularly superoxide anion, to form the stable peroxynitrite anion ($ONOO^-$).[15–17] Using a bioassay to detect endothelium-derived relaxing factor (EDRF) release from porcine aortic endothelial cells, Gryglewski et al[15] demonstrated that EDRF is protected by inactivation by superoxide dismutase (SOD), but not by catalase. Similarly, Rubanyi and Vanhoutte[16] demonstrated that superoxide anions suppress endothelium-dependent relaxation induced by acetylcholine (ACh) in canine coronary arteries. The reaction between NO and superoxide anion is extremely rapid, with a rate constant approximating $1.9 \times 10^{10}$ mol/L per second.[16] Thus, the availability of endothelium-derived NO is dependent both on production and on scavenging of superoxide anion by endogenous antioxidants such as SOD, glutathione (GSH), ascorbate, and $\alpha$-tocopherol.[18–21]

## Oxidative Stress and Atherosclerosis

Studies conducted in experimental models of atherosclerosis implicate enhanced oxidative degradation of endothelium-derived NO as a cause of endothelial dysfunction. Minor and coworkers[22] reported that endothelium-dependent vascular relaxation was diminished despite increased eNOS activity and NO production in cholesterol-fed rabbits, suggesting that decreased bioavailability of NO more likely is secondary to its degradation by oxygen-derived free radicals rather than decreased production. Consistent with this postulate, O'Hara and colleagues[23,24] reported that blood vessels from cholesterol-fed rabbits produced three- to fivefold more superoxide anion than those of control rabbits. In cholesterol-fed rabbits, treatment with SOD, oxypurinol, $\alpha$-tocopherol, or probucol has been shown to restore endothelium-dependent vasodilation.[23,25–29] Probucol (via its antioxidant properties) improves endothelium-dependent relaxation in atherosclerotic aortas of Watanabe rabbits.[30]

Evidence that oxygen radicals contribute to abnormal endothelium-dependent vasodilation in patients with atherosclerosis is compelling. Meredith et al assessed endothelium-dependent vasodilation of epicardial coronary arteries in response to ACh in patients with coronary artery disease (CAD) prior to and following the administration of SOD.[31] Intracoronary administration of SOD significantly attenuated the vasoconstrictive response to ACh in these atherosclerotic vessels, suggesting a role for superoxide anion as a mediator of abnormal endothelium-dependent vasodilation. Anderson et al[32] studied the effect of antioxidant therapy in conjunction with lipid-lowering therapy in patients with hypercholesterolemia and coronary disease. Patients were treated for 1 year with either a step 1 American Heart Association diet, a combination of lovastatin and cholestyramine to reduce the cholesterol level, or the combination of probucol plus lovastatin to both reduce the cholesterol level and provide an antioxidant effect. The strategy of combining a lipid-lowering and an antioxidant drug was the only treatment that significantly improved endothelium-dependent vasodilation. The susceptibility of a low-density lipoprotein (LDL) to oxidation was determined by measuring the lag phase of conjugated diene formation induced by $Cu^{2+}$. Prolongation of lag phase was increased significantly in patients randomized to probucol plus lovastatin; moreover, the vasomotor response to ACh related significantly to the lag phase of conjugated diene formation.[33]

# Methods to Measure Vascular Function in Humans

Studies in humans have utilized a variety of techniques to examine endothelium-dependent vasodilation. Each of these can provide important information regarding vasomotor tone and serve as a surrogate or bioassay for endothelium-derived NO. Venous occlusion strain gauge plethysmography has been used to measure forearm blood flow during intra-arterial administration of pharmacologic agents that induce endothelium-dependent or endothelium-independent vasodilation. This technique provides information regarding dilator function in resistance vessels, avoiding the confounding effects of atherosclerosis because resistance vessels are devoid of atheroma. During these experiments, endothelium-dependent agonists such as ACh or methacholine are infused into the brachial artery and dose-blood flow response curves are generated. Using this technique, the author's laboratory and others have found that endothelium-dependent vasodilation is impaired in patients with hypercholesterolemia, hypertension, and diabetes mellitus, and also that endothelium-dependent vasodilation decreases with each decade of aging.[34–38] (Figures 1 and 2).

Vascular ultrasonography has been employed as a noninvasive technique to assess flow-mediated endothelium-dependent vasodilation of a peripheral conduit artery, such as the brachial artery in humans, in vivo. Flow-mediated, endothelium-dependent vasodilation of the brachial artery occurs during re-

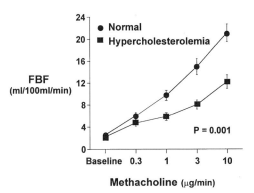

**Figure 1.** Forearm blood flow (FBF) dose-response curves to methacholine in hypercholesterolemic and normal subjects. Endothelium-dependent vasodilation to methacholine was attenuated significantly in hypercholesterolemic subjects compared with healthy age-matched control subjects. Reproduced with permission from Reference 49.

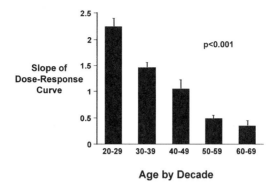

**Figure 2.** Slope of the methacholine dose-response for each of five decades between ages 20 and 69. Endothelium-dependent vasodilation declined with each decade. Values represent mean SEM. Reproduced with permission from Reference 38.

active hyperemia, as increased shear stress stimulates local release of endothelium-derived NO.[39] Reduced flow-mediated endothelium-dependent vasodilation of the brachial artery correlates with coronary endothelium-dependent vasodilation induced by ACh and is impaired in patients with CAD.[39,40] In addition, flow-mediated vasodilation is reduced in patients with risk factors for atherosclerosis, such as hypercholesterolemia, type I diabetes mellitus, cigarette smoking, and hyperhomocysteinemia.[41–44]

# Vitamin C as an Antioxidant

Vitamin C is the primary water-soluble antioxidant in human plasma. It is capable of scavenging superoxide anion and sparing other endogenous antioxidants from consumption.[45–47] The reaction rate constant between vitamin C and superoxide anion is $3 \times 10^5$ mol/L per second, approximately $10^4$ times slower than the reaction rate observed between superoxide anion and SOD, which is $2 \times 10^9$ mol/L per second. It has been estimated that an ascorbic acid concentration of approximately 10 mmol/L would be required for it to compete effectively with SOD as a scavenger of superoxide anion.[48]

# Hypercholesterolemia and Oxidant Stress

Endothelium-dependent vasodilation is reduced in patients with hypercholesterolemia.[35,49,50] The forearm blood flow response to intra-arterial methacholine, as assessed by venous occlusion plethysmography, is attenuated in young hypercholesterolemic patients compared with age-matched healthy subjects (Figure 1).[35,49] To determine whether superoxide anion contributes to this impairment in endothelium-dependent vasodilation, Ting et al.[49] measured endothelium-dependent vasodilation and endothelium-independent vasodilation of forearm resistance vessels of hypercholesterolemic patients prior to and during the coadministration of intra-arterial vitamin C. Vitamin C was administered at a constant dose of 24 mg/min to achieve a local forearm concentration of 1–10 mmol/L. In hypercholesterolemic subjects, endothelium-dependent vasodilation to methacholine was augmented by coinfusion of vitamin C (Figure 3). Endothelium-independent vasodilation was not affected by coinfusion of vitamin C. Moreover, vitamin C did not alter endothelium-dependent vasodilation in healthy subjects. These findings support a role for superoxide anion as a mechanism for reduced endothelium-dependent vasodilation in patients with hypercholesterolemia. However, two studies have not detected any beneficial effect of antioxidants on endothelium-dependent vasodilation in humans with hypercholesterolemia. Garcia et al found that SOD did not modify endothelium-dependent vasodilation in forearm resistance vessels; however the inability of Cu-Zn SOD to cross the cell membrane and scavenge intracellular sources of superoxide radicals may explain this negative finding.[51] Gilligan et al[52] found that 1-month treatment with vitamin C, vitamin E, and β-carotene, did not affect endothelium-dependent vasodilation in the forearm of hypercholesterolemic patients.

Lipids other than cholesterol may affect endothelial function. For example, free fatty acids impair endothelium-dependent vasodilation in humans. Steinberg et al[53] raised systemic free fatty acid levels by administering intralipid (20% fat emulsion) to healthy volunteers to achieve a 2- to10-fold increase in free fatty acid levels. This reduced endothelium-dependent vasodilation of leg resistance vessels. Raising triglyceride levels without increasing free fatty acid concentration did not affect endothelial function. Vogel et al.[54] reported that flow-mediated endothelium-dependent vasodilation in the brachial artery was reduced significantly for up to 6 hours following a high-fat meal, sufficient to increase triglyceride-rich lipoproteins and, presumably, free fatty acids. Thereafter, Plotnick et al[55] reported that pretreatment with antioxidant vitamins C (1 g) and E (800 IU) orally prevented the attenuation of endothelium-dependent vasodilation following a high-fat meal. Additional studies would be required to determine whether triglycerides per se or free

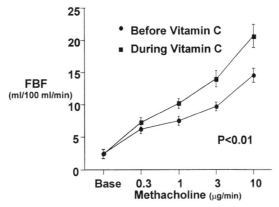

**Figure 3.** The effect of vitamin C on endothelium-dependent vasodilation in hypercholesterolemia. Vitamin C caused significant improvement in the forearm blood flow response to methacholine. Reproduced with permission from Reference 49.

fatty acids reduce endothelium-dependent vasodilation after fatty meals and to assess which component is affected by antioxidants.

## Oxidant Stress and Diabetes Mellitus

Endothelium-dependent vasodilation is impaired in patients with type I diabetes mellitus, whether assessed in forearm resistance vessels by venous occlusion plethysmography or the brachial artery by vascular ultrasonography.[37,42] In patients with type II diabetes mellitus, both endothelium-dependent vasodilation and endothelium-independent vasodilation are reduced, implicating either additional abnormalities in the NO signaling pathway, or other functional disturbances of the vascular smooth muscle inhibiting its ability to dilate.[56]

Inactivation of NO by oxygen-derived free radicals may be an important mechanism contributing to reduced endothelium-dependent vasodilation in diabetes. Several reactions may contribute to the formation of oxygen radicals in diabetes including glucose autooxidation, nonenzymatic protein glycation, and cyclooxygenase catalysis.[57] Autooxidation of glucose, as catalyzed by transition metals and glycosylation of proteins, can generate oxygen-derived free radicals.[58] Experimental hyperglycemia increases arachidonic acid metabolism and eicosinoid synthesis, which increases oxygen-derived free radical production.[58-60] Production of oxygen-derived free radicals is increased in circulating granulocytes and monocytes of patients with diabetes.[61,62] Also, levels of endogenous antioxidants such as SOD, catalase, and GSH-peroxidase (Px) are decreased in some animal models of diabetes.[63,64] Several studies have found decreased levels of vitamin C in patients with diabetes mellitus.[65-68] The duration of diabetes mellitus and the severity of hyperglycemia correlates inversely with endogenous levels of antioxidants.[69,70]

Scavengers of oxygen radicals improve endothelium-dependent relaxation in diabetic animals, both in vitro and in vivo.[71-74] These findings have been

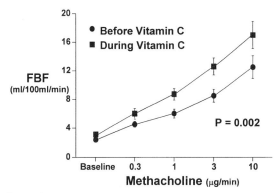

**Figure 4.** The effect of vitamin C on endothelium-dependent vasodilation in insulin-dependent diabetes mellitus. Vitamin C caused significant improvement in the forearm blood flow response to methacholine. Reproduced with permission from Reference 75.

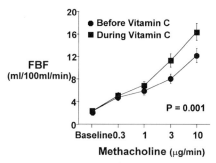

**Figure 5.** The effect of vitamin C on endothelium-dependent vasodilation in noninsulin-dependent diabetes mellitus. Vitamin C caused significant improvement in the forearm blood flow response to methacholine. Reproduced with permission from Reference 76.

extended to patients with type I diabetes mellitus and to those with type II diabetes mellitus. Timimi et al[75] found that intra-arterial administration of vitamin C improves endothelium-dependent vasodilation in patients with type I diabetes mellitus and Ting et al[76] found that intra-arterial administration of vitamin C improves endothelium-dependent vasodilation in forearm resistance vessels of patients with type II diabetes mellitus (Figures 4 and 5). Vitamin C did not affect endothelium-independent vasodilation in either study. Thus, oxygen radicals appear to reduce endothelium-dependent vasodilation in humans with diabetes.

Hyperglycemia is common to both type I and type II diabetes mellitus and is likely to contribute to oxidant stress and endothelial vasodilator dysfunction in both disorders. The reduction in endothelium-dependent vasodilation that occurs when normal rabbit aortic rings are incubated in a high-glucose medium is restored by oxygen radical scavengers.[77,78] In healthy humans, a 6-hour hyperglycemic clamp impairs endothelium-dependent vasodilation in forearm resistance vessels.[79] In a preliminary report, Beckman et al[80] observed that intra-arterial administration of vitamin C reversed the abnormal endothelium-dependent vasodilation that occurred in healthy patients during a hyperglycemic clamp.

## Oxidant Stress in Cigarette Smokers

Experimental studies also indicate a potential role of oxygen-derived free radicals in mediating abnormal endothelium-dependent vasodilation in cigarette smokers. Plasma levels of F2-isoprostanes, an index of lipid peroxidation, are increased in cigarette smokers.[81] Extract from cigarette smoke impairs endothelium-dependent vasodilation via superoxide anion production in isolated porcine coronary arteries.[82] Moreover, plasma levels of vitamin C are lower in smokers than nonsmokers.[83] Heitzer et al[84] assessed forearm vascular reactivity in smokers and nonsmokers prior to and during intra-arterial administration of vitamin C. ACh-induced endothelium-dependent vasodilation of forearm resistance vessels was less in smokers than nonsmokers. Intra-arterial vitamin C restored endothelium-dependent vasodilation in nonsmokers to a level comparable with that observed in smokers. In a subsequent study, Heitzer and colleagues[85] assessed endothelium-dependent vasodilation in forearm resistance vessels in healthy subjects, smokers, hypercholesterolemic patients, and hypercholesterolemic patients who smoked. Endothelium-dependent vasodilation was impaired in all three groups, most severely so in the hypercholesterolemic smokers in whom autoantibody titers against oxidized LDL were increased substantially.

# Oxidant Stress and Endothelial Function in Hypertension

Endothelium-dependent vasodilation is impaired in patients with hypertension.[34,36] In experimental models of hypertension, superoxide anion contributes to abnormalities in endothelium-dependent relaxation.[86–88] Taddei et al[89] studied the effects of intra-arterial vitamin C on endothelium-dependent vasodilation on forearm resistance vessels in patients with essential hypertension. Compared with normotensive subjects, endothelium-dependent vasodilation was reduced in the patients with essential hypertension. Endothelium-dependent vasodilation increased during coinfusion of vitamin C. The authors suggested the origin of oxidative stress was via the cyclooxygenase pathway, because indomethacin also restored endothelium-dependent vasodilation in patients with hypertension to the same degree as that observed during vitamin C administration, whereas there was no additive effect of vitamin C and indomethacin on endothelium-dependent vasodilation.

# Endothelial Dysfunction in Nonatherosclerotic Vessels of Patients with Cornary Artery Disease

As noted previously, endothelium-dependent vasodilation is impaired in nonatherosclerotic peripheral conduit arteries of patients with CAD.[39,40] The severity of peripheral artery endothelial dysfunction correlates with that of epicardial coronary arteries measured during intracoronary infusion of ACh.[40] Many patients with CAD have multiple risk factors for atherosclerosis, and these may be responsible for abnormal peripheral endothelium-mediated vasodilator activity. Therefore, it follows that oxidant stress may contribute to endothelial dysfunction in peripheral arteries of patients with CAD. Indeed, Levine et al.[90] reported that acute oral administration of vitamin C improved flow-mediated endothelium-dependent vasodilation in the brachial artery of patients with CAD. In addition to vitamin C, reduced GSH contributes to the regulation of the intracellular redox state. In patients with CAD, increasing levels of intracellular GSH by L-2-oxothiazolidine-4-carboxylic acid (which is converted to cysteine and then reduced to GSH intracellularly) improves impaired endothelium-dependent vasodilation in peripheral arterial beds.[91] In patients with risk factors, intravenous infusion of GSH improves endothelium-dependent vasodilation of angiographically normal coronary arteries.[92]

# Summary

Endothelium-dependent vasodilation is impaired in most, if not all, of the factors associated with atherosclerosis. Antioxidants improve endothelium-dependent vasodilation in patients with coronary atherosclerosis. Antioxidants also restore endothelium-dependent vasodilation in patients with diabetes, hypercholesterolemia, hypertension, and in smokers. Thus, inactivation of NO by oxygen-derived free radicals may be a theme common to atherosclerosis and its risk factors. Antioxidant therapy, by improving the bioavailability of NO, may not only improve vasomotor function and subsequently reduce adverse cardiovascular events in patients with atherosclerosis, but also has the potential to retard atherogenesis in patients with risk factors for atherosclerosis.

# References

1. Stamler JS, Loh E, Roddy M-A, et al. Nitric oxide regulates basal systemic and pulmonary vascular resistance in healthy humans. *Circulation* 1994;89:2035–2040.
2. Vallance P, Collier J, Moncada S. Effects of endothelium-derived nitric oxide on peripheral arteriolar tone in man. *Lancet* 1989;2:997–1000.
3. Ludmer PL, Selwyn AP, Shook TL, et al. Paradoxical vasoconstriction induced by acetylcholine in atherosclerotic coronary arteries. *N Engl J Med* 1986;315:1046–1051.
4. Zeiher AM, Drexler H, Wollschlager H, et al. Modulation of coronary vasomotor tone in humans. Progressive endothelial dysfunction with different early stages of coronary atherosclerosis. *Circulation* 1991;83:391–401.
5. Quyyumi AA, Kakak N, Mulcahy D, et al. Nitric oxide activity in the atherosclerotic human coronary circulation. *J Am Coll Cardiol* 1997;29:308–317.
6. Kubes P, Suzuki M, Granger DN. Nitric oxide: An endogenous modulator of leukocyte adhesion. *Proc Natl Acad Sci U S A* 1991;88:4651–4656.
7. Radomski MW, Palmer RM, Moncada S. An L-arginine/nitric oxide pathway present in human platelets regulates aggregation. *Proc Natl Acad Sci U S A* 1990;87:5193–5197.
8. Garg UC, Hassid A. Nitric oxide-generating vasodilators and 8-bromo-cyclic guanosine monophosphate inhibit mitogenesis and proliferation of cultured rate vascular smooth muscle cells. *J Clin Invest* 1989;83:1774–1777.
9. DeCaterina R, Libby P, Peng H-B, et al. Nitric oxide decreases cytokine-induced endothelial activation. *J Clin Invest* 1995;96:60–68.
10. Tsao PS, Wang BY, Buitrago R, et al. Nitric oxide regulates monocyte chemotactic protein-1. *Circulation* 1997;96:934–940.
11. Spiecker M, Peng HB, Liao JK. Inhibition of endothelial vascular cell adhesion molecule-1 expression by nitric oxide involves the induction and nuclear translocation of I-$\kappa$B$\alpha$. *J Biol Chem* 1997;272:30969–30974.
12. Moroi M, Zhang L, Tasuda T, et al. Interaction of genetic deficiency of endothelial nitric oxide, gender, and pregnancy in vascular response to injury in mice. *J Clin Invest* 1998;101:1225–1232.

13. Cayatte AJ, Palacino JJ, Horten K, et al. Chronic inhibition of nitric oxide production accelerates neointima formation and impairs endothelial function in hypercholesterolemic rabbits. *Arterioscler Thromb* 1994;14:753–759.

14. Cooke JP, Singer AH, Tsao P, et al. Antiatherogenic effects of L-arginine in the hypercholesterolemic rabbit. *J Clin Invest* 1992;90:1168–1172.

15. Gryglewski RJ, Palmer RMG, Moncada S. Superoxide anion is involved in the breakdown of endothelium-derived vascular relaxation factor. *Nature* 1986;320: 454–456.

16. Rubanyi GM, Vanhoutte PM. Oxygen-derived free radicals, endothelium, and responsiveness of vascular smooth muscle. *Am J Physiol* 1986;250:H815–H821.

17. Beckman JS, Beckman TW, Chen J, et al. Apparent hydroxyl radical production by peroxynitirite: implications for endothelial injury from nitric oxide and superoxide. *Proc Natl Acad Sci U S A* 1990;87:1620–1624.

18. Gotoh N, Niki E. Rates of interactions of superoxide with vitamin E, vitamin C and related compounds as measured by chemiluminescence. *Biochim Biophys Acta* 1992;1115:201–207.

19. Winterbourn CC, Metodiewa D. The reaction of superoxide with reduced glutathione. *Arch Biochem Biophys* 1994;314:284–290.

20. Nishikimi M. Oxidation of ascorbic acid with superoxide anion generated by the xanthine-xanthine oxidase system. *Biochem Biophys Res Commun* 1975;63:463–468.

21. Mügge A, Elwell JK, Peterson TE, et al. Release of intact endothelium-derived relaxing factor depends on endothelial superoxide dismutase activity. *Am J Physiol* 1991;260:C219–C225.

22. Minor RL Jr, Myers PR, Guerra R Jr, et al. Diet-induced atherosclerosis increases the release of nitrogen oxides from rabbit aorta. *J Clin Invest* 1990;86:2109–2116.

23. Ohara Y, Peterson TE, Harrison DG. Hypercholesterolemia increases endothelial superoxide anion production. *J Clin Invest* 1993;91:2546–2551.

24. Ohara Y, Peterson TE, Sayegh HS, et al. Dietary correction of hypercholesterolemia in the rabbit normalizes endothelial superoxide anion production. *Circulation* 1995;92:898–903.

25. Mügge A, Elwell JH, Peterson TE, et al. Chronic treatment with polyethyleneglycolated superoxide dismutase partially restores endothelium-dependent vascular relaxations in cholesterol-fed rabbits. *Circ Res* 1991;69:1293–1300.

26. Keaney JF Jr, Gaziano JM, Xu A, et al. Dietary antioxidants preserve endothelium-dependent vessel relaxation in cholesterol-fed rabbits. *Proc Natl Acad Sci U S A* 1993;90:11880–11884.

27. Keaney JF Jr, Gaziano JM, Xu A, et al. Low-dose alpha-tocopherol improves and high-dose alpha-tocopherol worsens endothelial vasodilator function in cholesterol-fed rabbits. *J Clin Invest* 1994;93:844–851.

28. Keaney JF Jr, Xu A, Cunningham D, et al. Dietary probucol preserves endothelial function in cholesterol-fed rabbits by limiting vascular oxidative stress and superoxide generation. *J Clin Invest* 1995;95:2520–2529.

29. White CR, Brock TA, Chang LY, et al. Superoxide and peroxynitrite in atherosclerosis. *Proc Natl Acad Sci U S A* 1994;91:1044–1048.

30. Simon BC, Haudenschild CC, Cohen RA. Preservation of endothelium-dependent relaxation in atherosclerotic rabbit aorta by probucol. *J Cardiovasc Pharmacol* 1993;21:893–901.

31. Meredith IT, Hoffmann KE, Anderson TJ, et al. Post-ischemic vasodilation in the human forearm is dependent on endothelium-derived relaxing factor. *Clin Res* 1993;41:192A.

32. Anderson TJ, Meredith IT, Yeung AC, et al. The effect of cholesterol-lowering and antioxidant therapy on endothelium-dependent coronary vasomotion. *N Engl J Med* 1995;332:488–493.

33. Anderson TJ, Meredith IT, Charbonneau F, et al. Endothelium-dependent coronary vasomotion relates to the susceptibility of LDL to oxidation in humans. *Circulation* 1996;93:1647–1650.

34. Creager MA, Roddy M-A. Effect of captopril and enalapril on endothelial function in hypertensive patients. *Hypertension* 1994;24:499–505.
35. Creager MA, Cooke JP, Mendelsohn ME, et al. Impaired vasodilation of forearm resistance vessels in hypercholesterolemic humans. *J Clin Invest* 1990;86:228–234.
36. Panza JA, Quyyumi AA, Brush JE, et al. Abnormal endothelium-dependent vascular relaxation in patients with essential hypertension. *N Engl J Med* 1990;320: 22–27.
37. Johnstone MT, Creager SJ, Scales KM, et al. Impaired endothelium-dependent vasodilation in patients with insulin-dependent diabetes mellitus. *Circulation* 1993;88:2510–2516.
38. Gerhard MG, Roddy M-A, Creager SJ, et al. Aging progressively improves endothelium-dependent vasodilation in forearm resistance vessels in humans. *Hypertension* 1996;27:849–853.
39. Lieberman EH, Gerhard MD, Uehata A, et al. Flow-induced vasodilation of the human brachial artery is impaired in patients <40 years of age with coronary artery disease. *Am J Cardiol* 1996;78:1210–1214.
40. Anderson TJ, Uehata A, Gerhard MD, et al. Close relationship of endothelial function in the human coronary and peripheral circulations. *J Am Coll Cardiol* 1995;26:1235–1241.
41. Celermajer DS, Sorensen KE, Gooch VM, et al. Non-invasive detection of endothelial dysfunction in children and adults at risk of atherosclerosis. *Lancet* 1992;340: 1111–1115.
42. Clarkson P, Celermajer DS, Donald AE, et al. Impaired vascular reactivity in insulin-dependent diabetes mellitus is related to disease duration and low density lipoprotein cholesterol levels. *J Am Coll Cardiol* 1996;28:573–579.
43. Celermajer DS, Sorensen KE, Georgakopoulos D, et al. Cigarette smoking is associated with dose-related and potentially reversible impairment of endothelium-dependent dilation in healthy young adults. *Circulation* 1993;88:2149–2155.
44. Tawakol A, Omland T, Gerhard M, et al. Hyperhomocyst(e)inemia is associated with impaired endothelium-dependent vasodilation in humans. *Circulation* 1997; 95:1119–1121.
45. Frei B, Stocker R, Ames BN. Antioxidant defenses and lipid peroxidation in human blood plasma. *Proc Natl Acad Sci U S A* 1988;85:9748–9752.
46. Frei B, England L, Ames BN. Ascorbate is an outstanding antioxidant in human blood plasma. *Proc Natl Acad Sci* 1989;86:6377–6381.
47. Retsky KL, Freeman MW, Frei B. Ascorbic acid oxidation production protect human low density lipoprotein against atherogenic modification. *J Biol Chem* 1993;268:1304–1309.
48. Jackson TS, Xu A, Vita JA, et al. Ascorbate prevents the interaction of superoxide and nitric oxide only at very high physiological concentrations . *Circ Res* 1998;83: 916–922. In process citation.
49. Ting HH, Timimi FK, Haley EA, et al. Vitamin C improves endothelium-dependent vasodilation in forearm resistance vessels of humans with hypercholesterolemia. *Circulation* 1997;95:2617–2622.
50. Casino PR, Kilcoyne CM, Quyyumi AA, et al. The role of nitric oxide in endothelium-dependent vasodilation of hypercholesterolemic patients. *Circulation* 1993;88: 2541–2547.
51. Garcia CE, Kilcoyne CM, Cardillo C, et al. Evidence that endothelial dysfunction in patients with hypercholesterolemia is not due to increased extracellular nitric oxide breakdown by superoxide anions. *Am J Cardiol* 1995;76:1157–1161.
52. Gilligan DM, Sack MN, Guetta V, et al. Effect of antioxidant vitamins on low density lipoprotein oxidation and impaired endothelium-dependent vasodilation in patients with hypercholesterolemia. *J Am Coll Cardiol* 1994;24:1611–1617.
53. Steinberg HO, Tarshoby M, Monestel R, et al. Elevated circulating free fatty acid levels impair endothelium- dependent vasodilation. *J Clin Invest* 1997;100:1230–1239.

54. Vogel RA, Corretti MC, Plotnick GD. Effect of a single high-fat meal on endothelial function in healthy subjects. *Am J Cardiol* 1997;79:350–354.

55. Plotnick GD, Corretti MC, Vogel RA. Effect of antioxidant vitamins on the transient impairment of endothelium-dependent brachial artery vasoactivity following a single high-fat meal [see Comments]. *JAMA* 1997;278:1682–1686.

56. Williams SB, Cusco JA, Roddy M-A, et al. Impaired nitric oxide-mediated vasodilation in patients with non-insulin-dependent diabetes mellitus. *J Am Coll Cardiol* 1996;27:567–574.

57. Tesfamariam B. Free radicals in diabetic endothelial cell dysfunction. *Free Radic Biol Med* 1994;16:383–392.

58. Wolff SP, Dean RT. Glucose autoxidation and protein modification. The potential role of 'autoxidative glycosylation' in diabetes. *Biochem J* 1987;245:243–250.

59. Tesfamariam B, Jakubowski JA, Cohen RA. Contraction of diabetic rabbit aorta caused by endothelium-derived $PGH_2$-$TxA_2$. *Am J Physiol* 1989;257:H1327–H1333.

60. Brown ML, Jakubowski JA, Leventis LL, et al. Elevated glucose alters eicosanoid release from porcine aortic endothelial cells. *J Clin Invest* 1988;82:2136–2141.

61. Wierusz-Wysocka B, Wysocki H, Siekierka H, et al. Evidence of polymorphonuclear neutrophils (PMN) activation in patients with insulin-dependent diabetes mellitus. *J Leukoc Biol* 1987;42:519–523.

62. Hiramatsu K, Arimori S. Increased superoxide production by mononuclear cells of patients with hypertriglyceridemia and diabetes. *Diabetes* 1988;37:832–837.

63. Dohi T, Kawamura K, Morita K, et al. Alterations of the plasma selenium concentrations and the activities of tissue peroxide metabolism enzymes in streptozotocin-induced diabetic rats. *Horm Metab Res* 1988;20:671–675.

64. Wohaieb SA, Godin DV. Alterations in free radical tissue-defense mechanisms in streptozocin-induced diabetes in rat. Effects of insulin treatment. *Diabetes* 1987;36:1014–1018.

65. Chen MS, Hutchinson ML, Pecoraro RE, et al. Hyperglycemia-induced intracellular depletion of ascorbic acid in human mononuclear leukocytes. *Diabetes* 1983;32:1078–1081.

66. Yue DK, McLennan S, Fisher E, et al. Ascorbic acid metabolism and polyol pathway in diabetes. *Diabetes* 1989;38:257–261.

67. Cunningham JJ, Ellis SL, McVeigh KL, et al. Reduced mononuclear leukocyte ascorbic acid content in adults with insulin-dependent diabetes mellitus consuming adequate dietary vitamin C. *Metabolism* 1991;40:146–149.

68. Som S, Basu S, Mukherjee D, et al. Ascorbic acid metabolism in diabetes mellitus. *Metabolism* 1981;30:572–577.

69. Sundaram RK, Bhaskar A, Vijayalingam S, et al. Antioxidant status and lipid peroxidation in type II diabetes mellitus with and without complications. *Clin Sci (Colch)* 1996;90:255–260.

70. Thornalley PJ, McLellan AC, Lo TW, et al. Negative association between erythrocyte reduced glutathione concentration and diabetic complications. *Clin Sci (Colch)* 1996;91:575–582.

71. Hattori Y, Kawasaki H, Abe K, et al. Superoxide dismutase recovers altered endothelium-dependent relaxation in diabetic rat aorta. *Am J Physiol* 1991;261:H1086–H1094.

72. Langestroer P, Pieper GM. Regulation of spontaneous EDRF release in diabetic rat aorta by oxygen free radicals. *Am J Physiol* 1992;263:H257–H265.

73. Diederich D, Skopec J, Diederich A, et al. Endothelial dysfunction in mesenteric resistance arteries of diabetic rats: role of the free radicals. *Am J Physiol* 1994;266:H1153–H1161.

74. Ammar RF Jr, Gutterman DD, Dellsperger KC. Topically applied superoxide dismutase and catalase normalize coronary arteriolar responses to acetylcholine in diabetes mellitus in vivo. *Circulation* 1994;90:I574.

75. Timimi FK, Ting HH, Haley EA, et al. Vitamin C improves endothelium-dependent vasodilation in patients with insulin-dependent diabetes mellitus. *J Am Coll Cardiol* 1998;31:552–557.

76. Ting HH, Timimi FK, Boles KS, et al. Vitamin C improves endothelium-dependent vasodilation in patients with non-insulin-dependent diabetes mellitus. *J Clin Invest* 1996;97:22–28.
77. Bohlen HG, Lash JM. Topical hyperglycemia rapidly suppresses EDRF- mediated vasodilation of normal rate arterioles. *Am J Physiol* 1993;265:H219–H225.
78. Tesfamariam B, Cohen RA. Free radicals mediate endothelial cell dysfunction caused by elevated glucose. *Am J Physiol* 1992;236:H321–H326.
79. Williams SB, Goldfine AB, Timimi FK, et al. Acute hyperglycemia atenuates endothelium-dependent vasodilation in humans in vivo. *Circulation* 1998;97:1695–1701.
80. Beckman JA, Goldfine AB, Woodcome ME, et al. Acute administration of vitamin C restores the endothelium-dependent vasodilation of forearm resistance vessels impaired by acute hyperglycemia. *Circulation* 1998;98:I176.
81. Morrow JD, Frei B, Longmire AW, et al. Increase in circulating products of lipid peroxidation (F2- isoprostanes) in smokers. Smoking as a cause of oxidative damage. *N Engl J Med* 1995;332:1198–1203.
82. Murohara T, Kugiyama K, Ohgushi M, et al. Cigarette smoke extract contracts isolated porcine coronary arteries by superoxide anion-mediated degradation of EDRF. *Am J Physiol* 1994;266:H874–H880.
83. Schectman G, Byrd JC, Gruchow HW. The influence of smoking on vitamin C status in adults [see Comments].. *Am J Public Health* 1989;79:158–162. Comments.
84. Heitzer T, Just H, Münzel T. Antioxidant vitamin C improves endothelial dysfunction in chronic smokers. *Circulation* 1996;94:6–9.
85. Heitzer T, Yla-Herttuala S, Luoma J, et al. Cigarette smoking potentiates endothelial dysfunction of forearm resistance vessels in patients with hypercholesterolemia. Role of oxidized LDL. *Circulation* 1996;93:1346–1353.
86. Grunfeld S, Hamilton CA, Mesaros S, et al. Role of superoxide in the depressed nitric oxide production by the endothelium of genetically hypertensive rats. *Hypertension* 1995;26:854–857.
87. Tschudi MR, Mesaros S, Luscher TF, et al. Direct in situ measurement of nitric oxide in mesenteric resistance arteries. Increased decomposition by superoxide in hypertension. *Hypertension* 1996;27:32–35.
88. Wei EP, Kontos HA, Christman CW, et al. Superoxide generation and reversal of acetylcholine-induced cerebral arteriolar dilation after acute hypertension. *Circ Res* 1985;57:781–787.
89. Taddei S, Virdis A, Ghiadoni L, et al. Vitamin C improves endothelium-dependent vasodilation by restoring nitric oxide activity in essential hypertension. *Circulation* 1998;97:2222–2229.
90. Levine GN, Frei B, Koulouris SN, et al. Ascorbic acid reverses endothelial vasomotor dysfunction in patients with coronary artery disease. *Circulation* 1996;93:1107–1113.
91. Vita JA, Frei B, Holbrook M, et al. L-2-Oxothiazolidine-4-carboxylic acid reverses endothelial dysfunction in patients with coronary artery disease. *J Clin Invest* 1998;101:1408–1414.
92. Kugiyama K, Ohgushi M, Motoyama T, et al. Intracoronary infusion of reduced glutathione improves endothelial vasomotor response to acetylcholine in human coronary circulation. *Circulation* 1998;97:2299–2301.

## Chapter 19

# Endothelium-Derived Nitric Oxide: An Antiatherogenic Molecule

*Shanthi Adimoolam, PhD, and John P. Cooke, MD, PhD*

## Introduction

Since the turn of the 20th century, cardiovascular diseases (CVDs) have been established as the leading cause of death in the United States. The American Heart Association (AHA) provides the surprising statistic that every 33 seconds, an American succumbs to heart disease. The primary cause of CVD is atherosclerosis,[1] a complex process believed to be initiated by a "response to injury" of the endothelium.[2] The mechanisms by which an "injury" precipitates atherogenesis are delineated incompletely, but certain risk factors have been identified: hypercholesterolemia, hypertension, diabetes mellitus, tobacco use, and a family history of premature atherosclerosis. In addition to these traditional risk factors, there is increasing evidence that elevated plasma levels of lipoprotein(a), homocysteine, and C-reactive peptide also may accelerate the process of atherosclerosis. Obesity, type A personality, and sedentary lifestyle also are predisposing factors.

The mechanisms by which these various risk factors precipitate and/or accelerate atherogenesis are not defined completely. However, most of them share one pathophysiological effect: an early impairment of endothelial vasodilator function. This impairment of endothelial function precedes evidence for structural changes in the vessel. We hypothesize that this early impairment in endothelial vasodilator function not only contributes to the adverse effects of these risk factors on vascular reactivity, but also plays an important role in the initiation and progression of atherosclerosis.

## Endothelium-Derived Nitric Oxide: A Pluripotential Factor

Our laboratory has focused on the role of the endothelium in the initiation of atherogenesis. The endothelium elaborates a number of substances that

From Panza JA, Cannon RO III (eds): *Endothelium, Nitric Oxide, and Atherosclerosis* ©Futura Publishing Co, Inc, Armonk, NY, 1999.

play a major role in the regulation of the tone and structure of the underlying vascular smooth muscle. One of these paracrine factors is endothelium-derived relaxing factor (EDRF). EDRF is now known to be nitric oxide (NO). NO synthase (NOS) metabolizes L-arginine to L-citrulline and NO.[3] NO is the most potent endogenous vasodilator known, and it functions similarly to exogenous nitrovasodilators such as nitroglycerin. Chemiluminescence bioassay studies have provided conclusive evidence that NO is synthesized by endothelial cells[4] and is the major causative agent for endothelium-dependent relaxation.

NO exerts its action by diffusing to the adjacent vascular smooth muscle layer, where it activates soluble guanylate cyclase, resulting in the production of cyclic guanosine monophosphate (cGMP). This cyclic nucleotide is the second messenger for the action of endothelium-derived NO (EDNO; as with the exogenous nitrovasodilators), which activates cGMP-dependent kinases and phosphatases mediating vascular smooth muscle relaxation.

EDNO is a potent regulator of systemic resistance. Inhibitors of the enzyme NOS result in an elevation of blood pressure, a consequence of an increase in systemic vascular resistance.[5,6] Also, the vasoconstrictor effects of norepinephrine, serotonin, vasopressin, and angiotensin II are modulated by their activation of endothelial NO (eNO) release.[7]

In addition to its role as a potent vasodilator, NO has inhibitory effects on circulating blood elements. NO inhibits platelet adherence and aggregation and together with prostacyclin, reduces platelet-vessel wall interaction.[8] The effects of NO are associated with the production of cGMP in the platelet. This in turn leads to phosphorylation of proteins that regulate platelet activation and adherence. NO also inhibits the adherence of leukocytes to the endothelium.[9] Monocytes binding to the endothelial cells in vitro is inhibited by exogenous NO in a dose-dependent manner.[10] Attempts to investigate the mechanism by which NO inhibits monocyte adherence and infiltration currently is under investigation in our laboratory.

NO has acute as well as chronic effects on endothelial adhesiveness. Experimentally, it has been shown that endothelial cells become more resistant to monocyte adherence within minutes of exposure to exogenous NO.[11] Because of the rapid time course of this inhibition, it is likely caused by a cGMP-dependent effect on adhesion signaling. In addition, chronic exposure to NO inhibits expression of genes for adhesion molecules and chemokines involved in monocyte adhesion and infiltration.[12,13] Inhibition of NO synthesis increases expression of endothelial proteins required for adhesion of monocytes.[12] NO appears to play a role here by preventing activation of specific transcriptional factors, for example, nuclear factor-kappa B (NF-$\kappa$B).[12,14]

There is accumulating evidence to indicate that NO exerts its effect on endothelial adhesiveness partially by controlling the activity of oxidant-responsive transcriptional pathways.[12,14] endothelial and vascular smooth muscle cells in the presence of cytokines or oxidized lipoproteins elaborate superoxide anion. The increase in reactive oxygen species is associated with increased monocyte-endothelial cell adhesion.[13] These observed effects are reversed by antioxidants or NO donors.[13,15]

It is well established that hypercholesterolemia reduces the bioactivity of EDNO.[16,17] With this reduction in NO activity, a cascade of events is activated, including increased superoxide anion generation, stimulation of oxidant-sensitive transcription, and activation of genes encoding proteins that regulate endothelial adhesiveness.[12,15]

The role of NO may be to reduce intracellular oxidative stress by one of several possible mechanisms. NO can act by scavenging the superoxide anion, forming peroxynitrite anion, a highly reactive free radical.[18] This free radical could be nitrosylated subsequently to form $S$-nitrosothiols,[18] a class of molecules known to induce vasodilation, inhibit platelet aggregation, and interfere with leukocyte adherence to the vessel wall.[19,20] Alternatively, NO may ameliorate oxidative stress by terminating the autocatalytic chain of lipid peroxidation that is initiated by oxidized low-density lipoprotein (ox-LDL) or intracellular generation of oxygen-derived free radicals. Finally, NO may directly suppress the generation of oxygen-derived free radicals by nitrosylating and thereby inactivating oxidative enzymes. Therefore, there is accumulating evidence that NO suppresses the expression of monocyte adhesion molecules and chemokines. The beneficial effects of NO appear to be effected by reducing intracellular oxidative stress, which in turn suppresses oxidant-triggered transcription.

NO also has an inhibitory action on the growth of vascular smooth muscle cells. This inhibitory effect has been confirmed in vitro using NO donors. This effect is mimicked by exogenous administration of 8-bromo-cGMP, which is a stable analog of the second messenger of NO action.[21] It has been shown in a number of disease states where the release of NO is reduced or abolished, such as restenosis, hypercholesterolemia, and hypertension, that there is an increase in the proliferation of vascular smooth muscle cells within the media and the intima.

## Nitric Oxide Inhibits Atherogenesis

Some of the critical events involved in atherogenesis are monocyte adherence and infiltration, platelet adherence and aggregation, and proliferation of vascular smooth muscle cells. EDNO has been shown to inhibit each of these processes, and thus we have proposed that NO is an endogenous antiatherogenic molecule.[22,23] It seems plausible that an endothelial injury or alteration that results in a reduction in NO activity could promote atherogenesis. Likewise, it has been demonstrated in a number of disorders associated with atherosclerosis that there also is an impairment in the ability of the endothelium to elaborate NO.[24] Thus an endothelial injury or alteration leading to a reduction in NO activity could promote atherogenesis. In support of this hypothesis, a number of disorders linked to atherosclerosis also are associated with an impairment in the ability of the endothelium to elaborate NO. Animal and human models of hypercholesterolemia, hypertension, homocysteinemia, diabetes mellitus, and exposure to tobacco are each associated with impaired NO-dependent vasodilation. The endothelial impairment precedes any structural changes of atherogenesis. This impairment in NO bioactivity is caused by a reduced synthesis and/or an increased degradation of NO.

It seems logical that, if reduction in the NO activity promotes atherogenesis, then restoration of its activity might be expected to retard progression of the disease. Indeed, a wide variety of interventions that inhibit the progression of atherosclerosis also are associated with improvements in NO-dependent vasodilation: lipid-lowering agents, antioxidants, estrogen, angiotensin-converting enzyme inhibitors, and L-arginine. Nevertheless, the improvements in endothelial function could be a secondary phenomenon and not imply causality. However, direct evidence now indicates that EDNO has a direct role as an antiatherogenic molecule.

If the above proposed role for NO in atherogenesis were true, then increasing the synthesis of NO by the vessel wall should inhibit a number of key processes in atherosclerosis and halt progression of the disease. Our group was the first to demonstrate that endothelial dysfunction induced by hypercholesterolemia could be reversed by intravenous administration of the NO precursor L-arginine. Subsequently, we demonstrated that chronic enhancement of endothelium-dependent NO-mediated vasodilation could inhibit atherogenesis. New Zealand white rabbits were fed either normal chow or a high-cholesterol diet; some of the animals on the high-cholesterol diet also received supplemental dietary arginine or methionine.[22] At 10 weeks, the thoracic aortae and coronary arteries were harvested for studies of vascular reactivity and histomorphometry. NO-dependent vasodilation to acetylcholine was inhibited in the hypercholesterolemic animals receiving vehicle. In contrast, hypercholesterolemic animals receiving L-arginine had an improvement in NO-dependent vasodilation. The L-arginine supplementation had a striking effect on vascular structure. A notable reduction in the surface area of the thoracic aorta involved by lesions was observed in the hypercholesterolemic animals receiving arginine (Figure 1).[22] The differences were even more pronounced in the left main coronary artery; no lesions at all were observed in the hypercholesterolemic animals receiving L-arginine.[25] The mechanism by which dietary arginine inhibits atherogenesis is likely multifactorial. Clearly, L-arginine appears to potently inhibit monocyte-endothelial cell adhesion. In comparison with the thoracic aortae from normal animals, these from hypercholesterolemic rabbits demonstrated a threefold increase in the number of adherent cells associated with an increase in vascular monocyte chemotactic protein 1 (MCP-1) expression as detected by Northern analysis. Administration of L-arginine increases vascular NO synthesis (as detected by chemiluminescence) and reduces endothelial adhesiveness in hypercholesterolemic animals.[26] Conversely, normocholesterolemic animals exposed to nitro-arginine (an antagonist of NOS) manifest a reduced vascular NO synthesis, an increase in endothelial adhesiveness, and an increased vascular expression of MCP-1.[26] Thus hypercholesterolemia leads to a reduction in NO activity, which is associated with increased monocyte-endothelial cell binding, possibly caused by the increased expression of specific chemokines and adhesion molecules. The expression of the chemokines and adhesion molecules is modulated by local NO activity.

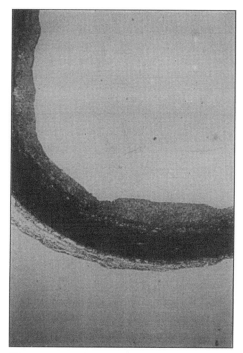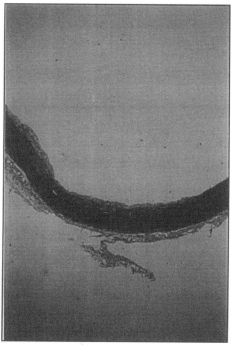

**Figure 1.** Photomicrographs of thoracic aortas from New Zealand white rabbits fed a high-cholesterol diet in the absence (**left panel**) or the addition (**right panel**) of dietary arginine. Reproduced with permission from Reference 22.

## Asymmetric Dimethylarginine: An Atherogenic Factor?

The mechanisms of the lipid-induced derangement in the NOS pathway are complex. Certainly, excess elaboration of superoxide anion contributes,[13,27] but there is clear evidence that there is a deficiency of bioactive NO that can be compensated for by increased NO synthesis.[26] Recently, asymmetric dimethylarginine (ADMA) has been identified as a competitive inhibitor of NOS (Figure 2).[28] The elevation of plasma and/or intracellular ADMA in hypercholesterolemia and atherosclerosis may explain the "arginine paradox." The paradox arose as a discrepancy between in vivo and in vitro observations. In vitro studies of the enzyme NOS indicated that its $K_m$ for L-arginine was in a micromolar range, whereas L-arginine existed in millimolar concentrations in plasma. Therefore, L-arginine should not be rate limiting. However, the original observations of our group revealed that under certain conditions (eg, hypercholesterolemia or atherosclerosis), administration of L-arginine could improve endothelium-dependent vasodilation.[24] Subsequently, this work was confirmed by other investigators, and ex vivo studies confirmed increases in vascular NO synthesis.[26,29] An endogenous inhibitor that is elevated under certain conditions may explain these observations. Other explanations of the arginine paradox include the observation that L-glutamine interferes with

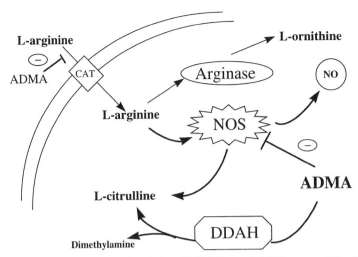

**Figure 2.** Asymmetric dimethylarginine (ADMA) can inhibit competitively the production of nitric oxide (NO) from NO synthase. ADMA is converted normally by the enzyme dimethylamino hydrolase (DDAH) to L-citrulline, which then is recycled back to L-arginine. ADMA also can decrease the uptake of L-arginine via the cationic transporters.

activation of NOS,[30] and the finding that eNOS is restricted largely to the cell membrane within caveolae and is associated there with the Y+ transporter for L-arginine.[31] Although these peculiarities of the NOS pathway may contribute to the sensitivity of NOS to local L-arginine concentrations, they do not explain the fact that L-arginine administration has little effect on normal endothelial function, but reverses the impairment of endothelial vasodilator function observed in hypercholesterolemia, tobacco exposure, aging, atherosclerosis, and perhaps hypertension and diabetes mellitus. Rather, the most parsimonious explanation for the arginine paradox is the existence of a circulating inhibitor, levels of which become elevated under certain conditions. A significant elevation in plasma levels of ADMA between normal ($1.0 \pm 0.1$ $\mu$mol/L) and hypercholesterolemic individuals ($2.2 \pm 0.2$ $\mu$mol/L) has been noted.[32] An increase in ADMA levels in elderly patients with peripheral arterial disease and atherosclerosis also is observed, ranging from 2.5 $\mu$mol/L to 3.5 $\mu$mol/L.[33] Boger et al[29] have demonstrated an elevation in plasma levels of ADMA in hypercholesterolemic rabbits, as well as in hypercholesterolemic and atherosclerotic humans,[32,33] in concordance with disrupted eNO elaboration.

The role of ADMA as an inhibitor of NOS has been confirmed in our lab by the incubation of ADMA with cultured cells. Over a period of 24 hours, concentrations of ADMA that are observed in patients with atherosclerosis were observed to inhibit NO synthesis. The deficit in NO synthesis was associated with a cascade of events: increased endothelial superoxide radical elaboration and NF-$\kappa$B activation, which resulted in enhanced MCP-1 expression and monocyte adherence to the endothelium. All these effects of ADMA were reversed by L-arginine, consistent with the hypothesis that ADMA acts as a competitive inhibitor in the NOS pathway.

ADMA is elevated in uremic patients,[34] and in chronic renal failure.[35] Accumulation of ADMA also has been shown to be associated with decreased NO production/release from regenerated endothelial cells.[36] ADMA levels also are higher in congestive heart failure[37] and experimental hypertension.[38] All of these conditions are associated with an endothelial vasodilator impairment that is reversible by L-arginine.[24]

As discussed in the previous sections, NO bioactivity is impaired in hypercholesterolemia and atherosclerosis. The effects of this reduced activity is manifested as attenuated endothelium-dependent vasodilatation, increased platelet aggregability, and monocyte adhesiveness for the endothelium, which in turn may contribute to the development and progression of atherosclerosis. To support this view, pharmacologic inhibition of NOS promotes atherosclerosis in animal models of hypercholesterolemia.[39,40] However, this effect of NO impairment can be overcome by L-arginine supplementation, which improves endothelial function, inhibits platelet activation and monocyte adhesiveness for the endothelium, and slows progression or even induces regression of lesions.[22,24–26]

The origin of ADMA is still an enigma. Dimethylarginines are most likely products of degradation of methylated proteins, rather than the methylation of free arginines.[41,42] The enzyme S-adenosyl methionine:protein arginine N-methyl transferase (protein methylase I) specifically methylates internal arginine residues in a variety of polypeptides, producing $N^G$-monomethyl-L-arginine (L-NAME), ADMA, and $N^G,N'^G$-dimethyl-L-arginine (SDMA) on degradation.[43] Fickling and coworkers[44] observed the release of ADMA and SDMA from human umbilical vein endothelial cells (HUVECs). Recent work from our lab has revealed that the stimulation of HUVECs with ox-LDL or cytokines increases ADMA accumulation in the media approximately fourfold. This increase in ADMA elaboration appears to be caused by reduced degradation, rather that augmented synthesis.

This local synthesis of ADMA in cells and tissues possibly could serve as a mechanism for regulation of NOSs. Exogenous ADMA concentrations between 1 and 10 $\mu$mol/L inhibit NOS in the vasculature of rat mesentery tissue[45] and rat brain.[46] Faraci et al[46] reported a $IC_{50}$ value of 1.8 $\mu$mol/L for the inhibition of NO production by ADMA in rat cerebellar homogenate. Fickling and colleagues[44] demonstrated that 2 and 10 $\mu$mol/L ADMA inhibited nitrite production by 17% and 33%, respectively, in lipopolysaccharide-stimulated I774 macrophages. These results, along with the recent observations from our lab, suggest that ADMA may be an autocrine regulator of eNOS.

## Mechanism of Asymmetric Dimethylarginine Elevation

The mechanism for elevation of ADMA levels could be caused by its increased synthesis and/or decreased degradation. The enzyme dimethylarginine dimethylamino hydrolase (DDAH) metabolizes ADMA (but not SDMA).[47] DDAH catalyzes the hydrolytic decrease of the methyl amino moiety of ADMA and forms citrulline and dimethylamine. ADMA synthesis appears to occur continuously in the vessel wall. When addition of $S$-2-amino-4 (3-methyl guanidino) butanoic acid (4124W), a synthetic inhibitor of DDAH, was added to an organ chamber, it causes a slowly developing, endothelium-dependent contraction of rat aortic rings, an effect that is reversed by L-arginine.[42] This reversal by L-arginine strongly suggests that the vasoconstrictor effect of DDAH inhibition is caused by accumulation of ADMA. ADMA may serve as an endogenous regulator of NO synthesis.

DDAH has been purified to homogeneity and characterized[48] and has been cloned in rats[49] and in humans (M. Kimoto, personal communication, 1998). Studies to determine the localization of this enzyme have revealed that DDAH mostly colocalizes with NOS.[50,51] Sites of DDAH expression in the rat kidney have all been shown to express some isoform of NOS.[52]

Preliminary results from our lab have indicated that cytokine or ox-LDL stimulation of HUVECs results in an increase in ADMA levels in the culture medium. Western blot analysis of these cell lysates using a monoclonal antibody against rat DDAH reveals no change in the expression levels of the protein before or after stimulation. However, activity assays for DDAH using ADMA as a substrate and measuring the formation of citrulline reveal that the enzyme activity is reduced to approximately 50% on stimulation. This reduction of function could be explained by an alteration of DDAH or an increased

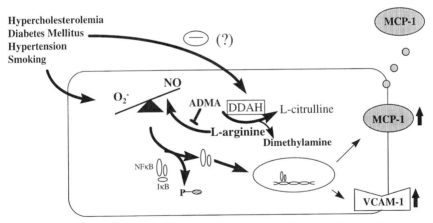

**Figure 3.** Atherosclerotic risk factors such as hypercholesterolemia, hypertension, tobacco, and diabetes mellitus lead to increased free-radical production and decreased NO activity in endothelial cells. This endothelial dysfunction not only has acute effects on vascular tone, but also chronic effects on vessel structure. Increased superoxide anion leads to activation of nuclear factor–kappa B (NF-$\kappa$B) via phosphorylation and degradation of the inhibitor protein I-$\kappa$B$\alpha$. Then NF-$\kappa$B is free to translocate into the nucleus to initiate transcription of proatherogenic genes such as vascular cell adhesion molecule 1 (VCAM-1) and mitotic-control protein 1 (MCP-1). NO can inhibit these processes by inhibiting superoxide production, directly scavenging superoxide anions, as well as increasing the transcription and activity of I-$\kappa$B$\alpha$. Moreover, because NO is a paracrine factor, it can have important inhibitory effects on circulating leukocytes and underlying smooth muscle cells. The increased ADMA found in these risk factors can inhibit NO production. Our current hypothesis for the increased ADMA is the lipid-induced inhibition of DDAH, the degradation enzyme for ADMA.

expression of an inhibitor of DDAH on stimulation (Figure 3). Currently, studies are underway in our lab to test these hypotheses. Transgenic animal models overexpressing DDAH also are under construction to study in depth the in vivo effects of this enzyme and its effect on hypercholesterolemia.

# Summary

The weight of the evidence strongly supports the view that NO is an endogenous antiatherogenic molecule. The injury to the endothelium that triggers atherogenesis may be an impairment of the NOS pathway. A deficit in NO bioactivity is characterized by an increase in intracellular oxidative stress and the activation of oxidant-responsive genes encoding adhesion molecules and chemokines. These changes facilitate interaction of circulating blood elements with the endothelium. Monocyte infiltration and foam cell formation are followed by platelet adherence and proliferation of vascular smooth muscle. NO has an inhibitory role in all these key processes in atherogenesis. Strong evidence now indicates that hypercholesterolemia and other metabolic disorders leading to atherosclerosis disrupt the NOS pathway. These metabolic disorders are associated with a decrease in NO bioactivity and elevated levels of ADMA. A detailed understanding of the mechanism of action of its degradative enzyme DDAH will shed further light on this issue. Owing to this strong correlation between endothelial dysfunction and atherosclerosis, basic insights into the mechanism of reduced NO bioactivity will lead to new therapeutic strategies to retard the progression or induce the regression of atherosclerosis.

# References

1. Mahley RW. Atherogenic lipoproteins and coronary artery disease: Concepts derived from recent advances in cellular and molecular biology. *Circulation* 1985;72:943–948.
2. Ross R. The pathogenesis of atherosclerosis. *N Engl J Med* 1986;314:488–500.
3. Moncada S, Higgs EA. Molecular mechanisms and therapeutic strategies related to nitric oxide. *FASEB J* 1995;9:1319–1330.
4. Palmer RMJ, Ferrige AG, Moncada S. Nitric oxide release accounts for the biological activity of endothelium derived relaxing factor. *Nature* 1987;327:524–526.
5. Rees DD, Palmer RMJ, Moncada S. Effects of endothelium derived nitric oxide in the regulation of blood pressure. *Proc Natl Acad Sci U S A* 1989;86:3375–3378.
6. Vallance P, Collier J, Moncada S. Effects of endothelium derived nitric oxide on peripheral arteriolar tone in man. *Lancet* 1989;2:997–1000.
7. Anggard EE, Botting RM, Vane JR. Endothelin. *Blood Vessels* 1990;27:269–281.
8. Cohen RA. The role of nitric oxide and other endothelium derived vasoactive substances in vascular disease. *Prog Cardiovasc Dis* 1995;XXXVIII:105–128.
9. Kubes P, Suzuki M, Granger DN. Nitric oxide: An endogenous modulator of leukocyte adhesion. *Proc Natl Acad Sci U S A* 1991;88:4651–4655.
10. Bath PMW, Hassall DG, Gladwin AM, et al. Nitric oxide and prostacyclin. Divergence of inhibitory effects on monocyte chemotaxis and adhesion to endothelium in vitro. *Arterioscler Thromb* 1991;11:254–260.
11. Tsao PS, Lewis NP, Alpert S, et al. Exposure to shear stress alters endothelial adhesiveness: Role of nitric oxide. *Circulation* 1995;92:3513–3519.

12. Tsao PS, Buitrage R, Chang JR, et al. Fluid flow inhibits endothelial adhesiveness: Nitric oxide and transcriptional regulation of VCAM-1. *Circulation* 1996;94:1682–1689.

13. Tsao PS, Wang BY, Buitrago R, et al. Nitric oxide regulates monocyte chemotactic protein-1. *Circulation* 1997;96:934–940.

14. Peng HB, Libby P, Liao JK. Induction and stabilization of I kappa B alpha by nitric oxide mediates inhibition of NF-kappa B. *J Biol Chem* 1995;270:14214–14219.

15. Marui N, Offerman MK, Swerlick R, et al. Vascular cell adhesion molecule-1 (VCAM-1) gene transcription and expression are regulated through an antioxidant sensitive mechanism in human vascular endothelial cells. *J Clin Invest* 1993;92:1866–1872.

16. Heistad DD, Armstrong MLI, Marcus ML, et al. Augumented responses to vasoconstrictor stimuli in hypercholesterolemic and atherosclerotic monkeys. *Circ Res* 1984;43:711–718.

17. McLenahan JM, Wilham JK, Fish RD, et al. Loss of flow mediated endothelium-dependent dilation occurs early in the development of atherosclerosis. *Circulation* 1991;84:1273–1278.

18. Radi R, Beckman JS, Bush KM, et al. Peroxynitrite oxidation of sulfhydryls. The cytotoxic potential of superoxide and nitric oxide. *J Biol Chem* 1991;266:4244–4250.

19. Stamler JS, Simon DI, Osborne JA, et al. *S*-nitrosylation of proteins with nitric oxide: Synthesis and characterization of biologically active compounds. *Proc Natl Acad Sci U S A* 1992;89:444–448.

20. Stamler JS, Mendelson ME, Amarante P, et al. *N*-acetylcysteine potentiates platelet inhibition by endothelium-derived relaxing factor. *Circ Res* 1989;65:789–795.

21. Garg UC, Hassid A. Nitric oxide-generating vasodilators and 8-bromocyclic guanosine monophosphate inhibit mitogenesis and proliferation of cultured rat vascular smooth muscle cells. *J Clin Invest* 1989;83:1774–1777.

22. Cooke JP, Singer AH, Tsao PS, et al. Anti-atherogenic effects of ʟ-arginine in the hypercholesterolemic rabbit. *J Clin Invest* 1992;90:1168–1172.

23. Cooke JP, Tsao PS. Is NO an endogenous anti-atherogenic molecule? *Arterioscler Thromb* 1994;14:653–655.

24. Cooke JP, Dzau VJ. Derangements of the nitric oxide synthase pathway, ʟ-arginine, and cardiovascular disease. *Circulation* 1997;96:379–382. Editorial.

25. Wang B, Singer AH, Tsao PS, et al. Dietary arginine prevents atherogenesis in the coronary artery of the hypercholesterolemic rabbit. *J Am Coll Cardiol* 1994;23:452–458.

26. Tsao PS, McEvoy LM, Drexler H, et al. Enhanced endothelial adhesiveness in hypercholesterolemia is attenuated by ʟ-arginine. *Circulation* 1994;89:2176–2182.

27. Ohara Y, Peterson TE, Harrison DG. Hypercholesterolemia increases endothelial superoxide anion production. *J Clin Invest* 1993;91:2546–2551.

28. Vallance P, Leone A, Calver A, et al. Endogenous dimethylarginine as an inhibitor of nitric oxide synthesis. *J Cardiovasc Pharmacol* 1992;20(suppl 12):60–62.

29. Bode-Boger SM, Boger RH, Kienke S, et al. Elevated ʟ-arginine/dimethylarginine ratio contributes to enhanced systemic NO production by dietary ʟ-arginine in hypercholesterolemia rabbits. *Biochem Biophys Res Commun* 1996;219:598–603.

30. Arnal JF, Munzel T, Venema RC, et al. Interactions between ʟ-arginine and ʟ-glutamine change endothelial NO production. An effect independent of NO synthase substrate availability. *J Clin Invest* 1995;95:2565–2572.

31. McDonald KK, Zharikov S, Block ER, et al. A caveolar complex between the cationic amino acid transporter 1 and endothelial nitric-oxide synthase may explain the "arginine paradox." *J Biol Chem* 1997;272:31213–31216.

32. Boger RH, Bode-Boger SM, Szuba A, et al. Asymetric dimethylarginine: A novel risk factor for endothelial dysfunction. *Circulation* 1997;96(suppl):I32.

33. Boger RH, Bode-Boger SM, Thiele W, et al. Biochemical evidence for impaired nitric oxide synthesis in patients with peripheral arterial occlusive disease. *Circulation* 1997;95:2068–2074.

34. Arese M, Strasly M, Ruva C, et al. Regulation of nitric oxide synthesis in uraemia. *Nephrol Dial Transplant* 1995;10:1386–1397.

35. Vallance P, Leone A, Calver A, et al. Accumulation of an endogenous inhibitor of nitric oxide synthesis in chronic renal failure. *Lancet* 1992;339:572–575.

36. Azuma H, Sato J, Hamasaki H, et al. Accumulation of endogenous inhibitors for nitric oxide synthesis and decreased content of L-arginine in regenerated endothelial cells. *Br J Pharmacol* 1995;115:1001–1004.

37. Feng Q, Lu X, Fortin AJ, et al. Elevation of an endogenous inhibitor of nitric oxide synthesis in experimental congestive heart failure. *Cardiovasc Res* 1998;37:667–675.

38. Matsuoka H, Itoh S, Kimoto M, et al. Asymmetrical dimethylarginine, an endogenous nitric oxide synthase inhibitor, in experimental hypertension. *Hypertension* 1997;29:242–247.

39. Cayatte AJ, Palacino U, Horten K, et al. Chronic inhibition of nitric oxide production accelerates neointima formation and impairs endothelial function in hypercholesterolemic rabbits. *Arterioscler Thromb* 1994;14:753–759.

40. Naruse K, Shimizu K, Muramatsu M, et al. Long term inhibition of NO synthesis promotes atherosclerosis in hypercholesterolemic rabbit thoracic aorta. *Arterioscler Thromb* 1994;14:746–752.

41. McDermott SR. Studies on the catabolism of $N^GO$-methylarginine, $N^G,N^G$-dimethylarginine and $N^G,N'^G$-dimethylarginine in the rabbit. *Biochem J* 1996;154:179–184.

42. MacAllister RJ, Parry H, Kimoto M, et al. Regulation of nitric oxide synthesis by dimethylarginine dimethylamino hydrolase. *Br J Pharmacol* 1996;119:1533–1540.

43. Rawal N, Rajpurohit R, Lischwe MA, et al. Structural specificty of substrate for S-adenosylmethionine:protein arginine N-methyl transferases. *Biochem Biopyhys Acta* 1995;1248:11–18.

44. Fickling SA, Leone AM, Nussey SS, et al. Synthesis of $N^G,N^G$-dimethylarginine by human endothelial cells. *Endothelium* 1993;1:137–140.

45. Kurose I, Wolfe R, Grisham MB, et al. Effects of an endogenous inhibitor of nitric oxide synthesis on post capillary venules. *Am J Physiol* 1995;268:2224–2231.

46. Faraci FM, Brian JE, Heistad DD. Response of cerebral blood vessels to an endogenous inhibitor of nitric oxide synthase. *Am J Physiol* 1995;269:1522–1527.

47. Mac Allister RJ, Fickling SA, Whitley GSJ, et al. Metabolism of methylarginines by human vasculature: Implications for the regulation of nitric oxide synthesis. *Br J Pharmacol* 1994;112:43–48.

48. Ogawa I, Kimoto M, Sasaoka K. Purification and properties of a new enzyme $N^G,N^G$-dimethylarginine, dimethylaminohydralase from rat kidney. *J Biol Chem* 1989;264:10205–10209.

49. Kimoto M, Sasakawa T, Tsuji H, et al. Cloning and sequencing of cDNA encoding $N^G,N^G$-dimethylarginine dimethylaminohydrolase from rat kidney. *Biochim Biophys Acta* 1997;1337:6–10.

50. Kimoto M, Whitley GSJ, Tsuji H, et al. Detection of $N^G,N^G$-dimethylarginine, dimethylaminohydrolase in human tissues using a monoclonal antibody. *J Biochem* 1995;117:237–238.

51. Kimoto M, Tsuji H, Ogawa I, et al. Detection of $N^G,N^G$-dimethylarginine, dimethylamino hydrolase in the nitric oxide generating systems of rats using monodonal antibody. *Arch Biochem Biophys* 1993;300:657–662.

52. Tojo A, Welch WJ, Bremer V, et al. Colocalization of dimethylating enzymes and NOS and functional effects of methylarginines in rat kidney. *Kidney Int* 1997;52:1593–1601.

## Chapter 20

# Hormone Therapy and Nitric Oxide Bioactivity in Postmenopausal Women

*Richard O. Cannon III, MD*

## Introduction

Cardiovascular disease caused by atherosclerosis is the leading cause of morbidity and mortality in women living in developed societies, as it is for men, although the clinically apparent onset of disease expression is shifted by approximately a decade later in women. This delay in disease expression relative to men may in part be a result of antiatherogenic effects of estrogen prior to failure of ovarian function during menopause. The Nurses' Health Study[1] reported an approximately 50% reduction in cardiovascular risk in postmenopausal women currently on estrogen therapy at the time of their most recent biennial follow-up evaluation compared with women who had never used hormone therapy. This beneficial effect of estrogen therapy in postmenopausal women (which remains to be proven in randomized clinical trials) may in part result from increases in high-density lipoprotein (HDL) cholesterol levels and reduction in low-density lipoprotein (LDL) cholesterol levels to a more favorable ratio, retarding atherogenesis. However, epidemiological studies question whether alteration in lipid profile alone can account for all of the apparent cardiovascular benefit of estrogen therapy.[2]

Animal studies have indicated that estrogen may have vascular effects independent of changes in lipoprotein profile. Thus, intravenous administration of estradiol-17$\beta$ to ovariectomized primates fed an atherogenic diet was found to reverse acutely the epicardial coronary artery response to acetylcholine (ACh) from constriction to dilation without any effect on nitroglycerin-mediated vasodilation, suggesting estrogen-mediated improvement in endothelial function independent of lipoprotein effects.[3] This study is consistent with the demonstration of estrogen-enhanced endothelium-dependent relaxation of rabbit femoral artery rings to ACh.[4] On the other hand, one group found estrogen at supraphysiological concentrations to have endothelium-

From Panza JA, Cannon RO III (eds): *Endothelium, Nitric Oxide, and Atherosclerosis* ©Futura Publishing Co, Inc, Armonk, NY, 1999.

independent dilator effects on arterial ring preparations from rabbit coronary arteries.[5]

# Acute Coronary Artery Effects of Estrogen in Humans

To determine the direct effects of estrogen at physiological concentrations on epicardial and microvascular coronary artery dynamics in postmenopausal women, we infused estradiol-17β into the coronary arteries of 20 postmeno-pausal women who were at least 2 months off hormone therapy, 7 of whom had angiographic evidence of atherosclerosis of the left coronary artery, with test-ing of endothelium-dependent and endothelium-independent dilator respon-siveness. Coronary artery diameters were measured by computer-assisted quantitative coronary angiography and blood flow velocity was measured with a Doppler wire positioned in the proximal left coronary artery, with the product of these values used to derive volume flow. ACh was infused at escalating doses (range 3–300 μg/min) as an endothelium-dependent agonist, and adenosine and sodium nitroprusside were infused as endothelium-independent agonists. The dose of intracoronary estradiol was selected to achieve physiological concentrations of estradiol in the coronary venous circu-lation (282 ± 121 pg/mL from 16 ± 11 pg/mL prior to infusion). Estradiol did not affect basal coronary artery diameter, blood flow, or resistance. However, epicardial coronary artery constriction induced by ACh infusion in the control study was prevented during repeat ACh infusion with concomitant estradiol administration (Figure 1). Estradiol also potentiated the vasodilator coronary microvascular response to ACh as manifest by significantly greater coronary

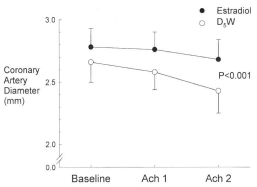

**Figure 1.** Plot of coronary artery diameter of proximal left coronary artery segments measured at the tip of the flow velocity wire with measurements at baseline, following that dose of acetylcholine (ACh) that resulted in the highest flow (ACh 1 median dose 30 μg/min) and the next higher concentration of ACh that resulted in a lesser increase in flow (ACh 2 median dose 100 μg/min), during the control study ($D_5$ W) and with repeat measurements during intracoronary infusion of estradiol 75 ng/mL for 15 minutes. Data are expressed as means ± SEM. Reproduced with permission from Reference 6.

flow and lower coronary resistance compared with the control study with ACh alone (Figure 2). The effect of estradiol on coronary dynamics was most prominent in women with the most impaired responses to ACh at both the epicardial ($r = -0.72$, $P < 0.001$) and microvascular ($r = -0.59$, $P = 0.006$) coronary artery levels. In contrast, estradiol did not affect the coronary epicardial or microvascular dilator responses to either adenosine or sodium nitroprusside. Thus, physiological concentrations of estradiol, although without effect on basal epicardial or microvascular coronary dynamics, enhanced the release of relaxing factors from the endothelium in response to ACh.

Consistent with these findings, Roque et al[7] recently reported that 15 postmenopausal women with normal coronary angiograms, who underwent measurement of coronary dynamic responses to escalating intracoronary doses of ACh and nitroglycerin, showed epicardial constriction at baseline and no constriction following 24 hours of estradiol administered as a transdermal patch (100 $\mu$g). Furthermore, the coronary flow response to ACh was enhanced significantly following 24 hours of estrogen treatment. In this brief study using a transdermal preparation of estrogen, lipoprotein changes that could have affected the coronary response to ACh would not be anticipated. Herrington et al[8] reported that four postmenopausal women chronically taking conjugated equine estrogens at conventional dosages had epicardial coronary dilator re-

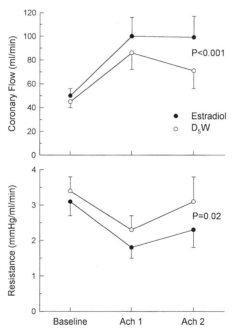

**Figure 2.** Plots of coronary flow (top) and resistance (bottom) at baseline and in response to that dose of ACh that produced the highest flow during the control study (ACh 1 median dose 30 $\mu$g/min) and the next higher concentration of ACh that resulted in a lesser increase in flow (ACh 2 median dose 100 $\mu$g/min) with measurements made during the control study ($D_5$ W) compared with repeat measurements at the same doses of ACh during intracoronary infusion of estradiol 75 ng/mL for 15 minutes. Data are expressed as means ± SEM. Reproduced with permission from Reference 6.

sponses to escalating doses of intracoronary ACh, as opposed to constrictor responses to the same concentrations of ACh noted in six untreated postmenopausal women, with similar dilator responses to nitroglycerin in the two groups. However, the specificity of these responses for estrogen is tempered by reduction in LDL and elevation in HDL cholesterol levels associated with chronic oral estrogen therapy, that might have contributed to improvement in endothelium-dependent vasodilator responsiveness.

## Systemic Vascular Effects of Estrogen

To determine the systemic microvascular responses to estrogen, we infused estradiol-17$\beta$ into the brachial arteries of 40 postmenopausal women achieving physiological concentrations in the brachial vein, with forearm flow measured by venous occlusion strain-gauge plethysmography.[9] The 20 women with risk factors for atherosclerosis had significantly reduced vasodilator responses to intra-arterial infusions of ACh and sodium nitroprusside compared with the responses of 20 postmenopausal women without risk factors. Compared with the forearm flow responses to escalating doses of ACh (range 7.5–30 $\mu$g/min for 2 minutes) prior to estrogen administration, infusion of estradiol-enhanced ACh-stimulated blood flow in the 20 women with risk factors for atherosclerosis and to a lesser degree in the 20 women without risk factors. Estradiol also potentiated slightly, but still significantly, the forearm vasodilator response to sodium nitroprusside in women with risk factors for atherosclerosis but not in the women without risk factors. Thus, acute administration of estradiol selectively potentiated endothelium-dependent microvascular dilation in forearms of healthy postmenopausal women and both endothelium-dependent and endothelium-independent vasodilator responsiveness in women with risk factors for atherosclerosis and evidence of impaired vascular function.

Estrogen also has beneficial effects on endothelium-dependent vasodilator responsiveness of large systemic arteries. In this regard, Lieberman et al[10] reported that 1 or 2 mg oral estradiol administered daily to 13 postmenopausal women for 9 weeks enhanced brachial artery flow-mediated dilator responses during postischemic hyperemia (measured by ultrasonography), compared with the placebo phase in this randomized, double-blind study and without potentiation of the vasodilator response to nitroglycerin. As flow-mediated dilation of the radial artery following ischemia is attenuated following infusion of an inhibitor of nitric oxide (NO) synthesis,[11] improvement in flow-mediated dilation of the brachial artery following an intervention or therapy generally is accepted as augmented endothelium-dependent NO bioactivity. As noted previously, the use of an oral estrogen preparation likely caused changes in lipoprotein levels that could have contributed to the improved endothelial function.

The acute vascular effects of estrogen may have accounted for the improvement in time to 1 mm ST segment depression and the total duration of treadmill exercise of 11 postmenopausal women with coronary artery disease

(CAD) after sublingual estradiol-17β administration, compared with exercise after placebo in a randomized, double-blind study.[12] Because the peak heart rate–systolic blood pressure was not augmented significantly by estradiol administration, systemic vasodilating effects of acutely administered estradiol may have accounted for improvement in exercise in this study. Whether similar anti-ischemic benefit can be achieved with chronic estrogen therapy is unknown at present.

## Vascular Effects of Combined Hormone Therapy

In clinical practice, a progestin compound usually is combined with estrogen to reduce the risk of uterine malignancy otherwise associated with prolonged estrogen therapy. However, animal studies suggest that concurrent progesterone therapy may significantly modify the beneficial effects of estrogen on vascular reactivity. Thus, progesterone was found to antagonize endothelium-dependent vasodilator responses to estrogen canine coronary arteries.[13] In ovariectomized monkeys with diet-induced atherosclerosis, the addition of medroxyprogesterone acetate diminished the beneficial effect of estrogen on endothelium-dependent coronary vasoreactivity.[14] Sorensen et al[15] studied brachial artery vasomotor function in 100 healthy postmenopausal women randomized to either estradiol combined with noresthistrone (46 women) or no hormone therapy (54 women) and followed for approximately 3 years. In addition, 30 healthy premenopausal women were studied as controls. Brachial artery flow-mediated dilation was reduced significantly to an equivalent degree in hormone-treated and -untreated postmenopausal groups relative to premenopausal controls, and suggesting absence of benefit from hormone therapy on vasodilator responsiveness. However, a nonrandomized, cross-sectional study of postmenopausal women on a variety of different hormone replacement therapies reported a small improvement in vascular reactivity on combined hormone therapy relative to untreated women.[16]

Gerhard et al[17] recently reported that 0.2 mg estradiol applied trandermally by patch twice weekly in addition to intravaginal micronized progesterone improved brachial artery flow-mediated dilation similar to estradiol alone in 17 healthy postmenopausal women in randomized, double-blind, placebo-controlled trial. Although estradiol decreased low-density cholesterol levels by ~10%, there was no association between the change in these values and the improvement in flow-mediated dilation relative to the placebo phase.

## Gender Differences in Vascular Effects of Estrogen

Vascular effects of estrogen in men may differ from effects reported in postmenopausal women, particularly if the cellular effects of estrogen are mediated through the estrogen receptor, the cellular density of which is greater in women than men. Kawano et al[18] measured flow-mediated brachial artery dilation after forearm ischemia and following nitroglycerin administration before and after estradiol-17β administered transdermally for 36 hours to 15 postmenopausal women and 15 men matched for age and risk factors for atherosclerosis. Estradiol augmented brachial artery flow-mediated dilation and serum levels of nitrogen oxides in women but not in men. The dilator response to nitroglycerin was not affected by estradiol treatment in either women or men. Similarly, Collins et al[19] reported that the acute administration of estradiol-17β improved the epicardial coronary artery response to ACh in women but not men with coronary artery disease. However, when New et al[20] compared the long-term effects of estrogen on vascular function in 14 male to female transsexuals, 14 aged-matched men, and 15 premenopausal women, they found that brachial artery flow-mediated dilation was similar in transsexuals and in women but greater than in men. McCrohon et al[21] measured brachial artery flow-mediated dilation in 15 male to female transsexuals receiving long-term high-dose estrogen therapy, and 15 healthy male subjects matched for age, smoking history, and vessel size. Flow-mediated dilation was significantly greater in the transsexuals than in controls, as was the nitroglycerin response, findings compatible with either increased NO release from the endothelium or increased responsiveness of vascular smooth muscle to NO. Thus, long-term treatment with high-dose estrogen is associated with enhanced arterial reactivity in genetic males.

# Estrogen and Nitric Oxide

Although the studies described above are consistent with augmentation of NO release from the endothelium by estrogen, the mechanism of the endothelial effects of estradiol in animal and human studies also could be a result of non-NO–mediated effects. Potentiation of ACh-stimulated flow by estrogen could result from vascular smooth muscle relaxation caused by enhanced production or release of prostacyclin or another vasodilating prostanoid, activation of a hyperpolarizing factor, or by inhibition of the release or activity of vasoconstrictor substances such as endothelin and angiotensin II. To assess the contribution of NO to the vascular effects of estrogen, we measured coronary epicardial and microvascular responses to intracoronary ACh (range 3–300 μg/min) before and after intracoronary estradiol-17β at a dose achieving physiological concentrations in the coronary sinus in 20 estrogen-deficient women, 16 of whom had angiographic evidence of atherosclerosis or risk factors for atherosclerosis.[22] This testing was repeated after inhibition of NO synthesis with intracoronary $N^G$-monomethyl-L-arginine (L-NMMA) 64 μg/min for 5 minutes. Estradiol increased ACh-stimulated coronary flow above levels achieved with ACh alone and tended to lessen the severity of ACh-induced epicardial coronary artery vasoconstriction (Figure 3). However, following L-NMMA infusion, estradiol no longer potentiated the effects of ACh on coronary flow dynamics, and ACh once again caused epicardial constriction. Thus, the effect of estradiol at physiological concentrations on endothelium-

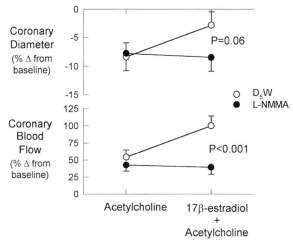

**Figure 3.** Epicardial coronary diameter (top) and coronary blood flow (bottom) responses to ACh are shown as relative changes from respective pre-ACh baseline values in 20 postmenopausal women. The dose of ACh represented on these graphs (100 μg/min) produced the coronary flow response that was enhanced maximally during coadministration of estradiol-17β. The effects of estradiol-17β (75 ng/min) on ACh-stimulated changes in coronary diameter and flow are shown before (●) and during (○) concomitant infusion of $N^{G}$-monomethyl-L-arginine (L-NMMA; 64 μmol/min), an inhibitor of nitric oxide (NO) synthesis. Data are expressed as means ± SEM. Probability values are for the significance of L-NMMA effects on coronary dynamics before and during estradiol infusion. Reproduced with permission from Reference 22.

dependent coronary vasodilator responsiveness in postmenopausal women is mediated through enhanced bioavailability of NO.

In a subsequent study, we compared the vascular effects of 0.625 mg daily oral conjugated equine estrogens to that of cholesterol-lowering therapy with 10 mg daily simvastatin in 28 hypercholesterolemic postmenopausal women (average LDL cholesterol levels 163 ± 36 mg/dL).[23] In addition to the individual administration of these therapies for 6 weeks, the combination of therapies was administered daily for 6 weeks in this randomized, double-blind, three-period study. All treatment schemes lowered total and LDL cholesterol levels from respective pretreatment values, with greater effects by simvastatin (−25% ± 14%) and by conjugated equine estrogens combined with simvastatin (−32% ± 14%) than for conjugated equine estrogens alone (−11% ± 11%). In contrast, only conjugated equine estrogens alone or combined with simvastatin increased HDL cholesterol levels (both 17% ± 15% from respective pretreatment values). Furthermore, only conjugated equine estrogens alone or combined with simvastatin lowered lipoprotein(a) from baseline values. Because the lipoprotein effects that might affect NO bioactivity differed between estrogen and statin therapies, and because estrogen may stimulate directly the release of NO by increased synthesis[24-26] or decreased oxidative inactivation[27] (because of antioxidant properties of estrogen[28]) as shown in endothelial cells in culture,[24-27] we reasoned that the effect of these therapies on endothelial NO bioactivity may differ. Furthermore, because the mechanism of the biological effects of these therapies differed, the combination of these therapies may be

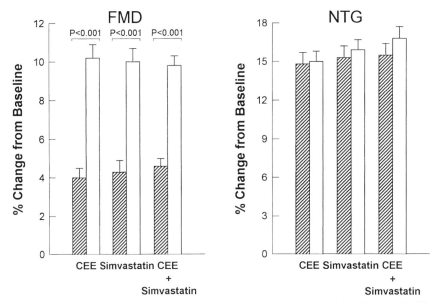

**Figure 4.** Flow-mediated (left panel) and nitroglycerin-induced (right panel) dilation before therapies (hatched bars) and following conjugated equine estrogens (CEE), 0.625 mg daily for 6 weeks (left); simvastatin, 10 mg daily for 6 weeks (center); and the combination of therapies daily for 6 weeks in 28 hypercholesterolemic postmenopausal women. Standard error of the mean is identified by the error bars. Reproduced with permission from Reference 23.

additive, an effect of potential importance to women at high risk for atherosclerosis or with established atherosclerotic disease. Despite the differing effects of these therapies on lipoprotein levels, flow-mediated dilation of the brachial artery improved on all three treatment schemes to a similar degree (Figure 4). None of these therapies improved the dilator response to nitroglycerin. Thus, estrogen and statin therapies both appear to improve vascular NO bioactivity in postmenopausal women but without additive effects.

## Effects of Estrogen on Markers of Inflammation

Therapies that enhance NO bioactivity may reduce vascular inflammation. In cell culture experiments, NO prevents activation of proinflammatory genes of the endothelium by limiting activation of an important nuclear transcription factor-kappa B (NF-$\kappa$B).[29–32] NF-$\kappa$B, normally maintained in an inactive state in the cytasol bound to an inhibitory subunit (I-$\kappa$B), is activated by many stimuli including cytokines, oxidized LDL, lipopolysacchrides, and infectious agents such as cytomegalovirus. Among the inflammatory proteins synthesized following gene activation are cell adhesion molecules, which are positioned across the endothelial cell membrane and bind to ligands on circulating inflammatory cells, facilitating their subsequent entry into the vessel wall. The effect of estrogen on this process is unclear: Estradiol-17$\beta$ was found in endothelial cell culture experiments to inhibit the expression of cell adhesion molecules in one study (with interleukin-1 as the proinflammatory stimulus)[33] but promote their expression in another study (with tumor necrosis factor–$\alpha$ as the proinflammatory stimulus).[34]

Experimental evidence suggests that cell adhesion molecules, once expressed on the endothelial cell surface, may be shed from the surface. Thus, E-selectin, intercellular adhesion molecule type 1 (ICAM-1), and vascular cell adhesion molecule type 1 (VCAM-1) have been detected in the culture supernatant within 4–6 hours of endothelial activation.[35] These same cell adhesion molecules have been measured in sera of humans using the same monoclonal antibody assay used to demonstrate adhesion molecules in the supernatant of activated endothelial cells in culture.[36,37] Serum concentrations of E-selectin, ICAM-1, and VCAM-1 have been reported to be higher in patients with CAD and dyslipidemia, compared with healthy subjects.[38,39] Although the biological function in sera remains unclear, the clinical relevance of the cell adhesion molecules has been suggested by several observational studies. Thus, E-selectin, ICAM-1, and VCAM-1 have been demonstrated in human coronary atherosclerotic arteries by immunohistochemistry.[40] In the Atherosclerosis Risk and Communities Study, higher serum of E-selectin and ICAM-1 were found in patients with coronary heart disease and carotid artery atherosclerosis than in healthy controls.[41]

Because conjugated equine estrogens and simvastatin, alone and in combination, increased vascular NO bioactivity in our study,[23] we reasoned that these therapies might reduce synthesis of cell adhesion molecules, based on the effects of NO in cell culture experiments.[29–32] However, despite equivalent effects of these therapies on NO bioactivity, we found that only therapies including conjugated equine estrogens significantly reduced E-selectin, ICAM-1, and VCAM-1 levels from respective pretreatment values (Figure 5).[23] These findings are consistent with the recent report of Caulin–Glaser et al,[42] who found that postmenopausal women not on hormone therapy who had CAD had higher levels of cell adhesion molecules in serum than women with CAD who were current users of hormone therapy.

The mechanisms by which estrogen therapy, but not simvastatin alone, reduced levels of cell adhesion molecules cannot be determined from our study, but may be independent of NO, as NO bioactivity as evidenced by improvement in brachial artery flow-mediated dilation was increased equally by simvastatin and conjugated equine estrogen therapies from respective pretreatment values. Of interest, a recent study showed that HDL, levels of which were increased significantly in our study by therapies that include conjugated equine estrogens but not simvastatin alone, dose dependently inhibits cytokine-induced expression of cell adhesion molecules in cultured endothelial cells.[43] Furthermore, we found that therapies including conjugated equine estrogens but not simvastatin alone,reduced levels of lipoprotein(a), a lipoprotein with structural similarity to LDL recently shown to stimulate the expression of ICAM-1 in cultured endothelial cells.[44]

However, in our study comparing the vascular effects of conjugated equine estrogens to simvastatin, although therapies including conjugated equine es-

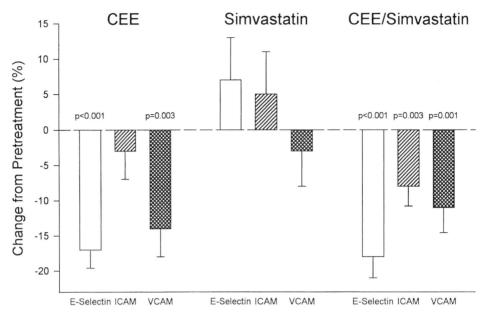

**Figure 5.** Percent change in E-selectin, VCAM-1, and ICAM-1 levels from respective pretreatment values following conjugated equine estrogens (CEE), 0.625 mg daily for 6 weeks (left); simvastatin, 10 mg daily for 6 weeks (center); and the combination daily for 6 weeks (right) in 28 hypercholesterolemic postmenopausal women.[23] Standard error of the mean is identified by the error bars. Differences in treatment effects on E-selectin were highly significant among therapies [$P < 0.01$ by analysis of variance (ANOVA)] as well as between therapies including CEE and simvastatin alone (both $P < 0.01$).

trogens increased levels of HDL cholesterol, we saw no correlation between the magnitude of increase in these levels [or decreases in levels of LDL cholesterol or lipoprotein(a)] and the decrease in levels of adhesion molecules (all $r <$ 0.164).[23] Furthermore, we have found previously that estrogen administered transdermally to avoid lipoprotein changes also reduces levels of cell adhesion molecules in postmenopausal women.[45] Accordingly, estrogen may inhibit directly inflammatory gene activation or gene product expression.

# Conclusions

In postmenopausal women, estrogen improves coronary and systemic endothelium-dependent vasomotor responsiveness, an effect associated with increased NO bioactivity. However, the mechanism of estrogenic stimulation of NO release—increased synthesis of NO versus protection of NO from oxidative degradation—in humans is unknown. Several studies suggest that the addition of progestin, necessary for combined hormone therapy in women with their uterus intact, may detract from the improvement in endothelium-dependent vasodilator responsiveness. However, the relevance of this finding, largely derived from animal studies, must be shown in humans. Estrogen reduces levels of cell adhesion molecules, especially E-selectin, with chronic use of oral therapy. This effect may be independent of NO, but the mechanism is unclear and is not replicated by statin therapy in hypercholesterolemic women. The biological and clinical relevance of this finding, suggestive of a vascular anti-inflammatory effect, remains to be defined.

*Acknowledgments:*   I greatly appreciate the intellectual contributions and hard work of my fellows past and present—Drs. David Gilligan, Michael Sack, Victor Guetta, Kwang Kon Koh, and Arnon Blum—and the many contributions of my colleagues Drs. Arshed Quyyumi and. Julio Panza. I also thank William Schenke for technical assistance; Londa Hathaway, RN, and Rita Mincemoyer, RN, for their management of clinical research protocols; and Toni Julia for typing the manuscript.

# References

1. Stampfer MJ, Colditz GA, Willett WC, et al. Postmenopausal estrogen therapy and cardiovascular disease: Ten-year follow-up from the Nurses' Health Study. *N Engl J Med* 1991;325:756–762.
2. Bush TL, Barrett-Connor E, Cowan LD, et al. Cardiovascular mortality and non-contraceptive use of estrogen in women: Results from the Lipid Research Clinics Program Follow-up Study. *Circulation* 1987;75:1102–1109.
3. Williams JK, Adams MR, Herrington DM, et al. Short-term administration of estrogen and vascular responses of atherosclerotic coronary arteries. *J Am Coll Cardiol* 1992;20:452–457.
4. Gisclard V, Miller VM, Vanhoutte PM. Effect of 17β-estradiol on endothelium-dependent responses of the rabbit. *J Pharmacol Exp Ther* 1988;244:19–22.
5. Jiang C, Sarrel PM, Lindsay DC, et al. Endothelium-independent relaxation of rabbit coronary artery by 17β-oestradiol in vitro. *Br J Pharmacol* 1991;104:1033–1037.
6. Gilligan DM, Quyyumi AA, Cannon RO III. Effects of physiological levels of estrogen on coronary vasomotor function in postmenopausal women. *Circulation* 1994;89:2545–2551.
7. Roque M, Heras M, Riog E, et al. Short-term effects of transdermal estrogen replacement therapy on coronary vascular reactivity in postmenopausal women with angina pectoris and normal results on coronary angiograms. *J Am Coll Cardiol* 1998;31:139–143.
8. Herrington DM, Braden GA, Williams JK, et al. Endothelium-dependent coronary vasomotor responsiveness in postmenopausal women with and without estrogen therapy. *Am J Cardiol* 1994;73:951–952.
9. Gilligan DM, Bader DM, Panza JA, et al. Acute vascular effects of estrogen in postmenopausal women. *Circulation* 1994;90:786–791.
10. Lieberman EH, Gebhard MD, Uehata A, et al. Estrogen improves endothelium-dependent, flow-mediated vasodilation in postmenopausal women. *Ann Intern Med* 1994;121:936–941.
11. Joannides R, Haefeli WE, Linder L, et al. Nitric oxide is responsible for flow-dependent dilation of human peripheral conduit arteries in vivo. *Circulation* 1995;91:1314–1319.
12. Rosano GMC, Sarrel PM, Poole-Wilson PA. Beneficial effect of oestrogen on exercise-induced myocardial ischemia in women with coronary artery disease. *Lancet* 1993;342:133–136.
13. Miller VM, Vanhoutte PM. Progesterone and modulation of endothelium-dependent responses in canine coronary arteries. *Am J Physiol* 1991;21:R1022–R1027.
14. Williams JK, Honore EK, Washburn SA, et al. Effects of hormone replacement therapy on reactivity of atherosclerotic coronary arteries in cynomolgus monkeys. *J Am Coll Cardiol* 1994;24:1757–1761.

15. Sorensen KE, Dorup I, Hermann AP, et al. Combined hormone replacement therapy does not protect women against the age-related decline in endothelium-dependent vasomotor function. *Circulation* 1998;97:1234–1238.
16. McCrohon JA, Adams MR, McCredle RJ, at al. Hormone replacement therapy is associated with improved arterial physiology in healthy postmenopausal women. *Clin Endocrinol* 1996;45:435–441.
17. Gerhard M, Walsh BW, Tawakol A, et al. Estradiol therapy combined with progesterone and endothelium-dependent vasodilation in postmenopausal women. *Circulation* 1998;98:1158–1163.
18. Kawano H, Motoyama T, Kugiyama K, et al. Gender difference in improvement of endothelium-dependent vasodilation after estrogen supplementation. *J Am Coll Cardiol* 1997;30:914–919.
19. Collins P, Rosano GM, Sarrel PM, et al. 17β-estradiol attenuates acetylcholine-induced coronary arterial constriction in women but not men with coronary heart disease. *Circulation* 1995;92:24–30.
20. New G, Timmins KL, Duffy SJ, et al. Long-term estrogen therapy improves vascular function in male to female transsexuals. *J Am Coll Cardiol* 1997;29:1437–1444.
21. McCrohon JA, Walters WAW, Robinson JTC, et al. Arterial reactivity is enhanced in genetic males taking high dose estrogens. *J Am Coll Cardiol* 1997;29:1432–1436.
22. Guetta V, Quyyumi AA, Prasad A, et al. The role of nitric oxide in coronary vascular effects of estrogen in postmenopausal women. *Circulation* 1997;96:2795–2801.
23. Koh KK, Cardillo C, Bui MN, et al. Vascular effects of estrogen and cholesterol-lowering therapies in hypercholesterolemic postmenopausal women. *Circulation* 1999;99:354–360.
24. Hishikawa K, Nakaki T, Marumo T, et al. Up-regulation of nitric oxide synthase by estradiol in human aortic endothelial cells. *FEBS Lett* 1995;360:291–293.
25. Hayashi T, Yamada K, Esaki T, et al. Estrogen increases endothelial nitric oxide by a receptor-mediated system. *Biochem Biophys Res Commun* 1995;214:847–855.
26. Caulin-Glaser T, Garcia-Cardena G, Sarrel P, et al. 17β-estradiol regulation of human endothelial cell basal nitric oxide release independent of cytosolic $Ca^{2+}$ mobilization. *Circ Res* 1997;81:885–892.
27. Arnal JF, Clamens S, Pechet C, et al. Ethinylestradiol does not enhance the expression of nitric oxide synthase in bovine endothelial cells but increases the release of bioactive nitric oxide by inhibiting superoxide anion production. *Proc Natl Acad Sci U S A* 1996;93:4108–4113.
28. Sack MN, Rader DJ, Cannon RO III. Oestrogen and inhibition of oxidation of low-density lipoproteins in postmenopausal women. *Lancet* 1994;343:269–270.
29. De Caterina R, Libby P, Peng H-B, et al. Nitric oxide decreases cytokine-induced endothelial activation. Nitric oxide selectively reduces endothelial expression of adhesion molecules and proinflammatory cytokines. *J Clin Invest* 1995;96:60–68.
30. Peng H-B, Rajavashisth TB, Libby P, et al. Nitric oxide inhibits macrophage-colony stimulating factor gene transcription in vascular endothelial cells. *J Biol Chem* 1995;270:17050–17055.
31. Zeiher AM, Fisslthaler B, Schray-Utz B, et al. Nitric oxide modulates the expression of monocyte chemoattractant protein 1 in cultured human endothelial cells. *Circ Res* 1995;76:980–986.
32. Tsao PS, Wang B-Y, Buitrago R, et al. Nitric oxide regulates monocyte chemotactic protein-1. *Circulation* 1997;96:937–940.
33. Caulin-Glaser T, Watson CA, Bender JR. Effects of 17β-estradiol on cytokine-induced endothelial cell adhesion molecule expression. *J Clin Invest* 1996;98:36–42.
34. Cid MC, Kleinman HK, Grant DS, et al. Estradiol enhances leukocyte binding to tumor necrosis factor (TNF)-stimulated endothelial cells via an increase in TNF-induced adhesion molecules E-selectin, intercellular adhesion molecule type 1, and vascular cell adhesion molecule type 1. *J Clin Invest* 1994;93:17–25.

35. Pigott R, Dillon LP, Hemingway IH, et al. Soluble forms of E-selectin, ICAM-1 and VCAM-1 are present in the supernatants of cytokine activated cultured endothelial cells. *Biochem Biophys Res Commun* 1992;187:594–589.
36. Rothlein R, Mainolfi EA, Czajkowski M. A form of circulating ICAM-1 in human serum. *J Immuno.* 1991;147:3788–3793.
37. Newman W, Beall LD, Carson CW, et al. Soluble E-selectin is found in supernatants of activated endothelial cells and is elevated in the serum of patients with septic shock. *J Immunol* 1993;150:644–654.
38. Haught WH, Mansour M, Rothlein R, et al. Alterations in circulating intercellular adhesion molecule-1 and L-selectin: Further evidence for chronic inflammation in ischemic heart disease. *Am Heart J* 1996;132:1–8.
39. Hackman A, Abe Y, Insull W Jr, et al. Levels of soluble cell adhesion molecules in patients with dyslipidemia. *Circulation* 1996;93:1334–1338.
40. Nakai K, Itoh C, Kawazoe K, et al. Concentration of soluble vascular cell adhesion molecule-1 (VCAM-1) correlated with expression of VCAM-1 mRNA in the human atherosclerotic aorta. *Coron Art Dis* 1995;6:497–502.
41. Hwang J-J, Ballantyne CM, Sharrett R, et al. Circulating adhesion molecules VCAM-1, ICAM-1, and E-selectin in carotid atherosclerosis and incident coronary heart disease cases. The Atherosclerosis Risk in Communities (ARIC) Study. *Circulation* 1997;96:4219–4225.
42. Caulin-Glaser T, Farrell WJ, Pfau SE, et al. Modulation of circulating cellular adhesion molecules in postmenopausal women with coronary artery disease. *J Am Coll Cardiol* 1998;31:1555–1560.
43. Cockerill GW, Rye K-A, Gamble JR, et al. High-density lipoproteins inhibit cytokine-induced expression of endothelial cell adhesion molecules. *Arterioscler Thromb Vasc Biol* 1995;15:1987–1994.
44. Tamaki S, Yamashita S, Kihara S, et al. Lipoprotein(a) enhances the expression of intercellular adhesion molecule-1 in cultured human umbilical vein endothelial cells. *Circulation* 1998;97:721–728.
45. Koh KK, Bui MN, Mincemoyer R, et al. Effects of hormone therapy on inflammatory cell adhesion molecules in postmenopausal healthy women. *Am J Cardiol* 1997;80:1505–1507.

## Chapter 21

# Clinical Trials Using Angiotensin-Converting Enzyme Inhibition to Alter Endothelial Dysfunction in Coronary Patients

G. B. John Mancini, MD, FRCP(C), FACP, and Eric W. Hamber

## Introduction

Angiotensin-converting enzyme (ACE) inhibitors are indicated in the therapy of hypertension, congestive heart failure (CHF), postmyocardial infarction, and to prevent progression of nephropathy.[1] Detailed analysis of some of the heart failure trials showed unexpected benefits in the prevention of ischemic events.[2-5] In the past several years postulated reasons for this benefit have focused on the effects of these agents on endothelial function.[6-8] The presumed linkage between endothelial function and the amelioration in ischemic clinical events was based on the myriad pathogenetic mechanisms that are subserved by the vascular endothelium and that also are known to play a role in the genesis of ischemic events. Thus, the combination of vulnerable atherosclerotic plaques, abnormal vasospasm, platelet aggregation, and clotting reactions are all known to contribute to ischemic events. They also are affected by the state of endothelial function. ACE inhibitors can alter these processes through effects on the endothelium, which by virtue of enhancing the bioavailability of nitric oxide (NO), may in the short term facilitate vasodilation, prevent platelet activation, and, perhaps over the long term, exert an antiatherosclerotic effect as well. Thus, it is conceivable that ACE inhibitors may play a significant role in patients with coronary disease by improving endothelial dysfunction. The purpose of this chapter is to review the emerging, clinical trial information that is pertinent to this issue and that may have a bearing ultimately on clinical practice guidelines. Studies employing acute intravenous or single oral doses of ACE inhibitors are not reviewed here.

From Panza JA, Cannon RO III (eds): *Endothelium, Nitric Oxide, and Atherosclerosis* ©Futura Publishing Co, Inc, Armonk, NY, 1999.

## Trial on Reversing Endothelial Dysfunction

The Trial On Reversing Endothelial Dysfunction (TREND) was a 6-month, multicenter, randomized, double-blind, placebo-controlled study of the effects of quinapril on endothelial dysfunction in coronary arteries of patients referred for coronary intervention procedures.[9] Endothelial function was assessed by serial intracoronary acetylcholine (ACh) infusions that assess stimulated NO production. Quantitative coronary angiography was used to assess the effects on the proximal conduit vessels, especially in those segments responding most abnormally to the ACh infusion during the randomization phase ("target" segments). To minimize confounding factors that might modulate the mechanisms of action of ACE inhibitors, patients were excluded if they were cardiomyopathic, hypertensive, hyperlipidemic, or diabetic. TREND patients also had to have at least one major coronary artery that was relatively patent (<40% diameter stenosis) and that had not been subjected to an interventional procedure. Patients were enrolled if in the baseline study an abnormal re-

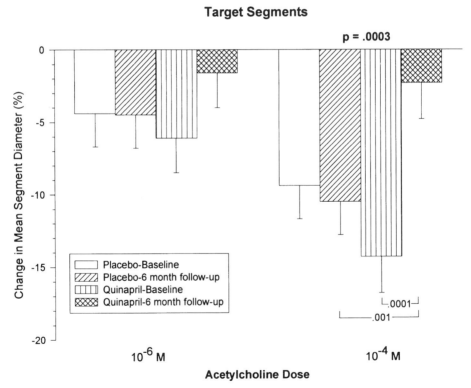

**Figure 1.** Percent changes in mean segment diameter in the target segment in each group at baseline and follow-up. Data are grouped on the basis of the concentration of ACh. At the lower dose, the quinapril group shows improvement (overall $P = 0.0003$). The constrictor response within the quinapril group at this dose level also is significantly improved ($P < 0.0001$), as is the difference in follow-up constrictive responses between the placebo and quinapril groups ($P < 0.001$). Reproduced with permission from Reference 9.

sponse (either frank constriction or lack of dilatation) could be documented by quantitative angiography. Thirteen patients within this cohort also were studied by using intracoronary Doppler flow wires to assess the effects on coronary blood flow velocity in response to both ACh and adenosine.[10] This was used to determine if quinapril had salutary effects on resistance vessels as well as epicardial vessels.

Figures 1 and 2 show the main results of TREND. In the target segments, at baseline, ACh induced a dose-related vasoconstrictor response that defined the presence and degree of endothelial dysfunction. After 6 months of double-blind, randomized therapy with placebo or oral quinapril at a dose of 40 mg/d, only the group assigned to quinapril showed improved responses to the ACh stimulation test. Less vasoconstriction was noted, implying improvement in the overall bioavailability of ACh-stimulated NO release. As expected, diameter or percent stenosis changes did not occur in the coronary arteries over the 6 months. In keeping with this, vascular sensitivity to NO donors (nitroglycerin) was not altered in either the placebo group or the quinapril group. Thus, the ACh effects appeared to be solely caused by alterations in endothelium-mediated pathways. Moreover, these effects were demonstrated in the absence of any major blood pressure or lipid changes. Of great interest is the observation that the differences between the groups were shown after cessation of the placebo or quinapril for an interval of 72 hours. It is conceivable that even greater effects would have been shown if the treatment group had been restudied while still ingesting quinapril.

The primary end point of the study was the net change in the diameter responses between baseline and follow-up. These results are shown in Figure 2. Positive net changes imply improvement in endothelial function and negative changes imply deterioration. The primary end point, based on analysis of

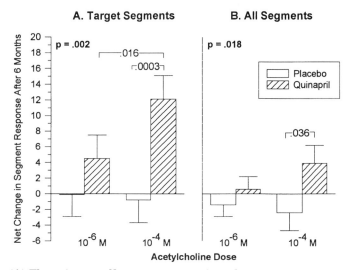

**Figure 2.** (**A**) The primary efficacy parameter (net change in segment response after 6 months in the target segment, expressed as percent ± SEM, plotted on *y* axis) for two concentrations of acetylcholine (ACh) (*x* axis). (**B**) Analysis of all segments. Reproduced with permission from Reference 9.

the target segments (ie, those constricting the most during the prerandomization, baseline ACh study) is positive, but so too is the more conservative analysis, which includes all segments, irrespective of the prerandomization response to ACh. At least a 5% improvement in target segment response was noted in 28% or 15/54 segments in the placebo group versus 53% or 27/51 segments in the quinapril group ($P < 0.008$). There also were multiple target segments that showed a baseline constrictor response, which at follow-up had reversed to a normal, dilatory response (7.1% or 3/42 segments in the placebo group versus 22% or 9/41 in the quinipril group, $P < 0.002$). Using stepwise regression analysis methods, we could not identify any clinical or demographic feature that predicted the positive results other than assignment to the active, quinapril arm of the trial.

Figure 3 shows the results of the substudy assessing the coronary microcirculation with the use of Doppler velocity measurements.[10] The placebo group showed no change in the ratio of ACh-stimulated flow expressed as a ratio of adenosine-stimulated flow (ie, endothelium-dependent flow vs nonendothelium-dependent flow). In contrast, the five patients randomized to quinapril showed an improvement in this measurement after 6 months of therapy. Thus, improved endothelial function at the microcirculatory level is improved in concert with the improvement of endothelial function noted in the conduit arteries.

As already stated, the only independent predictor of improved endothelial dysfunction in the TREND study was randomization to the active quinapril arm. Even so, data were reanalyzed with respect to patient subgroups to see if any new insights regarding mechanisms of action might arise. Figure 4 shows the response seen in smokers and nonsmokers.[11] ACE inhibition was effective in both groups. The improvement induced by quinapril in the smokers is accentuated mainly by the tendency toward net deterioration in the endothelial function that occurred over the 6 months in the smokers in the placebo

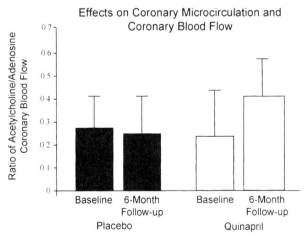

**Figure 3.** Results of a Doppler velocity substudy are demonstrated. Endothelium-mediated increases in flow were noted in the quinapril group but not the placebo group. Adapted with permission from Reference 10.

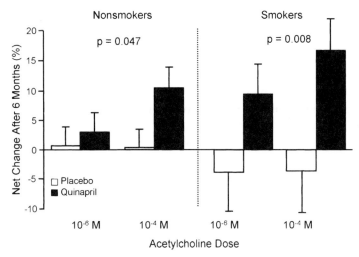

**Figure 4.** Efficacy of quinapril for improving endothelial dysfunction is shown in the same format as Figure 2. Quinapril responses were similar in both groups. However, there was a tendency in smokers to show some deterioration in endothelial function during the 6 month tudy. Adapted with permission from Reference 11.

group. No indication of rapid deterioration was noted in the placebo patients who were nonsmokers.

Pitt et al[12] examined the effects of quinapril on endothelial function stratified on the basis of the low-density lipoprotein (LDL) level, even though

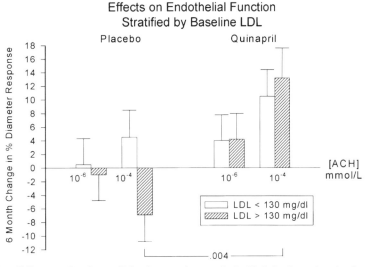

**Figure 5.** Efficacy of quinapril for improving endothelial dysfunction is shown in the same format as Figures 2 and 4. Quinapril shows similar efficacy irrespective of the level of low-density lopoprotein (LDL). However, patients in the placebo group with a higher LDL showed a tendency toward deterioration of endothelial function during the 6-month study. Adapted with permission from Reference 12.

these patients were not markedly hyperlipidemic. Figure 5 shows this analysis using an LDL value of 130 mg/dL to stratify the patients. This value is close to the median LDL value noted in the trial. Quinapril was equally effective in inducing a net improvement in the constrictor response, irrespective of the LDL level. However, as was the case with the smokers, the placebo patients with LDL 130 mg/dL showed a marked tendency toward deterioration of endothelial function during the 6 months of observation. At the high dose of ACh infusion, the difference between the placebo responses and the quinapril responses achieved statistical significance. Both the smoking and the LDL post hoc analyses suggest that even though quinapril is efficacious in both patient subsets, the presence of underlying risk factors may greatly enhance the ability to demonstrate the value of ACE inhibition in preserving or enhancing endothelial function. These findings are consistent with the notion that the impact of ACE inhibition in coronary patients may be modulated by the underlying absolute risk profile of the patient.

# Brachial Artery Normalization of Forearm Flow Study

Anderson and coworkers[13] recently have presented the results of the Brachial Artery Normalization of Forearm Flow (BANFF) study, which was an open-label, randomized trial in coronary patients with a similar profile as those reported in the TREND study. These investigators examined the effects of quinapril, enalapril, losartan, and amlodipine on flow-mediated dilatation of the brachial artery induced by brachial artery occlusion. In a crossover study, each patient was subjected to the study drugs in sequences lasting for 2 months per drug. After 2 months of therapy and even after discontinuation of the active drug for 72 hours before retesting, the quinapril group showed amelioration of endothelial dysfunction. In contrast, the other agents did not induce any significant improvement in flow-mediated, conduit artery dilatation. These results confirm the results of TREND in so far as quinapril was able to induce a measureable improvement in endothelial dysfunction even after cessation of the agent for 72 hours before retesting. Uniquely, improvements were achieved after only 2 months and at one-half the dose (20 mg) compared with the 6-month interval of therapy using 40 mg in TREND. Furthermore, enalapril at a dose of 10 mg/d was not effective. This raises important questions regarding the relative efficacy of differing ACE inhibitors in the clinical arena when used for the purpose of altering endothelial dysfunction. Unique pharmacodynamic properties of each agent may lead to consideration of different oral dosing levels to achieve these effects in patients. Moreover, the time at which testing is performed after dosing may influence results disparately when different agents are used. The TREND and BANFF studies suggest that quinapril can ameliorate endothelial function after chronic therapy with doses between 20–40 mg/d when assessed 72 hours after the last oral dose and provided that chronic therapy has been undertaken for at least 2 months. Whether enalapril or other agents would show similar results at higher doses, if earlier testing had been undertaken or if a more protracted treatment period had been selected, is unknown at this time.

## Angiotensin-Converting Enzyme Inhibitor Studies Using Other Endothelium-Modulated End Points in Coronary Patients

The endothelium plays a critical role in maintaining a thromboresistant, intimal surface. This feature has been assessed in some studies by measuring systemic levels of plasminogen activator inhibitor-1 (PAI-1) activity and antigen, tissue-plasminogen activator (tPA) activity, and von Willebrand factor and their responses to ACE inhibitors.[8] For example, Wright and coworkers[14] examined the fibrinolytic status of patients that had suffered an acute myocardial infarction 2 months earlier. Patients were treated in a randomized, double-blind, crossover protocol, which started with either placebo or captopril for 1 month before crossover to the alternate therapy. Measurements were made of tPA antigen as well as PAI-1 antigen and activity. Levels of these substances also were compared with values in normal men. The results indicated that captopril normalized the high values found in the coronary patients as compared with values seen in normal subjects.

More recently, Vaughan et al[15] reported the results in 120 subjects participating in the Healing And Early Afterload Reduction Therapy (HEART) study. This was a prospective, randomized, double-blind, placebo-controlled, parallel study. A placebo-treated group was compared with two ramipril-treated groups—one given 0.625 mg and the other given 10 mg of ramipril per day. After only 2 weeks of therapy, ramipril lowered the PAI-1 measurements but not the tPA measurements. Similarly, Oshima et al[16] showed that after acute myocardial infarction, imidapril given for 2 weeks induced a hastened reduction in PAI-1 activity as compared with levels seen in patients randomized to placebo. These studies are compatible with the notion that ACE inhibitors improve thromboresistant properties and these changes may be mediated at least in part through the effects of the ACE inhibitor on the endothelium. If this is the case, it may well be that other aspects of endothelial function, such as ACh-induced or shear-induced conduit vasodilatation also may have been improved within the 2 weeks of initiation of ACE inhibitor therapy. This conjecture is important to investigate because there may be significant time differences in the ability to detect change in endothelial function when differing index parameters are used.

## Establishing the Role of Angiotensin-Converting Enzyme Inhibition in Clinical Care of Uncomplicated Coronary Patients

Recently, Pepine has summarized the ongoing trials that are evaluating the role of ACE inhibitors in patients with coronary disease and preserved left ventricular function.[17,18] Ongoing quantitative coronary angiography studies, using outcomes that are based on ischemia detection, will assess various ACE inhibitors over the short to long term (0.5–5 years) in the following: (1) ambulatory monitoring, (2) B-mode ultrasound measures of progression of carotid intima medial thickness, and (3) progression of coronary artery disease. The question of whether ACE inhibitor therapy is superior to, additive to, or synergistic with concomitant therapy using antioxidants or lipid-lowering agents also will be addressed by some of these studies.

Clearly, however, clinical outcome trials will dictate clinical practice moreso than studies showing surrogate outcomes. Quinapril Ischemic Event Trial (QUIET) was a long-term study designed to monitor the incidence of ischemic events in uncomplicated coronary patients defined as per the TREND criteria.[19] The final ischemic event results of QUIET have not been published but they appear to be negative, possibly related to methodological problems such as a high rate of dropout, nonprotocol use of ACE inhibitors, and use of "soft" clinical end points. However, Cashin–Hemphill et al[20] have looked at the antiatherosclerotic effects of quinapril, which were examined in a subset of the patients enrolled in QUIET. This has been examined in relation to postangioplasty restenosis and also with respect to the underlying LDL level.[21] There were 453 angiographic substudy patients and 164 (36%) of them had restenosis. The rate of restenosis was the same in the placebo and in the treated group (78 patients in the quinapril arm and 86 in the placebo arm). The overall incidence of progression (defined as a 0.40-mm diminution in minimum lumen diameter in a diseased, nonintervened vessel) was the same in the patients that suffered restenosis as in the patients who had no restenosis, and it was not lessened by the use of quinapril. Of greater interest was the apparent effect of ambient LDL on the angiographic results. Figure 6 shows that the overall rate of progression in the placebo group was worse if LDL was ≥130 mg/dL. This rate of progression was significantly greater than the rate noted in patients with similarly increased LDL who were treated with quinapril. Thus, the ability to demonstrate the value of quinapril was modulated by the effect of LDL on the natural, absolute rate of progression of atherosclerosis.

Other clinical event studies, enrolling over 25 000 patients in aggregate currently are underway in uncomplicated coronary patients.[17,18] This database, in conjunction with the results from QUIET, will determine whether there is a definite role for ACE inhibition as secondary prevention therapy in uncomplicated coronary patients. These clinical end point studies will address the issue of additiveness, synergy, or superiority of combinations of ACE inhibitors with either antioxidants or lipid-lowering drugs.

This line of investigation provides an interesting parallel to lipid-lowering trials. In the lipid-lowering arena one of the most important outcomes has been the effect on reducing recurrent ischemic events early after aggressive lipid lowering at a time when few, if any, morphologic changes in the coronary tree would be contemplated. However, morphological changes are demonstrable 2 or 3 years later based on angiographic follow-up. These observations led to the speculation that lipid lowering could improve abruptly endothelial dysfunction to account for some of the early reduction in clinical events, whereas the longer term benefits on atheroma burden took place more slowly. Treasure[22] and

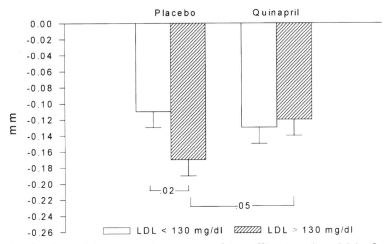

Change in Mean MLD Per Patient
Stratified by Baseline LDL

**Figure 6.** Angiographic progression measured in millimeters ($y$ axis) is shown. The segment minimum lumen diameter (MLD) was used to perform these analyses. Note the greater progression in the placebo group patients who have LDL $\geq$ 130 mg/dL. Quinapril was able to curtail this significantly whereas the less pronounced progression in the patients with very LDL was not improved by quinapril therapy. Adapted with permission from Reference 21.

Anderson[23] provide direct evidence that reversal of endothelial dysfunction can occur in the short term and that this phenomenon is likely to be of central importance in explaining both the short- and long-term clinical and angiographic benefits of aggressive lipid lowering. The same reasoning is applicable to ACE inhibitors but data to substantiate this are in a state of evolution.

In summary, the studies reviewed in detail in this chapter suggest that various aspects of endothelial function can be ameliorated with ACE inhibitor therapy in patients with relatively uncomplicated coronary disease, perhaps within a period of time as short as 2 weeks and sustainable for at least 6 months. Uncomplicated coronary patients—that is, those who do not have severe hyperlipidemia, CHF, uncontrolled hypertension, or diabetes with microalbuminuria—constitute a very large group. The clinical challenge is to determine whether such amelioration can be sustained for a longer period in these patients and whether a sustained effect can be correlated with an improvement in their clinical outcomes.

# References

1. Brown NJ, Vaughan DE. Angiotensin-converting enzyme inhibitors. *Circulation* 1998;97:1411–1420.
2. Yusuf S, Pepine CJ, Garces C, et al. Effect of enalapril on myocardial infarction and unstable angina in patients with low ejection fractions. *Lancet* 1992;340:1173–1178.
3. Rutherford JD, Pfeffer MA, Moyé LA, et al. Effects of captopril on ischemic events after myocardial infarction: Results of the Survival and Ventricular Enlargement Trial. *Circulation* 1994;90:1731–1738.

4. Lonn EM, Yusuf S, Jha P, et al. Emerging role of angiotensin-converting enzyme inhibitors in cardiac and vascular protection. *Circulation* 1994;90:2056–2069.

5. Flather MD, Kober L, Pfeffer MA, et al. Meta-analysis of individual patient data from trials of long-term ACE-inhibitor treatment after acute myocardial infarction (SAVE, AIRE, and TRACE Studies). *Circulation* 1997;98:I706. Abstract.

6. Mancini GBJ. Emerging concepts: Angiotensin-converting enzyme inhibition in coronary artery disease. *Cardiovasc Drugs Ther* 1996;10:609–612.

7. Mancini GBJ. Role of angiotensin-converting enzyme inhibition in reversal of endothelial dysfunction in coronary artery disease. *Am J Med* 1998;105(suppl A):40S–47S.

8. Drexler H. Endothelial dysfunction: Clinical Implications. *Prog Cardiovasc Dis* 1997;39:287–324.

9. Mancini GBJ, Henry GC, Macaya C, et al. Angiotensin-converting enzyme inhibition with quinapril improves endothelial vasomotor dysfunction in patients with coronary artery disease: The TREND (Trial on Reversing Endothelial Dysfunction) Study. *Circulation* 1996;94:258–265.

10. Schlaifer JD, Wargovich TJ, O'Neill B, et al. Effects of quinapril on coronary blood flow in coronary artery disease patients with endothelial dysfunction. *Am J Cardiol* 1997;80:1594–1597.

11. Schlaifer JD, Mancini GBJ, O'Neill BJ, et al. Influence of smoking status on angiotensin-converting enzyme inhibition-related improvement in coronary endothelial function. *Eur Heart J* 1997;18:15. Abstract.

12. Pitt B, Pepine C, O'Neill B, et al. Modulation of ACE inhibitor efficacy on coronary endothelial dysfunction by low density lipoprotein cholesterol. *J Am Coll Cardiol* 1997;29:70A. Abstract.

13. Anderson TJ, Overhiser RW, Haber H, et al. A comparative study of four antihypertensive agents on endothelial function in patients with coronary disease. *J Am Coll Cardiol* 1998;31(suppl A):327A.

14. Wright RA, Flapan AD, Alberti KGMM, et al. Effects of captopril therapy on endogenous fibrinolysis in men with recent uncomplicated myocardial infarction. *J Am Coll Cardiol* 1994;24:67–73.

15. Vaughan DE, Rouleau J-L, Ridker PM, et al. Effects of ramipril on plasma fibrinolytic balance in patients with acute anterior myocardial infarction. *Circulation* 1997;96:442–447.

16. Oshima S, Ogawa H, Mizuno Y, et al. The effects of the angiotensin-converting enzyme inhibitor imidapril on plasma plasminogen activator inhibitor activity in patients with acute myocardial infarction. *Am Heart J* 1997;134:961–966.

17. Pepine CJ. Ongoing clinical trials of angiotensin-converting enzyme inhibitors for treatment of coronary artery disease in patients with preserved left ventricular function. *J Am Coll Cardiol* 1966;27:1048–1052.

18. Pepine CJ. Potential role of angiotensin-converting enzyme inhibition in myocardial ischemia and current clinical trials. *Clin Cardiol* 1997;20(suppl II):58–64.

19. Lees RS, Pitt B, Chan RC, et al. Baseline clinical and angiographic data in the Quinapril Ischemic Event (QUIET) Trial. *Am J Cardiol* 1996;78:1011–1016.

20. Cashin-Hemphill L, Dinsmore RE, Chan RC, et al. Atherosclerosis progression in subjects with and without post-angioplasty restenosis in QUIET. *J Am Coll Cardiol* 1997;29:418A. Abstract.

21. Cashin-Hemphill L, Dinsmore RE, Chan RC, et al. LDL cholesterol and angiographic progression in the QUIET Trial. *J Am Coll Cardiol* 1997;29:85A. Abstract.

22. Treasure CB, Klein JL, Weintraub WS, et al. Beneficial effects of cholesterol-lowering therapy on the coronary endothelium in patients with coronary artery disease. *N Engl J Med* 1995;332:481–487.

23. Anderson TJ, Meredith IT, Yeung AC, et al. The effect of cholesterol-lowering and antioxidant therapy on endothelium-dependent coronary vasomotion. *N Engl J Med* 1995;332:488–493.

## Chapter 22

# Nitrate Therapy in Cardiovascular Disease

*Jonathan Abrams, MD*

## Introduction

Nitroglycerin (NTG) and the long-acting nitrates have been prescribed by physicians for over a century. The earliest report of NTG for the treatment of angina pectoris by Murrell occurred in 1879; initially, isoamyl nitrate had been used by Brunton some years earlier. NTG was synthesized first by Sobrero and was used subsequently by Alfred Nobel in the munitions industry in the late 19th century. Nitrates enjoyed considerable popularity in the United States during the early part of this century as part of the homeopathic tradition, nicely discussed in an historical overview by Fye.[1] Although these drugs were used initially for angina pectoris, when synthetic long-acting nitrates became available these agents were administered for the treatment of hypertension; however, it is unlikely that oral nitrates could be very beneficial in hypertension because of attenuation or tolerance to the systolic blood pressure–lowering effects of these agents, a phenomenon documented by Crandall in 1931.[2] Nevertheless, a French study suggested that these drugs may be effective for systolic hypertension of the elderly.[3]

### The Modern Era

Nitrate therapy encountered major ups and downs in the 1960s and 1970s. Needleman[4] had an important negative influence on the acceptance of long-acting oral nitrate compounds; by extending his observations in rats to humans, he suggested that oral nitrate therapy could not be effective clinically, because rapid hepatic metabolism of orally administered nitrates would preclude achieving therapeutic blood levels. However, these agents continued to be prescribed, and when transdermal NTG was introduced in the early 1980s, interest in nitrate therapy was enhanced considerably. Furthermore, nitrates were administered in the early development of vasodilator therapy for congestive heart failure and were found to be effective.[5] Thus, by the mid-1980s,

From Panza JA, Cannon RO III (eds): *Endothelium, Nitric Oxide, and Atherosclerosis* ©Futura Publishing Co, Inc, Armonk, NY, 1999.

long-acting nitrates enjoyed considerable popularity as well as a resurgence of physician acceptance that they were useful clinically.

The last 15 years have been characterized by the development of new nitrate formulations [isosorbide 5-mononitrate (ISMN or 5-ISMN); transmucosal, transdermal, and oral spray NTG; commercially available intravenous NTG; and in Europe, intravenous isosorbide dinitrate (ISDN)], and the recognition that nitrate tolerance to continued or repetitive nitrate administration is a common phenomenon and can interfere clearly with the clinical benefits of these drugs. A great deal of controversy has been engendered by the tolerance issue, and it took a number of years for investigators, clinicians, and industry to come to the mutual conclusion that attenuation or tolerance to the beneficial effects of nitrates in patients with angina pectoris or congestive heart failure is a major problem. Most well-designed contemporary studies of nitrate tolerance have demonstrated consistently loss of effectiveness of nitrates when these drugs are administered in a tolerance-inducing fashion. Thus, sustained administration of transdermal NTG patches, intravenous NTG, or frequent doses of oral long-acting nitrates readily result in a decrease in nitrate effects, often with complete abolition of hemodynamic action.[6] Very recent data, in fact, suggest that in the presence of nitrate tolerance, there actually may be a vasoconstrictor milieu in the coronary vasculature that could have adverse consequences in patients with coronary artery disease.[7] Furthermore, it has been established that during the nitrate-free interval with intermittent NTG patch therapy, there is a possibility of rebound vasoconstriction that could be important clinically. Episodes of patch-off nocturnal angina, reduction of early morning exercise test performance (the 0-hour effect), and an increase in angina have been demonstrated,[8] although these are not always observed and remain somewhat controversial. A preliminary report suggests that chronic therapy with iISDN may be detrimental in postmyocardial infarction (post-MI)-subjects.[9]

During the 1980s and 1990s, the use of organic nitrates for the acute coronary syndromes of MI and unstable angina expanded greatly in the United States and around the world. Although the limited data in unstable angina are positive, there are relatively few randomized placebo-controlled studies assessing nitrate efficacy in this clinical syndrome. Nevertheless, the most current guidelines call for the routine use of intravenous NTG in hospitalized patients with unstable angina, and this is the accepted clinical approach throughout the United States and Canada. A number of older studies utilizing intravenous NTG during acute MI (AMI) in animals and humans stimulated considerable interest, suggesting that NTG may reduce morbidity and even mortality in this setting.[10,11] An influential meta-analysis suggested a substantial survival advantage when intravenous NTG was administered early in AMI.[12] Limited data also suggested a favorable effect on left ventricular (LV) remodeling in the postinfarction state.[11,13] These observations led to the inclusion of a nitrate arm in two European megatrials, the Fourth International Study of Infarct Survival (ISIS-4) and Gruppo Italiano per lo Studio Della Sopravvivenza nell' Infarcto Miocardico (GISSI 3).[14,15] Unfortunately, although these studies are flawed (primarily because of the widespread use of open-label nitrates in patients not given nitrate by protocol), no benefit was found for routine nitrate

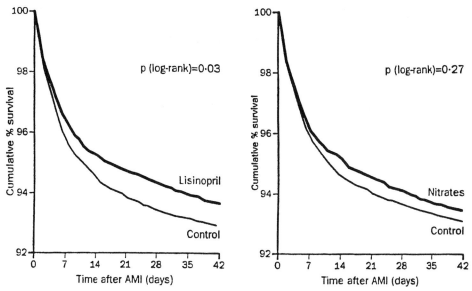

**Figure 1.** Six-week survival in lisinopril, nitrate, and respective controls in 19,000 patients admitted with MI. Reproduced with permission from Reference 15.

administration beginning in the first 24 hours after infarction and continuing for 5–6 weeks. No harm was noted, and there was a trend toward benefit, although somewhat less than that for the administration of angiotensin-converting enzyme (ACE) inhibitors in the same study population[14,15] (Figure 1). The GISSI-3 investigators also reported a significant early survival advantage with the combination of an ACE inhibitor and a nitrate.[15]

Over the past 5 years, the major advances of nitrate therapy have focused on the conundrum of nitrate tolerance (see following text). A wide variety of basic and clinical investigations have been carried out to examine how and why blood vessels lose their responsiveness to organic nitrates on repetitive or continued nitrate administration. The most promising recent hypotheses regarding nitrate tolerance include endothelial cell production of oxygen free-radical anions, as well as enhanced vascular smooth muscle cell sensitivity to a variety of endogenous vasoconstrictors. Nevertheless, the only practical way to diminish or eliminate the appearance of nitrate tolerance is to use a dosing regimen that includes a nitrate-free interval of 10–14 hours, as well appropriate use of nitrate formulations, to avoid continued exposure of vascular smooth muscle to administered nitrate over a 24-hour period. The downside of this approach is that it leaves the patient unprotected from the beneficial actions of nitrates for a period of up to 12 hours; furthermore, there is the possibility of rebound vasoconstriction, particularly with intermittent NTG patch therapy.[7,8]

## Clinical Status of Nitrates

There is considerable agreement as to the cardiovascular syndromes for which nitrates are beneficial (Table 1). Nitrate therapy for AMI and congestive

**Table 1**
**Clinical Indications for Nitrates**

| Condition | Comments |
|---|---|
| • Acute attacks of angina pectoris | Highly effective |
| • Prophylaxis of chronic stable angina | Comparable efficacy to calcium and beta blockers. Tolerance a problem |
| • Unstable angina | NTG very useful |
| • AMI | |
|   -Control of chest pain and ischemia | Often effective: use sublingual, intravenous NTG. Caution to avoid hypotension |
|   -Hypertension, acute heart failure | Very useful; intravenous or high-dose topical |
|   -Routine 24–48 hour infusion of intravenous NTG | Little positive data; consider in large anterior MI |
| • Post-MI left ventricular remodeling | Limited positive data. Uncertain benefits |
| • Chronic congestive heart failure | Useful adjunct to ACE inhibitors—can use with hydralazine. Consider for all symptomatic subjects on ACE inhibitors and digitalis |
| • Acute heart failure/pulmonary edema | Highly effective—especially intravenous NTG |
| • Hypertension | Useful in intravenous formulation. Limited positive data in systolic hypertension of the elderly in oral formulation |

Reproduced with permission from Reference 43.

heart failure remains a subject of some disagreement. Stable angina pectoris remains to be the most common condition for which nitrates are administered.

# Pharmacology of Organic Nitrates

Although a variety of organic nitrate compounds have been utilized over the years, at the present time only three nitrate moieties are recommended for use in the United States. These are NTG, ISDN, and fISMN or 5-ISMN, all available in a variety of formulations (Table 2). Older compounds, such as pentaerythritol tetranitrate, rarely are used in clinical practice. Furthermore, oral NTG capsules, in vogue for many decades, virtually have no clinical trial support for efficacy, and although still available in some pharmacies, should not be prescribed.

## Nitroglycerin

NTG, the classic nitrate, is available in many formulations. The NTG molecule is rather malleable, allowing for transdermal, oral, submucosal, and intravenous administration. NTG has a very rapid half-life of 1.5–2 minutes.

Table 2
**Nitrate Formulations: Dosing Recommendations and Pharmacokinetic**

|  | Usual Dose (mg) | Onset of Action (mins) | Effective Duration of Action |
|---|---|---|---|
| Sublingual NTG | 0.3–0.6 | 2–5 | 20–30 mins |
| Sublingual ISDN | 2.5–10.0 | 5–20 | 45–120 mins |
| Buccal NTG | 1–3 pm or tid | 2–5 | 30–300 mins* |
| Oral ISDN | 10–60 bid-tid | 15–45 | 2–6 h |
| Oral ISDN-SR | 80–120 once daily | 60–90 | 10–14 h |
| Oral ISMN | 20 bid[†] | 30–60 | 3–6 h |
| Oral ISMN-SR | 60–120 once daily | 60–90 | 10–14 h |
| NTG ointment | 0.5–2.0 inch tid | 15–60 | 3–8 h |
| NTG patch | 0.4–0.8 mg/h[‡] | 30–60 | 8–12 h |

Therefore, if long-acting or prophylactic administration is required, topical, transmucosal, or oral sustained release dosing is necessary.

## Isosorbide Dinitrate

This popular compound has been utilized worldwide for decades. It is highly effective; numerous clinical trials have used ISDN and have demonstrated convincingly efficacy in patients with angina pectoris as well as congestive heart failure. ISDN has a half-life of 40–80 minutes and should be administered no more than 2–3 times daily, dosing in standard formulation. ISDN is metabolized in blood vessels and the liver to two compounds, the 2-ISMN and 5-ISMN molecules. The latter is active pharmacologically, representing perhaps 50% of the overall hemodynamic effect of an administered dose of ISDN. The potency of the 2-ISMN molecule is uncertain and probably is modest. When ISDN is given in any formulation, most of the early effects, perhaps the first 30–90 minutes, are likely to be related to the parent compound itself. By 1–2 hours, plasma concentrations of 5-ISMN are increasing, and it is believed that this metabolite is responsible for the sustained or late effects following ISDN administration. ISDN is manufactured in a variety of formulations (see Table 2); in Europe, oral spray and intravenous ISDN are available, and in Japan, an ISDN plastic wrap has been used.

When ISDN is administered orally, there is extensive hepatic first-pass clearance of the compound, resulting in no more than 20%–25% bioavailability of ISDN itself. This has led to the mistaken impression that ISDN may not be an effective compound, whereas this formulation is quite active; its pharmacologic actions are derived from ISDN itself (early effects) as well as the 5-ISMN metabolite (later effects).

## 5-Isosorbide Mononitrate

This synthetic molecule has enjoyed considerable popularity in the United States since its initial release in standard formulation. More recently, an extended release tablet has become available for once daily dosing. The latter probably is the ideal oral nitrate on the market; administration produces rapidly rising plasma concentrations, which taper off over a 24-hour period, resulting in low plasma concentrations 18–24 hours after administration. This decrease in nitrate plasma levels is sufficient to provide for a nitrate-responsive vasculature and the avoidance of nitrate tolerance. 5-ISMN is completely bioavailable; plasma concentrations after dosing demonstrate much less scatter than with oral ISDN. This pharmokinetic profile makes the formulation quite attractive for clinical use. However, there are no data suggesting a greater clinical efficacy for 5-ISMN as opposed to ISDN in either standard or sustained release formulation. The half-life of 5-ISMN is 5–6 hours; it is believed that this compound is responsible for the prolonged effects of both ISDN and 5-ISMN.

Table 2 summarizes pertinent pharmacologic features of available short- and long-acting nitrates.

## Evolution Of Nitrate Therapy

The standard clinical uses for organic nitrates are listed in Table 1. The major role for these compounds is the acute treatment of chest pain or anginal attacks (sublingual, oral spray, transmucosal NTG; sublingual ISDN or prophylactic/preventive long-acting nitrate therapy for chronic angina pectoris). Numerous placebo-controlled trials have demonstrated efficacy of oral or topical nitrates in patients with stable angina, with an increase in overall exercise duration as well as time to chest pain and/or ischemia compared with placebo in the absence of nitrate tolerance[16] (Figure 2). Several recent clinical experiments utilizing sophisticated technology, such as positron emission testing tomography (PET) or quantitative thallium imaging, have documented objective evidence for decreased myocardial ischemia in patients with stable angina pectoris[17,18] (Figure 3). Intravenous NTG remains the drug of choice for the therapy of unstable angina, in conjunction with aspirin and heparin. The clinical usefulness of intravenous NTG is well known to physicians who work in emergency rooms or intensive care units and care for patients with acute coronary syndromes.

The role of organic nitrates in AMI remains somewhat uncertain. During the midlate 1980s and early 1990s, it was believed that intravenous NTG and possibly other nitrate formulations were effective in decreasing morbidity and even mortality when given early during AMI.[10–12] However, the European trials ISIS-4 and GISSI-3 appeared to have quenched enthusiasm for the routine administration of a nitrate in MI[14,15] (Figure 1). Data in animals and humans suggest that nitrates are effective in preventing or attenuating the LV cavity expansion, known as remodeling, that often occurs after large or transmural infarction.[11,13,19] However, there is a relatively limited database confirming benefit in this situation. At present, an ACE inhibitor is the drug of choice to prevent LV remodeling, whereas nitrates are a reasonable alternative for patients who cannot tolerate these drugs. The effectiveness of a nitrate and

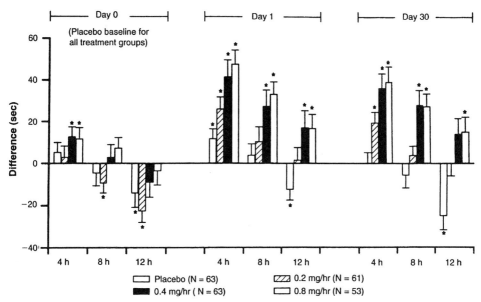

**Figure 2.** Intermittent transdermal NTG therapy. Change in treadmill walking time (mean ± SEM) to moderate angina compared with hour 0. Single-blind placebo patch application on day 0; double-blind patch application on days 1 and 30. *$P \leq 0.04$ (compared with hour 0). Note three different doses of active patch versus placebo. Reproduced with permission from Reference 36.

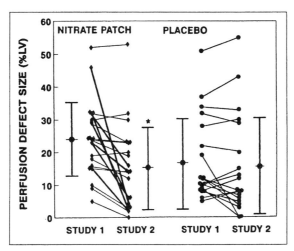

**Figure 3.** NTG patch efficacy in reducing exercise-induced ischemia in patients with angina. Mean and individual patient changes in exercise-induced LV perfusion defects from study 1 (baseline placebo patch) to study 2 (active nitrate vs placebo patch). NTG patch therapy significantly reduced the mean quantitative thallium perfusion defect size compared with placebo therapy (*$P = 0.04$). Bold lines indicate the seven patients receiving active patch therapy who reduced their perfusion defect size by ≥10% (absolute). Reproduced with permission from Reference 17.

ACE inhibitor together on post-MI remodeling is unknown; a recent study confirms modest benefits in subjects receiving both an ACE inhibitor and NTG patch therapy.[19] Left ventricular functions were better with combination therapy in GISSI-3[15]

# Mechanisms of Action

## Hemodynamic

The organic nitrates act primarily through vasodilatation of the vasculature, including the veins, arteries, and arterioles.[20] Resistance vessel relaxation is seen only at very high nitrate concentrations. There is considerable evidence, but no clinical proof, that nitrates also exert their favorable actions by interfering with platelet aggregation and the subsequent development of thrombus. The vasodilation induced by the organic nitrates is greatest in the venous or capacitance circulation. In fact, many physicians incorrectly believe that nitrates do not have a dilating effect on the arteries. An interesting observation from Australia suggests that brachial artery measurements of arterial pressure actually may underestimate the effects of nitrates on central aortic pressure because of the failure of the administered nitrate to diminish sufficiently the peripheral reflectance wave of arterial pulse transmission.[21] In any case, reduction in LV preload (decreased LV cavity size, decreased LV diastolic, and systolic pressure) and afterload (decreased systemic resistance, decreased arterial systolic pressure, and decreased LV size) results in a smaller heart operating at lower systolic and diastolic pressures with reduced LV wall stress or afterload. Thus, myocardial oxygen demands are decreased. At the same time, nutrient coronary blood flow may be enhanced through direct epicardial coronary artery vasodilatation, coronary artery stenosis dilatation, enlargement of coronary collaterals with enhanced collateral flow, and a reduction in LV diastolic pressure, all of which could improve coronary artery flow to zones of ischemia. Although the major efficacy of nitrates probably is caused by decreased myocardial oxygen consumption, one cannot rule out nitrate-induced increases in regional coronary blood flow to prevent or relieve myocardial ischemia in subsets of patients with stable angina or acute coronary syndromes.

## Cellular

NTG and the organic nitrates essentially are pro-drugs that are converted enzymatically to nitric oxide (NO) in the cytoplasm of vascular smooth muscle cells and platelets[22] (Figure 4). The enzyme(s) responsible for conversion of the parent molecule to NO have not been characterized fully; this occurs near the plasma membrane of the cell. The biotransformation of the parent nitrate moiety to NO appears to be a direct process, although prior views of the biochemical conversion process have implicated a variety of intermediate products, including the production of nitrosothiols. Nitrosothiols may be a

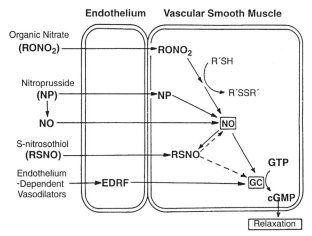

**Figure 4.** Nitrovasodilators, endothelium-dependent vasodilators, and vascular smooth muscle relaxation.Abbreviations: EDRF, endothelium-derived relaxing factor; GC, guanylate cyclase; GTP, guanosine triphosphate; NO, nitric oxide; R′SH and RSH, two distinct pools of intracellular sulfhydryl groups; R′SSR′, disulfide groups. Reproduced with permission from Reference 22.

byproduct of intracellular nitrate metabolism; these compounds can directly generate NO. NO activates the enzyme guanylate cyclase, responsible for the conversion of guanosine triphosphate to cyclic guanosine monophosphate (cGMP). The cGMP is a second messenger responsible for orchestrating the intracellular actions of administered nitrate, including vascular vasodilatation and antiaggregatory effects in platelets. Vascular smooth muscle relaxation occurs as a result of transient decreases in intracellular calcium ion, triggered by increases in GMP. The conversion of organic nitrates to NO is more active in veins as opposed to arteries, and uptake of nitrate by venous tissue is greater than in the arterial wall;[23] this presumably accounts for the potent venodilating capacity of organic nitrates. At high doses and concentrations, nitrates may relax the arteriolar or resistance vessels.

Japanese investigators have utilized a platelet assay of cGMP and demonstrated correlation of platelet cGMP levels and the physiological effects of administered nitrate.[24] They have used this assay to assess various strategies to prevent or reverse nitrate tolerance and recently have demonstrated that in the presence of nitrate tolerance, platelet cGMP concentrations are reduced, concordant with a decrease in vasodilator responses to nitrates in coronary arteries.[24] Recent experiments by Watanabe et al as well as others,[25–29] suggest that vitamin C and vitamin E may prevent nitrate tolerance, presumably through antioxidant actions. However, one preliminary report was unable to prevent tolerance with vitamin C.[30] More work clearly is required in this area.

Other NO donors, such as sodium nitroprusside and synthetic nitrosothiols, release NO primarily through nonenzymatic mechanisms and actually may be more potent than NTG with respect to vasodilation and the rapidity of onset. There are differences among the various nitrovasodilators with respect to the amount of NO that can be generated from different compounds. There is little evidence that nitroprusside induces vascular tolerance, suggesting that the direct release of NO from this compound may offer clues as to the mechanism(s) of tolerance.

## Platelet Effects

It has been known for some time that NTG and other organic nitrates have antiplatelet activity. Initially, this was somewhat controversial, because published data were inconsistent. Discrepancies among studies may have been caused in part by problems related to assay methods used to assess platelet aggregation. Most recently, there has been convincing evidence that nitrates impair the aggregation of platelets and the development of platelet thrombus.[31–33] In the Folts dog model, nitrates decrease cyclic flow variations by diminishing the thrombus burden.[32] Thus, in ex vivo systems, organic nitrates interfere with normal platelet action. Although it is difficult to establish that these observations are relevant to patients with coronary artery disease, it is reasonable to speculate that the efficacy of intravenous NTG in unstable angina in part is caused by decreasing the platelet-thrombus burden. Recent uncontrolled and preliminary data suggest that patients taking long-acting nitrates who subsequently develop an acute coronary syndrome may be more likely to manifest unstable angina as opposed to AMI,[34] indicating that chronic NTG use may favorably modify the platelet-thrombotic process that contributes to AMI. Thus, erosion or fissuring of vulnerable plaque may be more likely to result in a nonobstructive clot, resulting in unstable angina or non-Q MI. More data are required to confirm this hypothesis.

# Clinical Use of Nitrates

## Stable Angina Pectoris

Sublingual NTG remains the worldwide gold standard for treatment or prevention of acute attacks of angina pectoris. The extremely rapid onset of effect correlates with abolition of chest pain, which typically begins within several minutes after sublingual NTG administration. Oral NTG spray is a reliable alternative to sublingual tablets. Although sublingual ISDN has been used to treat angina, it has a significantly slower onset of action (although a longer duration of activity) and therefore should not be used for urgent therapy of angina. All of these short-acting formulations are useful for angina prophylaxis; thus, individuals with relatively predictable anginal discomfort during a specific activity may decrease the likelihood of or eliminate an anginal attack by taking a short-acting nitrate several minutes prior to engaging in physical exertion, such as golfing, sex, climbing stairs, etc.

Long-acting nitrates are prescribed by physicians throughout the world to prevent or decrease anginal episodes in patients with chronic stable angina. A multiplicity of exercise studies have demonstrated consistently increased exercise duration and augmented time to chest pain and onset of ischemic ST changes with long-acting nitrates.[8,16,17,35–37] (Figures 2 and 3) Unfortunately, nitrate tolerance will eliminate this benefit when nitrates are taken in an inappropriate fashion, such as the continuous application of transdermal NTG or four times daily oral ISDN.[6,35]

There are limited data to suggest that nitrates are either less or more effective than β-blockers or calcium channel antagonists for the prevention of angina. Individuals who demonstrate a typical response to sublingual NTG should be given a long-acting nitrate to control angina attack rates, either as monotherapy or in combination with a β-adrenergic blocker or calcium antagonist. Some have suggested that nitrates should not be used as monotherapy because of the problem of tolerance and absence of protective coverage during the nocturnal nitrate-free interval. I do not agree, and successfully have used nitrates as the only antianginal agent in a large number of patients who have relatively infrequent stable angina. It is common for physicians to underdose nitrates (as well as other antianginal agents); thus, it is important to push nitrate dosage to the limit of side effects to control the anginal syndrome. On the other hand, larger doses are more likely to induce nitrate tolerance.

Combination antianginal therapy is used commonly in patients with chronic stable angina, although only limited data confirms the efficacy of utilizing two or three different drugs together. The combined use of nitrates with a β-blocker is particularly attractive, in that the two agents complement each other; β-blockers attenuate the tachycardia induced by nitrates, whereas nitrates may diminish the negative contractility effects of β-blockers, as well as a propensity toward LV enlargement. Nitrates can be used with calcium channel blockers, although the use of two potent hypotensive agents together can cause problems in some patients. Nitrates should be considered for individuals who appear to have episodes of coronary vasoconstriction or spasm, which may be suggested by frequent rest pain, variable angina threshold, emotion-related angina, and nocturnal symptoms. These agents should be considered for postinfarction angina. Several recent studies have documented objective evidence of decreased ischemia in patients with coronary disease and angina with the use of an NTG patch. Using PET, a Canadian group has demonstrated beneficial metabolic alterations in zones of myocardial ischemia.[18] An exercise study from Baylor College of Medicine utilizing quantitative thallium imaging demonstrated a decrease in the total size of the induced ischemic defect with a 0.4-mg NTG patch[17] (Figure 3). These data are reassuring, confirming the results of a large number of exercise testing studies, and are concordant with the multiplicity of actions by which organic nitrates decrease myocardial ischemia. The mechanisms of angina induction may be different from one patient to the next; the diverse effects of nitrates offer a variety of mechanisms of action that can decrease or prevent ischemia.

## Unstable Angina Pectoris

Although relatively few studies utilizing nitrates for unstable angina are available, several older trials have been positive.[38,39] The polypharmacy typically used in unstable angina has increased over the years and now includes aspirin, heparin, IIb-IIIa platelet receptor inhibitors, intravenous NTG, and often the use of a β-blocker and/or calcium channel agent. Physicians who treat individuals with acute coronary syndromes are well aware of the predictable effect of intravenous NTG in controlling rest angina. Concerns have been raised regarding a possible heparin-intravenous NTG interaction.[40] Our recent review of the existing data has lead us to conclude that this is not an important issue.[41] Intravenous NTG should be used promptly in patients with unstable angina and gradually tapered as the syndrome comes under control; the infusion rate can be rapidly increased or decreased. Although one must presume that nitrate tolerance will occur with the continuous infusion of NTG, there are limited data documenting this. Nevertheless, it is imperative that physicians do not abruptly discontinue an intravenous NTG infusion because of theoretical concerns about tolerance. Rebound vasoconstriction and recurrence of chest pain is common when intravenous NTG is stopped suddenly. In patients who are responsive to intravenous NTG, conversion to oral or topical nitrates can begin within the first 24−48 hours of admission or when the syndrome appears to be under control.

## Acute Myocardial Infarction

Intravenous NTG is used commonly during the first 24–36 hours of an AMI. Older human and animal data have documented significant reductions in ST segment elevation and infarct size with NTG when administered early in AMI.[10,11,13] Furthermore, a number of these studies appeared to confirm a beneficial effect of nitrates on morbidity and mortality in AMI.[10,12] A meta-analysis published in 1988 suggested a substantial survival benefit in patients treated with intravenous NTG.[12] In addition, data from Jugdutt and colleagues in animals and humans have indicated a benefit in LV remodeling when nitrates are used during the early hours after AMI.[11,13] Although there are clear-cut indications for nitrate use in AMI (Table 3), the promise of increased survival and/or decreased morbidity suggested by the earlier trials and the meta-analysis has dissipated with publication of the European megatrials, ISIS-4 and GISSI-3.[14,15] These studies were undertaken because of the favorable nitrate data cited above; the trials enrolled in the aggregate of 77,000 subjects, but were unable to confirm a benefit for the routine administration of a nitrate beginning in the first 24 hours of AMI and continuing for 5–6 weeks. There was a favorable trend for those individuals receiving nitrates, which was not statistically significant, although only slightly less beneficial than an ACE inhibitor (Figure 1). In the Italian trial, the combination of nitrates and an ACE inhibitor substantially reduced early and late mortality.[15,42] No individual subsets, such as anterior infarction, appeared to benefit from nitrates. The conclusion derived from this enormous database is that standard or routine therapy with nitrates beginning early in the infarct period and extending for 5–6 weeks does not alter the natural history of AMI. Nevertheless, it is common for physicians to use intravenous NTG in this setting. Furthermore, it should be pointed out that in the European trials, nonstudy use of nitrates

Table 3
**Indications for Nitrates in Acute Myocardial Infarction**

Established
  Relief of acute chest pain and/ or myocardial ischemia
  Prophylaxis and treatment of recurrent chest pain and/or ischemia
  Treatment of pulmonary edema and congestive heart failure
  Rapid control of hypertension (intravenous NTG)
Unproven
  Routine or prophylactic administration to reduce morbidity and mortality
  Selected use in extensive, anterior or recurrent MI
  Reduction of severity of mitral regurgitation
Note
  Intravenous NTG is the preferred formulation
  Avoid hypertension. Do not use instead of narcotics for infarction pain.
  Extreme caution in inferior MI, especially with right ventricular involvement

exceeded 50%, attenuating the chances of detecting a favorable effect of nitrate therapy. It is possible that intravenous NTG could be beneficial in large infarctions accompanied by extensive myocardial damage, as suggested by the early trials, which were undertaken before the advent of routine aspirin and thrombolytic therapy. Furthermore, the widespread use of ACE inhibitors after AMI, even for low-risk subsets, could minimize a substantive role for nitrates to prevent LV remodeling. Although the data from GISSI-3 in patients given a nitrate and an ACE inhibitor suggest a favorable effect on preventing LV damage as well as cavity expansion,[15,42] a specific recommendation to use nitrates for this purpose cannot be made; however, a recent report is consistent of benefit with this combination.[19]

In conclusion, nitrate therapy, particularly intravenous NTG, in the setting of AMI remains clinically indicated for a variety of indications (see Table 3). Recently published American College of Cardiology—American Heart Association (ACC—AHA) guidelines for the treatment of AMI support the use of intravenous NTG. However, there are no convincing data to support a routine prophylactic policy of nitrate administration to decrease morbidity or mortality. If used carefully, avoiding central hypotension, nitrate therapy is safe in the setting of AMI, although it must be used with caution, particularly in right ventricular infarction or subjects with borderline hypotension.

## Congestive Heart Failure

Although the Food and Drug Administration has never approved nitrates for use in heart failure, there is considerable published experience utilizing these agents for acute and chronic heart failure.[5,43–47] The most important effect of nitrates in symptomatic congestive heart failure is a predictable decrease in LV preload, with reductions in left atrial pressure as well as a decrease in pulmonary artery and right atrial pressures. The arterial (and at high doses, arteriolar) dilating effects of these agents "unload" the left ventricule, which is beneficial in the setting of LV systolic impairment. Thus, in contradistinction to the normal circulation where nitrate administration lowers stroke volume and cardiac output, in the presence of heart failure and a decreased ejection fraction, nitrates may increase stroke volume. This fact is not well recognized by clinicians.

Large doses of nitrates are required to induce vascular relaxation in heart failure. I believe that nitrates should be considered as adjunctive therapy for patients with heart failure who have not had an optimal response to ACE inhibitors and diuretics. A tolerance-avoidance regimen should be used. Finally, the Veterans Administration Heart Failure Trials (V-HeFT) have confirmed a survival advantage with the combination of ISDN and hydralazine in patients with moderate heart failure.[46,47] Although it is possible that hydralazine was responsible for some or all of the benefits in this trial, most experts believe that the nitrate (ISDN) was the key agent. Recent preliminary data suggest that hydralazine may prevent nitrate tolerance,[48] an intriguing observation that needs confirmation by larger studies.

# Problems with Nitrate Therapy

One of the major attributes of NTG and long-acting nitrates is the familiarity physicians have had with these agents over many decades. There are very few drug interactions. Other than hypotension, there is no serious adverse effect known related to the use of nitrates. Withdrawal of nitrates, particularly high-dose and/or intravenous NTG administration, may lead to a rebound vasoconstrictor state. Limited observations suggest a decreased angina threshold as well as a propensity for patch-off angina during the nitrate-free period while the NTG patches have been removed;[8] this has not been noted in all studies.[36] Older literature relating to the industrial use or manufacture of NTG compounds suggests that rebound vasoconstriction is a potential problem.[49] Clinically, such events are very uncommon. Most recently, an important interaction with organic nitrates and sildenafil (Viagra) has been documented, whereas sildenafil can potentiate significantly nitrate hypotension.[50,51] Sildenafil, a phosphodiesterase-5 inhibitor, may result in substantial enhancement of nitrate-induced hypotension. This compound presumably augments vascular cGMP concentrations, which, in conjunction with nitrate stimulation of guanylate cyclase and a resultant increase in cGMP production, induces sustained and robust vascular relaxation. Sildenafil is contraindicated absolutely in individuals who use organic nitrates, including sublingual NTG.[52]

The other major problem regarding nitrate therapy is the rapid development of attenuation or tolerance to nitrate actions. Recognition that nitrate tolerance is a relevant clinical issue dates back to no more than 15–20 years. It is now generally accepted that to avoid nitrate tolerance, a carefully prescribed dosing strategy must be employed, with a prolonged nitrate-free interval on a daily basis. The search for the mechanism(s) responsible for nitrate tolerance has preoccupied investigators for many years and, as of this writing,

Table 4
**Problems with Nitrate Therapy**

| | |
|---|---|
| • Headache | Common |
| • Nausea, vomiting | Uncommon |
| • Dizziness, presyncope | Occasional |
| • Hypotension | Occasional |
| • Exaggerated hypotensive response when used with Sildenafil (Viagra) | |
| • Possible heparin-intravenous NTG interaction | |
| • Nitrate tolerance | |
| • Rebound coronary vasoconstriction | |

it remains uncertain as to how precisely nitrate tolerance is initiated and sustained. A promising new hypothesis suggests that increased free-radical production by endothelial cells is induced in the presence of tolerance, and may be related causally to attenuation of nitrate hemodynamic effects.[53] In this setting, augmented vasoconstrictor responses to angiotensin II (Ang II), norepinephrine, and endothelin (ET) occur within the vascular wall.[53,54] A coronary angiography study appears to support this concept.[7] One recent study confirmed that captopril was able to block tolerance-induced supersensitivity to vasoconstrictors in patients with coronary artery disease.[55] Recent investigations have emphasized a potential role for antioxidants to prevention tolerance.[25–29] It is still too early to know whether this approach will be effective clinically; one study utilizing oral vitamin C was negative.[30]

Table 4 lists the common problems related to nitrate therapy.

## Side Effects

The major side effect of nitrates is the common appearance of headache, particularly in patients who have not been exposed previously to nitrates. The headache may be mild to severe: nitrate headaches limit the ability of approximately 15%–20% of individuals to tolerate these drugs. In general, as patients use these drugs over longer periods of time, the headache tends to disappear. The use of aspirin or acetaminophen may be useful. In addition, nausea and vomiting are seen occasionally. Importantly, significant hypotension, particularly in the upright position, in patients initially exposed to NTG may be a problem, resulting in dizziness, presyncope, and even overt fainting spells. The sildenafil interaction, discussed above, has become a critical matter for men with coronary disease who have erectile dysfunction and use nitrates. A vagally mediated paradoxic bradycardia with sublingual NTG has been observed, and may contribute to the hypotension caused by nitrates. Some individuals experience palpitations with nitrates, presumably related to reflex increases in heart rate.

## Nitrate Tolerance

The history of tolerance is a long complex story that remains unresolved as of this writing. The interested reader is referred to several recent comprehensive reviews of nitrate tolerance.[6,56,57] A wide variety of theories have been advanced to explain the phenomenon of tolerance (Table 5). Inadequate intracellular thiol availability, neurohormonal activation with increases in Ang II and aldosterone, plasma volume expansion, and impaired guanylate cyclase activity have all been postulated. Most of these concepts have not resulted in successful strategies designed to prevent or reverse tolerance. Neurohormonal activation and sulfhydryl group depletion have been the most carefully studied hypotheses; the published data regarding the benefits of thiol donors, ACE inhibitors, and diuretics have not been consistently convincing, although a recent positive trial using captopril is promising.[55] Inadequate intracellular thiol groups do not appear to be the cause of tolerance.[58]

An enhanced arterial vasoconstrictor state has been identified in the presence of nitrate tolerance, with augmented constrictor responses to endogenous neurohormones such as norepinephrine or Ang II.[53–55] Enhanced ET expression by endothelial cells has been noted[54] Adverse clinical sequels may be related to this phenomenon.[8,9] Furthermore, the failure of nitrates to result in a decrease in important hard clinical end points in many studies also could be related to the inherent downside of chronic nitrate administration related to vasoconstrictor forces. These alterations may be related in part to exuberant

---

Table 5
**Theories to Explain Tolerance**

| Tolerance | Theory |
|---|---|
| Sulfhydryl depletion | Inadequate generation of reduced sulfhydryl or cysteine groups required for organic nitrate biotransformation to nitric oxide |
| Impaired nitroglycerin transformation | Causes uncertain |
| Desensitization of soluble Guanylate cyclase | Impaired activity of the enzyme guanylate cyclase |
| Increase In Phosphodiesterase Activity | Enhanced cyclic guanosine monophosphate breakdown |
| Counterregulatory Neurohormonal Activation | Nitrate-induced increases in catecholamines, arginine vasopressin, plasma renin aldosterone, endothelin, and angiotensin II activity, with resultant vasoconstriction and fluid retention |
| Increased endothelial cell Production of Superoxides ($O_2{}^-$) | Activation of protein kinase C resulting in increased sensitivity to circulating and local vasoconstrictors, such as angiotensin II and endothelin-1 |
| Plasma volume shift | Increased intravascular blood volume related to decreased capillary pressure |

Reproduced with permission from Abrams J. Nitrates, Cardiology Clinics: Annual of Drug Therapy 1:37.

free-radical anion production by vascular endothelial cells in the presence of tolerance.[53] In this setting, nitrate-induced NO may be metabolized to form peroxynitrite, which itself is a weak free radical. These observations have led to trials of antioxidants to prevent or reverse tolerance. Although initial data are promising;[25–29] evaluation of the antioxidant hypothesis has yet to be explored in large clinical trials.

# Conclusions

NTG and the organic nitrate continue to play a significant beneficial role in cardiovascular medicine. These agents are useful to all of the ischemic cardiac syndromes, usually as adjunctive therapy. There is no better therapy for the treatment of acute episodes of anginal pain or unstable angina. If the conundrum of nitrate tolerance can be resolved, nitrates should enjoy an even larger place as part of our therapeutic armamentarium.

# References

1. Fye WB. Nitroglycerin: A homeopathic remedy. *Circulation* 1986;73:21–29.
2. Crandall LA, Leake CD, Loevenhart AS, et al. Acquired tolerance to and cross tolerance between the nitrous and nitric acid esters and sodium nitrite in man. *J Pharmacol Exp Ther* 1931;41:103–119.
3. Duchier J, Iannascoli F, Safar M. Antihypertensive effect of sustained release isosorbide dinitrate for isolated systolic sytemic hypertension in the elderly. *Am J Cardiol* 1987;60:99–102.
4. Needleman P. Efficacy of long-acting nitrates. *Am J Cardiol* 1976;38:400–402.
5. Franciosa JA, Blank RC, Cohn JN. Nitrate effects on cardiac output and left ventricular outflow resistance in chronic congestive heart failure. *Am J Med* 1978; 64:207–213.
6. Abrams J, Elkayam U, Thadani U, et al. Tolerance: An historical overview. *Am J Cardiol* 1998;81:3A–14A.
7. Caramori PA, Adelman AG, Azevedo ER, et al. Therapy with nitroglycerin increases coronary vasoconstriction in response to acetylcholine. *J Am Coll Cardiol* 1998;32:1969–1974.
8. Demots H, Glasser SP. Intermittent transdermal nitroglycerin therapy in the treatment of chronic stable angina. *J Am Coll Cardiol* 1989;13:786–788.
9. Kanamasu K, Takenika T, Hayashi T, et al. Increased incidence of cardial events in post-myocardial infarction patients treated with long-term oral isosorbide dinitrate. *Circulation* 1998;98(suppl):I637. Abstract.
10. Flaherty JT. Role of nitrates in acute myocardial infarction. In: Abrams J, Pepine C, Thadani U, eds. *Medical Therapy of Ischemic Heart Disease*. Boston, MA: Little Brown;, 1992:309–328.
11. Jugdutt BI, Warnica JW. Intravenous nitroglycerin therapy to limit myocardial infarct size, expansion and complications. Effect of timing dosage and infarct location. *Circulation* 1988;78:906–919.
12. Yusuf S, Collins R, MacMahon S, et al. Effect of intravenous nitrates on mortality in acute myocardial infarction: An overview of the randomized trials. *Lancet* 1988; i:1088–1092.
13. Jugdutt BI. Nitrates and left ventricular remodeling. *Am J Cardiol* 1998;81:57A–67A.

14. ISIS-4 (Fourth International Study of Infarct Survival) Collaborative group ISIS- 4. A randomized factorial trial assessing early oral captopril, oral mononitrate and intravenous magnesium sulphate in 58 050 patients with suspected myocardial infarction. *Lancet* 1995;345:669–685.

15. Gruppo Italiano per lo Studio Della Sopravvivenza nell' Infarcto Miocardico. GISSI-3 effects of lisinopril and transdermal trinitrate singly and together on 6-week mortality and ventricular function after acute myocardial infarction. *Lancet* 1994;343:1115–1122.

16. Abrams J. Use of nitrates in ischemic heart disease. *Curr Prob Cardiol.* 1992;17: 483–542.

17. Mahmarian JJ, Fenimore NL, Marks GF, et al. Transdermal nitroglycerin patch therapy reduces the extent of exercise-induced myocardial ischemia: Results of a double-blind, placebo-controlled trial using quantitative thallium-201-tomography. *J Am Coll Cardiol* 1994;24:25–32.

18. Fallen EL, Nahamia SC, Scheffel A, el al. Redistribution of myocardial blood flow with topical nitroglycerin in patients with coronary arterial disease. *Circulation* 1995;91:1381–1388.

19. Mahmarian JJ, Moye LA, Chiady DA, et al. Transdermal nitroglycerin patch therapy improves left ventricular function and prevents remodeling after acute myocardial infarction. *Circulation* 1996;97:2017–2024.

20. Abrams J. Mechanisms of action of the organic nitrates in the treatment of myocardial ischemia. *Am J Cardiol* 1992;70:30B–42B.

21. Kelly RP, Gibbs HH, Morgan JJ, et al. Nitroglycerin has more favorable effects on left ventricular afterload than apparent from measurements of pressure in peripheral artery. *Eur Heart J* 1990;11:138–144.

22. Fung H-L, Chung S-J, Baer JA, et al. Biochemical mechanism of organic nitrate action. *Am J Cardiol* 1992;70:4B–10B.

23. Fung H-L, Sutton SC, Kamiya A. Blood vessel uptake and metabolism of organic nitrates in the rat. *Pharmacol Exp Ther* 1984;228:334–341.

24. Watanabe H, Kakihana M, Ohtsuka S, et al. Platelet cyclic GMP: A potentially useful indicator to evaluate the effects of nitroglycerin and nitrate tolerance. *Circulation* 1993;88:29–36.

25. Watanabe H, Kakihana M, Ohtsuka S, et al. Randomized, double-blind, placebo-controlled study of supplemental vitamin E on an attenuation of the development of nitrate tolerance. *Circulation* 1997;96:2545–2550.

26. Watanabe H, Kakihana M, Ohtsuka S, et al. Randomized, double-blind, placebo controlled study of ascorbate on the preventive effects of nitrate tolerance in patients with congestive heart failure. *Circulation* 1998;97:886–891.

27. Watanabe H, Kakihana M, Ohtsuka S, et al. Randomized double-blind, placebo controlled study of the preventive effect of supplemental oral vitamin C on attenuation of development of nitrate tolerance. *J Am Cardiol* 1998;31:1323–1329.

28. Bassenge E, Fink N, Skatchkov M, et al. Dietary supplement with vitamin C prevents nitrate tolerance. *J Clin Invest* 1998;102:67–71.

29. Urabe Y, Kubo T, Suzuki S, et al. Vitamin E attenuates the development of nitrate tolerance in human epicardial arteries. *Circulation* 1998;98(supp):I637. Abstract.

30. Milone SD, Pace-Asciak CR, Azevedo ER, et al. Transdermal nitroglycerin therapy is not associated with biochemical markers of oxidative stress. *J Am Coll Cardiol* 1998;31:395A. Abstract.

31. Loscalzo J. Antiplatelet and antithrombotic effects of organic nitrates. *Am J Cardiol* 1992;70:18B–22B.

32. Folts JD, Stamler J, Loscalzo J. Intravenous nitroglycerin infusion inhibits cyclic blood flow responses caused by periodic platelet thrombus formation in stenosed canine coronary arteries. *Circulation* 1991;83:2122–2127.

33. Diodati J, Theroux P, Latour J-G, et al. Effects of nitroglycerin at therapeutic doses on platelet aggregation in unstable angina pectoris and acute myocardial infarction. *Am J Cardiol* 1990;66:683–688.

34. Garcia-Dorado D, Permanyer-Miralda G, Brotons C, et al. Attenuated severity of new acute ischemic events in patients with previous coronary heart disease receiving long-acting nitrates. *Clin Cardiol* 1999;22:303–308.

35. Parker JD, Parker JO. Nitrate therapy for stable angina pectoris. *N Engl J Med* 1998;338:520–531.

36. Parker JO, Amies MH, Hawkinson RW, et al. Intermittent transdermal nitroglycerin therapy in angina pectoris. Clinically effective without tolerance or rebound. *Minitran Efficacy Study Group Circulation* 1995;91:1368–1374.

37. Chrysant SG, Glasser SP, Bittar N, et al. Efficacy and safety of extended release isosorbide mononitrate for stable effort angina pectods. *Am J Cardiol* 1993;172:1249–1256.

38. Horwitz JD. Role of nitrates in unstable angina pectoris. *Am J Cardiol* 1992;64B–71B.

39. Curfman GD, Heinsimes JA, Lozner EC, et al. Intravenous nitroglycerin in the treatment of spontaneous angina pectoris: A prospective randomized trial. *Circulation* 1983;67:276–282.

40. Habbab M, Haft J. Heparin resistance induced by intravenous nitroglycerin: A word of caution when both drugs are used concomitanlty. *Arch Int Med* 1987;147:856–860.

41. Chavez J, Abrams J. The nitroglycerin heparin interaction. Submitted. In press.

42. GISSI Investigators. Six month effects of early treatment with lisinopril and transdermal gylceryl trinitrate singly and together withdrawn six weeks after acute myocardial infarction: The GISSI-3 trial. *J Am Coll Cardiol* 1996;27:334-341.

43. Elkayam U. A symposium: Nitrates in congestive heart failure: New mechanisms and rationale for use. *Am J Cardiol* 1996;77:1C–51C.

44. Elkayam U. Nitrates in the treatment of congestive heart failure. *Am J Cardiol* 1996;77:41C–51C.

45. Parker M, Lee WH, Kessler PD, et al. Prevention and reversal of nitrate tolerance in patients with congestive heart failure. *N Eng J Med* 1987;317:799–804.

46. Cohn JN, Archibald DG, Ziesche S, et al. Effect of vasolidator therapy on mortality in chronic congestive heart failure: Results of a Veterans Administration Cooperative Study. *N Engl J Med* 1986;314:1542–1547.

47. Cohn JN, Johnson G, Ziesche S, et al. A comparison of enalapril with hydralazine-isosorbide-dinitrate in the treatment of chronic congestive heart failure. *N Eng J Med* 1991;325:303–310.

48. Elkayam U, Canetti M, Wani OR, et al. Hydralazine-induce prevention of nitrate tolerance: Experimental and clinical evidence and potential mechanisms. *Am J Cardiol* 1998;81:44A–48A.

49. Abrams J. Nitroglycerin tolerance and dependence. *Am Heart J* 1980;99:113–123.

50. Webb D, Boolell M, Murhead G. Cardiovascular effects of phosphodiestrease type 5 inhibition with concomitant nitrate therapy. *Circulation* 1998;98(suppl):I637. Abstract.

51. Webb DJ, Murhead G. Viagra (sildenafil citrate) potentiates the hypotensive effects of nitrates in men with stable angina. *J Am Coll Cardiol* 1999;(March). In press.

52. Cheitlin MD, Hutter AM, Brindis RG, et al. Use of Sildanefil (Viagra) in patients with cardiovascular disease. American College of Cardiology—American Heart Association Expert Consensus Document. *J Amer Coll Cardiol* 1999;33:273–282. Review.

53. Munzel T, Sayegh H, Freeman BA, et al. Evidence for enhanced vascular superoxide anion production in nitrate tolerance. A novel mechanism underlying tolerance and cross-tolerance. *J Clin Invest* 1995;95:187–194.

54. Munzel T, Glaid A, Kurz S, et al. Evidence for a role of endothelin 1 and protein kinase C in nitroglycerin tolerance. *Proc Natl Acad Sci U S A* 1995;92:5244–5248.

55. Heitzer T, Just H, Brockhoff C, et al. Long-term nitroglycerin treatment is associated with supersensitivity to vasoconstrictors in men with stable coronary artery disease; prevention by concomitant treatment with captopril. *J Am Cardiol* 1998;31:83–88.

56. Elkayam U. Tolerance to organic nitrates: Evidence, mechanisms, clinical relevance, and strategies for prevention. *Am Intern Med* 1991;114:667–677.
57. Thadani U. Nitrate tolerance, rebond, and their clinical relevance in stable angina pectoris, unstable angina and heart failure. *Cardiovasc Drug Ther* 1996;10:735–742.
58. Boesgaard S, Nielsen-Kudsk JE, Laursen JB, et al. Thiols and nitrates: Reevaluation of the thiol depletion theory of nitrate tolerance. *Am J Cardiol* 1998;81:21A–29A.
59. Abrams, J. Nitrates. *Cardiology Clinics:* Annual of Drug Therapy; I:37.

# Index

313